BETWEEN A SHOT
AND A HARD PLACE

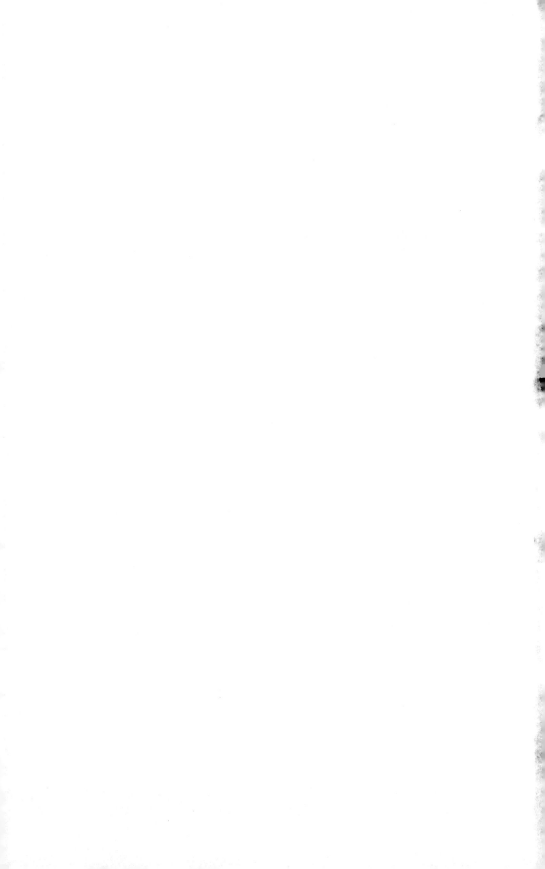

BETWEEN A SHOT AND A HARD PLACE

TACKLING DIFFICULT VACCINE QUESTIONS WITH BALANCE, DATA, AND CLARITY

JOEL WARSH, MD, MSC

EDITED BY:
MADIHA SAEED, MD
ALEXANDER SERBANESCU MD, MSC, CCFP, DIPLOMATE ABFM
SARAH INTELLIGATOR, ESQ.

gatekeeper press™
Tampa, Florida

ISBN (paperback): 9781662959714
eISBN: 9781662959721

Library of Congress Control Number: 2024952156

For information about custom editions, special sales, and premium purchases, please contact IPM@integrativepediatrics.com

Cover art and design by Sarah Intelligator

To all the parents, caregivers, and advocates who tirelessly seek a healthier, brighter future for their children—even when the path is unclear. To everyone who feels unheard, you are seen, you are valued, and your voice matters. May this book be a step toward a world where all concerns are heard, all voices are respected, and all children are given the foundation they need to thrive.

Here's to a future where we strive for and find balance, understanding, and resilience together.

TABLE OF CONTENTS

OPENING STATEMENT

(YOU'LL DEFINITELY WANT TO READ THIS BEFORE DIVING IN)

Human progress is neither automatic nor inevitable. Every step toward the goals requires sacrifices, suffering, and struggle; the tireless exertions and passionate concern of dedicated individuals.

—MARTIN LUTHER KING JR.

Over the past decade, it has become increasingly challenging to openly discuss vaccines. This subject has been relegated to whispers behind closed doors. The fear of judgment, censorship, or misinterpretation has promulgated a speakeasy atmosphere around the topic; seeking permission through secretive glances, many no longer know with whom they can discuss it and what, if anything, they can safely say. It feels a little bit like *Fight Club*—except the first rule of vaccines is you *don't* talk about vaccines. And *that* was my impetus for writing this book. It's not just about vaccines; it's about reclaiming the ability to participate in honest, thoughtful, and transparent discourse on a profoundly important topic that affects us all.

Although not its intention, this book will inevitably ruffle feathers. Despite having always been the type of guy who shies away from controversy, I know there is no way to broach this topic without inciting passion. Rather than continue to cautiously tiptoe around this subject, we must coax it out from the shadows. We must raise the volume from mere whispers to a level that's audible.

I won't proselytize or impose my beliefs. My aim is simply to invite conversation. You may disagree with parts of this book. That is perfectly fine. Disagreement fosters healthy debate and, ultimately, engenders progress.

1

Let the best ideas emerge in the public square through engagement, not suppression. Silencing opposing views merely deepens mistrust and stifles growth. I stand humbly willing to be proven wrong. I concede there will be areas where my understanding can evolve. I don't know everything there is to know about vaccines. Nor do I purport to. I am not a chemist or a biologist. I don't claim to be. I am a pediatrician and a parent who is deeply curious.

I have done my best to explore the available research, synthesize it thoughtfully, and approach this topic with an open mind. This book seeks to make sense of the vast and often overwhelming world of vaccine information. I believe the only pathway forward is through respectful conversation, *not* censorship.

Between a Shot and a Hard Place is not the definitive answer but (I hope) the beginning—a first step in a better direction.

I recognize that as experts and professionals engage with this material, they may offer insights and resources I might have overlooked or misunderstood. My perspective is just one of many in this complex and developing field. I welcome the opportunity to learn and grow. Given the divisive nature of this topic, I am committed to continuing the discussion well beyond these pages.

To keep the conversation alive, stay informed and explore additional resources, scan the QR code, or go to the website below.

You will find updates, corrections, references, and more on the book's website. Let's continue to learn together.

Join the conversation at www.theshotbook.com.

PROLOGUE

You must be the change you wish to see in the world.

—MAHATMA GANDHI

The way I got here is really one of those funny stories . . . like not how I got *here* on planet Earth (we all know how that happened). No, I am talking about the way I arrived at authoring a book on what I always considered a majorly off-limits subject.

It's a story that fatefully begins. . .

"Once upon a time, I met Sarah at a hockey game."

She was seated next to me. A fight broke out in the stands during intermission. We both stood up to investigate the hubbub when she turned to me and said, "Gotta love hockey."

And I do! I'm Canadian. Asking me whether I love hockey is like asking a fish if it loves water. I got her number, we went on our first date, and we hit it off. Little did I know then the serendipitous path on which this single pivotal moment would lead me. I would never have imagined that, eleven years after I maybe not so randomly attended a hockey game, I—a conventionally trained physician, steadfast in my Western predilections— would be writing *this* book.

For our second date, I got tickets to a hockey game—in the ninth row, no less. (I know, I'm a real Prince Charming.) The morning of our second date, Sarah sent a text message. This is what it said:

> *Listen Joel, after I got off the phone with you, I thought about a few things that you said during our conversation that actually made me a bit uncomfortable. It is not my style to bail, but I also think it would be far more unfair to you if I went to the game knowing that I don't feel as though we are on the same page.*

3

Yes, this is the *actual* message romantically fossilized in the cloud for posterity. I was confused. So of course, as I am prone to do when something doesn't make sense to me, I questioned. I called Sarah and asked what she meant. You see, Sarah grew up eating healthy foods at a time when healthy foods still tasted like cardboard. When Sarah was a child, her mom took her to acupuncturists, chiropractors, and other alternative health-care practitioners. On the rare occasion she visited a Western medical doctor, her views were often met with extreme skepticism and even laughed at.

As a divorce attorney, Sarah was keenly aware that her more "alternative" lifestyle choices ran contrary to those of a Western medical doctor—or so she thought. While we were obviously not discussing marriage (heck, we hadn't even gone on a second date), Sarah did not want to become emotionally invested in someone who would ultimately disrespect her views. If the relationship led to marriage and then children, Sarah believed that we would seek to raise our children differently and that our diametrically opposing viewpoints would inevitably lead to divorce. She went on to author a book on relationships in which she notes that the cornerstone of a successful relationship is shared fundamental values. Sarah knew that if I, like my peers, disparaged alternative perspectives, our relationship would fail. She wasn't wrong. She was just wrong about *me*. Sarah mistakenly lumped me in with the medical establishment that had been so dismissive of her choices.

The morning of what was to be our second date, Sarah and I had a lengthy, earnest, and respectful conversation. She unapologetically shared her position, and I listened. I was genuinely interested. She agreed to go on that second date with me, and then a third, and a fourth . . .

Over the course of the next several months, Sarah and I engaged in a number of healthy debates. (Have you ever tried debating with an attorney?) Mostly, Sarah left our discussions frustrated. She held deep conviction in her beliefs. I, on the other hand, was inspired. At that point, my training had been exclusively in Western medicine. The thought that medical interventions existed outside those penned in my textbooks was unthinkable. The prospect that someone may actually decline to give his or her child something I firmly knew to be lifesaving seemed preposterous.

It was around this same time—when I was still in my residency program—that Sarah also started preparing healthy, home-cooked, gluten-free meals for me, using organic produce and meat that wasn't factory-farmed. (I know, this may be the most Los Angeles sentence ever written.)

Before meeting Sarah, I routinely dined at the hospital cafeteria. I had no time to exercise. Occasionally, I was required to work nights and slept in several-hour increments during the daytime. It was compulsory that I work thirty-hour shifts—yes, *thirty hours*—catching brief naps wherever possible. I was not particularly health conscious. I grew up eating sugary snacks and even fast food.

After several weeks and months of eating the food Sarah prepared, not only did I lose weight, I felt better. My digestion improved. For me, this was that aha moment when I first made the connection between diet and health. Sarah also introduced me to various supplements to support my body at a time when it was undergoing such extreme stress. The guinea pig of my own zany science experiment, I personally experienced the benefits of healthy eating and "alternative" modalities.

Marry her? Well, as we nineties kids used to say, "Duh."

That is the way *this* chapter of the story ends. Yet it is also where the chapter of the Dr. Joel "Gator" story begins. My mind had been opened, but I had to be open-minded. As you read this book, I ask just that you, too, keep *your* mind open. *The health of our children depends on it.*

George Bernard Shaw said, "Those who cannot change their minds cannot change anything."

And change is, indeed, imperative.

Today parents are more skeptical of modern medicine than ever before. Not surprisingly, our children are sicker than ever before. Maybe, there is a correlation between the two. According to the results of a 2024 study published in the *Journal of the American Medical Association* (*JAMA*), public trust in physicians and hospitals has sharply declined from 71.5% in April 2020 to just 40.1% in January 2024. This data was not plucked from some small, fringe study. The decline in trust of 31.4 percentage points was based on an analysis of twenty-four online surveys conducted between April 2020 and January 2024 using responses from 443,455 adults across the United States. The public's trust in medicine is sadly at an all-time low. This is true across the globe as well.

I attribute this, in large part, to the fact that the medical community ostensibly suppresses any discussion around interventions that are routinely given. Parents who dare ask a question about a substance injected into their newborn babies are made to feel like pariahs *unless* they shut their mouths and trust the age-old mantra: "It's safe and effective." If we want to restore trust in medicine, we must be willing to engage in difficult conversations. We must be open to questioning long-held beliefs and remain transparent about the science—or lack thereof—behind our recommendations.

You may feel passionately one way or another. As you read this book, you may feel upset. That's great! It means you care deeply. Whether you fall into the militantly pro or staunchly anti-vax camps, we are all strangely unified by our shared zeal for children's health—we simply hold different ideas about the way health is achieved.

Admittedly, there are few topics more divisive than vaccines. Recently, my office received a call from the purported mother of a former patient. She asked whether the office still administers vaccines. When my staff member replied, "Yes," this mother's tone instantly switched from sweet to indignant as she chided:

"Good luck working with the devil, and I hope your office burns in hell."

Vaccines indubitably awaken strong emotions. When I informed my amazing literary agent that I planned to write this book, she politely declined to represent me. I was off to a good start. Before this book was even written, it already encountered harsh criticism. My agent asked what qualified *me* to write a book on vaccines and pointed out that I am not a vaccine researcher or a PhD. I'm glad she posed this question so that I can answer it for you, dear reader:

I am the *very* person who is entrusted to administer vaccines to my patients on a daily basis. I am told the Centers for Disease Control and Prevention (CDC) schedule *is* the standard of care. I am an integrative pediatrician who has extensive conventional medical training and also acknowledges the benefits of alternative modalities. I am not "pro-vax" or "anti-vax." I straddle both worlds with objectivity and healthy scrutiny. In earning my master's degree in epidemiology, I was tasked with extensively performing and synthesizing research. Frankly, I'm not quite sure who better to write this book than *I*.

While this book presents an exhilarating opportunity to promote healthy and meaningful discourse, it will simultaneously attract criticism, ridicule, and censorship. I have no doubt it will prove itself a Pyrrhic victory for me, both personally and professionally. I'm no stranger to this though. On a daily basis, I encounter name-calling and judgment—from complete strangers, no less. However, the conversations this book will invite are imperative and long overdue.

When, on December 23, 2013, I unsuspectingly sat in seat 9, row 3, of section 316 at an LA Kings' game, my life forever changed. I hope this single fateful moment for me also marked the moment that forever changed the trajectory of children's health in this country and even the world. As I embark upon this critical yet terrifying journey, I am prepared for the invariable personal and professional backlash that follows. This next, and perhaps most important, chapter starts with respectful dialogue. I vow to do my best to present all information—on both sides of the debate—with objectivity and candor. I ask merely that you receive it with an open mind. Our children are counting on it.

1

INTRODUCTION

TO JAB OR NOT TO JAB—THAT IS THE QUESTION . . . YOU SHOULD DEFINITELY NOT ASK

I think we ought to read only the kind of books that wound and stab us. If the book we are reading doesn't wake us up with a blow on the head, what are we reading it for?

—FRANZ KAFKA

They are going to call me an "anti-vax conspiracy theorist." They will brand me a "snake oil salesman," guilty of spreading "faux-scientific alarmism." Without reading this book, they will condemn me for "promoting vaccine hesitancy." As they predictably do to invalidate any narrative that deviates from theirs, they will malign me for "spreading"—*gasp!*—"misinformation."

Who are "they"? *They* are the ones who flip through the pages of their playbook, plucking every cliché aspersion routinely used to denounce anyone who asks questions that don't fit the script. The ubiquitous "they" may come after me professionally for so much as mentioning the word *nobody*—particularly a medical doctor—dare say unless it's mechanically uttered in the same breath as "safe and effective."

Vaccine.

There, I said it. Let the floodgates open . . .

Here's the thing. *I am not anti-vax. I am not a conspiracy theorist. I am not a tinfoil-hat-wearing crackpot.* (No offense to tinfoil hats. They're an undeniably cool fashion statement.) *I am* not *"woo-woo." I am a board-certified pediatrician. I earned a master's degree in epidemiology. I graduated*

9

from a reputable American medical school. I attended one of the top pediatric residency programs in the country.

Not only do I have extensive training in infectious disease, but my formal education is predominantly—if not virtually exclusively—in *conventional* Western medicine. My credentials ideally position me to speak on an intervention I regularly administer to my patients. Despite this, I have cautiously tiptoed around the subject of vaccines in fear of jeopardizing my reputation and facing undeniable public and professional censure.

These days the word *vaccine* ignites a war—or rather, a losing battle. When I talk about children's health but neglect to (or deliberately skirt) any metnion of vaccines, I incur the wrath of militant anti-vaxers. Conversely, if I—a pediatrician who is already dismissed as "fringe" because I include the descriptor *integrative* in my title—so much as whisper the word *vaccine*, I am chastised by the medical community.

I can't win. I have been careful not to align myself with either position, though this has not stopped both sides from voraciously taking to social media with their proverbial pitchforks to vilify me. It's frustrating. I'm frustrated. I firmly believe that when it comes to children's health, there is only *one* side—keeping our children healthy. The pathway to achieving this *mutual* goal is through respectful dialogue, not divisive rhetoric.

If you ask the off-limits questions, your child's doctor may acerbically raise an eyebrow and judgmentally scoff at you, before branding you a member of that ever-so-infamous "cult of Jenny McCarthy." You will be made to feel ignorant. Parents who choose to deviate from the "recommendations" are frequently booted from their pediatrician's practice—begging the question whether the word *recommendations* is, in fact, a misnomer. These so-called cult members come to my office and tearfully share such demoralizing experiences.

I'm disappointed that doctors behave this way, though I don't entirely blame them. Doctors spend far too many thankless years training *because* they are so passionate about helping others. Most of them are genuinely good people who care deeply about their patients. Still, some militant "anti-vaxers" attribute nefarious motives to doctors insisting that the impetus for giving vaccines is profit, not health.

This is *absurd* for a myriad of reasons, not the least of which is that for pediatricians, there is relatively little profit in vaccines. Of course, just as any business is compensated for rendering services to its customers, medical offices are compensated for administering vaccines. However, vaccines come with tremendous overhead costs. Vaccines are expensive, and medical offices are required to advance payment when they purchase vaccines in bulk. Medical offices must also pay skilled staff to administer vaccines.

Perhaps the most compelling counter to the myth that doctors are financially motivated to give vaccines is that most doctors are salaried employees who are paid the same salary regardless of whether or not they vaccinate their patients. The reality is that for most doctors, the paramount concern is the health and safety of patients. Doctors champion vaccines as one of the greatest inventions of modern medicine.

Doctors recite the Hippocratic oath, which, in part, states: "First, do no harm." The majority of doctors genuinely believe their failure to administer vaccines violates this oath and *results in harm* to their patients. *We doctors have seen firsthand the devastating outcomes of RSV, whooping cough, and measles, among others; we have tragically watched children in the ICU lose their lives to vaccine-preventable diseases; we have held hands with despondent parents, as we grapple with our inability to reassure them of their child's prognosis. These experiences inform our practice.* The pedagogy resoundingly equates vaccines with optimal health care.

Maybe, the problem is not with doctors but, in a broader sense, the shortcomings in medical education. As I reflect on my own training, I recognize that we were generally taught about vaccines and their common minor reactions. Yet comprehensive instruction on vaccine safety was conspicuously minimal.

A 2014 study published in the *Journal of Vaccine* surveyed ninety-two pediatric residency directors, and 59% of them reported that their programs lacked formal vaccine safety training for residents. If pediatricians are not learning about vaccine safety, who is?

So let's be clear: Doctors are not *giving vaccines to harm people or pad their pockets. From their perspective, they are giving vaccines to prevent devastating and even fatal diseases, consistent with the standard of care and published scientific literature.*

I get it. Vaccines are a hot-button subject. Nevertheless, we cannot deny their contribution to public health. We can, or at least should, all agree that vaccines have had remarkable health implications. They have played a part in eradicating diseases that historically decimated populations. They have protected and continue to protect human beings against debilitating diseases such as measles and polio—to name a small few. The benefits of a "perfectly working vaccine" are largely irrefutable.

Simultaneously true is that vaccines *do* come with risks. One would be hard-pressed to encounter an advertisement for *any* medication without being concurrently warned of the litany of potential side effects that may come along with it. To tout any medical intervention as entirely "without risk" is misleading and, frankly, irresponsible. You would not undergo heart surgery without first considering the risks and benefits with your doctor. A parent would not administer a medication like acetaminophen or steroids to his or her child without weighing the advantages against the potential reactions.

But we are asked—nay, *directed*—to blindly roll up our child's sleeve, stick out their arm, "trust the science" (when we are not actually told what that science is), and take countless jabs without scrutiny. When it comes to *this* particular medical intervention, parents are made to feel as though they cannot weigh the benefits versus the possible risks. For some reason, they are reassured there are "no risks." If there are truly "no risks," then why are parents chastised for asking questions?

The etymology of the words *science* and *doctor* are noteworthy:

Science derives from the Latin word *scire*, meaning, "to know." *Science* quite literally refers to the study of the physical and natural world through observation, experimentation, and testing theories in the pursuit of knowledge. Our understanding of the physical and natural world fluctuates as we obtain data, formulate new theories, and most importantly, continue to question.

Well-respected scientists believed the world was flat until it was proven to be round. Cigarettes were deemed "safe" and even prescribed by doctors until proven extremely harmful. Paint contained lead until it didn't, and car manufacturers were not required to install seat belts until 1967. You get the picture: The beauty of science is that it humbly provides for its own evolution.

However, when it comes to vaccines, we are told the science is "settled," which is a highly suspect oxymoron. Hell, it's an egregious red flag! Science, by its very definition, is never "settled."

We have seemingly forgotten that the word *doctor* comes from the Latin word *docere*—meaning "to teach." A doctor's job is *not* to force treatments on his or her patients. A doctor's job is to teach patients by providing them with the most accurate information available. Each patient should be empowered to make the best *informed* health-care decision for himself or herself.

For most of my career, I have strived to teach others about health and wellness while dancing around and even actively avoiding any discussion of vaccines on social media, podcasts, and all media platforms.

In retrospect, I am ashamed. Candidly, I was afraid—afraid of losing my platform, afraid of facing backlash from the medical establishment, afraid of losing friends. *I now recognize that it was cowardly to hide.* As a member of the medical community, I felt pressured to silently follow in lockstep with my peers. Although medicine is a science, ironically, I, a scientist, had been trained not to question a medical intervention I am expected to give to my patients. Why? I feel that we physicians are not in the position to answer many questions posed to us by our patients because we ourselves are discouraged from making any inquiry into this singular forbidden topic.

As I watched others like Robert F. Kennedy Jr., Elon Musk, Joe Rogan, Dr. Phil, Jordan Peterson, and Casey and Calley Means risk their livelihoods and reputations to crusade for health and freedom, I became inspired.

Hunter Thomson said, "The Edge . . . there is no honest way to explain it because the only people who really know where it is are the ones who have gone over."

After careful discussion with my wife and with the acute understanding of the potential (and inevitable) personal and professional repercussions to me . . . and us, I came to the conclusion that I cannot stay silent any longer—*not* for *me* but for my children and for the future health and wellness of *all* our children.

With fingers pressed together tightly over my eyes, I jumped over the "edge" into the uninviting waters and started advocating for our children.

In my practice and on social media, vaccines are the singular topic every parent seemingly clamors to discuss with me—more than all other topics combined. In fact, most patients choose my practice over others *because* they know I am—to the best of my ability with the information available today— willing to respectfully answer their questions without shaming them.

They want to be heard. Most of them intend to and, in fact, do vaccinate their children. They simply want to participate in a dialogue beforehand. They deserve it. Our children deserve it. Just as we expect full transparency with any medical intervention, we should expect transparency regarding *this* medical intervention.

With increasing regularity, patients and strangers alike share with me their intensifying distrust of modern medicine. They are hesitant to bring their child to a medical doctor, take a medication, or vaccinate. These are not just "crunchy" or "woo-woo" parents, though they are quickly labeled as such. These are caring parents, from all walks of life, who, like any good parent, want to weigh the risks and benefits prior to giving their healthy child a medical intervention.

According to a recent Pew Research Center poll, 28% of adults believe that parents should have the right to opt their children out of school vaccine mandates—this, up from 16% in 2019. Based on a Gallup poll, this one from 2024, the proportion of Americans who believe childhood vaccines are either "extremely" or "very" important amounted to just 69%—down from 94% in 2001. There is no denying that parents are more concerned about vaccines, and their apprehensions are not being addressed. Many of these individuals feel that modern medicine and Big Pharma are more interested in profits than health.

Modern medicine is missing the gargantuan, flashing warning sign. Western medicine's public relations team failed. Simply regurgitating the words *safe and effective* and commanding, "Just do it because we say so," are no longer enough—*and should never have been enough.* Parents demand candor. They want assurance that the vaccines and medications they give their beautiful babies improve health as opposed to adversely impacting it.

Once upon a time, doctors and scientists were among the most trusted and respected professions. I would venture to say that now we doctors are very low on the totem pole of esteemed professions. Frankly, given the current climate, I'm not really certain I want to continue practicing medicine. Doctors and patients have been pitted against each other—by Big Pharma, by Big Food, by Big Insurance, and by Big Corporate America. Doctors are no longer viewed by their patients as allies but as enemies. Doctors and patients are *not* adversaries though. Our common adversary is *them.* Doctors and their patients are on the same team; we share the same goals. If we feel like we are opponents, we can change that. We must change it. Our health is suffering, and our children are paying the price. We simply cannot afford the cost.

To facilitate such change, we must fundamentally acknowledge that *vaccines can be lifesaving and, at the same time, cause severe harm.* These propositions are not mutually exclusive. One may believe that vaccines are miraculous and every individual should receive the doses recommended by the Centers for Disease Control and Prevention (CDC). One can simultaneously recognize that Big Pharma may not always be transparent with its research or that its motives may be predominantly financial. One may *also* agree that we should continue to refine vaccine technology because someday, a deadly disease epidemic may necessitate a lifesaving intervention.

The unfortunate reality is that financial incentives can and do overshadow health. Big corporations may prioritize profit over your well-being, promulgating understandable distrust. Given this, there may be some value to conceding that, possibly, vaccines are not infallible—that just maybe, there is room for improvement and change.

In light of this apparent conflict between profit and health, the medical community cannot expect to regain the public's trust without addressing the gigantic elephant in the room:

Where are the long-term studies on vaccines comparing vaccinated to unvaccinated children? Where are the studies using inert placebos as controls? Where are the studies that show giving multiple and a rising number of vaccines simultaneously is safe?

For the most part, this information either does not exist or, at the very least, is not accessible. Much of the readily available information places vaccines on a pedestal, typically presenting an unchallenged and overly optimistic view of them. When parents don't know or can't predict the risk of side effects ten years from now, let alone over a lifetime, they can't make truly informed decisions. We are entitled to this rudimentary information before making decisions that could have serious repercussions (both good and bad) for our children's health.

Not surprisingly, avoiding this conversation has had the inverse intended effect. *By refusing to answer basic questions, issuing edicts, and rendering medical directives, doctors are, quite ironically, promoting vaccine hesitancy.*

An October 2024 report released by the CDC shows that between the 2019 and 2022 school years, the national kindergarten coverage with state-required vaccinations declined from 95% to approximately 93%. During the 2023 school year, coverage declined to less than 93% for all reported vaccines. The exemption rate increased from 3% to 3.3% from the year prior. The exemption rate was just 2.6% the year before that. Highlighting this incontrovertible trend, the exemption rate increased in forty-one jurisdictions, and in fourteen of those jurisdictions, the exemption rate exceeded 5%.

During the COVID-19 pandemic, when doctors confidently asserted that the new COVID-19 vaccines were "safe and effective"—even in the absence of long-term studies—we lost credibility as a profession.

In my humble opinion, doctors and our institutions should have, instead, said, "From our current research, the benefits of the vaccine appear to outweigh the known short-term risks of the vaccine."

If we are not honest with patients, why would they trust us? When doctors will happily discuss any medical intervention except one, they must understand that skepticism will invariably ensue. Instead of deflecting blame and pointing an accusatory finger at me or others like me, perhaps medicine should take a long, hard look in the mirror. The answer to vaccine hesitancy lies right there in the reflection.

In this book, I am going to be completely honest and attempt to stay as objective as possible. I will be vulnerable. I have no ulterior motive. My only "agenda" is healthy children. *If this leads to hesitancy, then the problem is* not *that I am shining a spotlight on the facts and the data but the facts and the data themselves.*

By now many of you will infer my position. *Whatever you think it is, you're* wrong. *You may assume my political predilection. You are also wrong.*

My political leanings should not matter though. Children's health is *not* tethered to a political ideology. Conflating politics with children's health succeeds merely in further dividing us. It does nothing to resolve the grave issues plaguing our children. Things aren't always black-and-white. Oftentimes, the nuance can be found in the many shades of gray in between. Indeed the vaccine debate is one that very much occupies the nebulous gray area. For some, this may seem incomprehensible. Today's society favors absolutism.

While I will share my thoughts, I also respect yours. I urge you to read this book through its conclusion to formulate your own opinion. As you do, I ask only that you check your bias at the door and remain open-minded. Every book in the vaccine lexicon—whether in favor of or staunchly opposed to—seemingly takes a side. *The current (and only) vaccine books on the market cherry-pick research, shaping narratives to neatly conform to the author's bias and comport with an agenda. This approach does not promote conversation or bridge the chasm. It further feeds the culture of absolutism.*

With such a wealth and variety of studies, authors are free to select whatever data supports *their* position, without addressing the data that runs contrary to it. Just by way of example, one needs to read the hepatitis B vaccine section in a book authored by Neil Miller or Robert F. Kennedy Jr. and then read the CDC website or the hepatitis B section in Gary Marshall's *The Vaccine Handbook*. The flagrant discrepancies would lead any reasonable person to conclude the authors are describing two completely different products. *True* informed consent requires access to the research and studies from *both* sides—a balanced, middle-of-the-road perspective.

The aim of *this* book is to synthesize information, ask questions (as any scientist should), analyze the data in an accessible format, engage in respectful discourse and allow you, dear reader, to draw *your own* conclusions—to empower you to make *your own informed* choices. *Much to the chagrin of many and the relief of others, I will not disparage vaccines—albeit I will surely be accused of "promoting vaccine hesitancy." That is not my purpose. In fact, it could be said that by facilitating transparent conversation, this book will do quite the opposite.* At the same time, this book will not venerate vaccines or anoint them our lord and savior.

I will not *decree vaccines good or bad*. I refuse to drive a deeper wedge. I will leave that to social media. Undoubtedly, this will anger both camps. Pro-vaxers will accuse me of condoning vaccine hesitancy. Anti-vaxers will brand me a coward. They want me to emphatically proclaim vaccines bad—to outright say, "Don't vaccinate."

I politely remind them, you can't have it both ways. You cannot be upset when doctors command you to vaccinate yet expect me to command people not to vaccinate.

These are both edicts that eliminate personal choice. The point is, doctors should educate their patients, not command them to do anything.

This book is the crossroads where science, personal choice, and individual health considerations converge and harmoniously coexist. I vow to winnow through the murky waters of vaccines with an open mind, a tinge of humor, and a whole lot of science. Specifically, I will attempt the following:

1. Present the full range of scientific data on vaccines, to the best of my ability
2. Facilitate a healthy and transparent conversation on a topic that has faced altogether too much censorship

3. Ask unanswered questions with scientific curiosity to, hopefully, invite answers
4. Demand greater accountability from the pharmaceutical and medical industries
5. Pave a symbiotic pathway forward that ensures the future health of our children

My aim is to foster a dialogue that has been silenced for too long. I want you to feel informed, respected, and empowered to ask questions of your medical doctor so that you can make the right choices—yes, *choices*—for yourself and your children.

This book will explore and analyze the vast gamut of literature— from the American Academy of Pediatrics (AAP) guidelines to Robert F. Kennedy Jr.'s research, from the CDC Schedule and *The Vaccine Handbook* to The *Vaccine Friendly Plan* and *Turtles All the Way Down*—to name a select few.

I *cannot* and *will not* tell you what to do. I don't have all the answers. I *will* engage in sincere discourse scientifically and holistically. In accordance with the scientific method, I will pose questions to which there are seemingly no answers. *I hope to extricate this topic from the clandestine shadows and nudge it into the mainstream. No topic should be "off-limits" when it comes to the health of our children, particularly when, in the United States, almost one in every two children now suffers from chronic disease.* This is an astounding and devastating statistic that none of us should accept.

The great David Bowie said, "If you feel safe in the area you're working in, you're not working in the right area. Always go a little further into the water than you feel you're capable of being in. Go a little bit out of your depth. And when you don't feel that your feet are quite touching the bottom, you're just about in the right place to do something exciting." Up until now, I've played it safe. I'm ready now . . . *we* are ready—ready to venture to that intimidating and uncomfortable place where our feet don't quite touch the bottom. It feels exciting.

On my first day of medical school, I stood up and took an oath to "first, do no harm."

Those words resonated deeply with me then; they continue to daily guide the decisions I make as a physician. Every choice, every recommendation I offer to my patients is rooted in this fundamental principle of medicine. It's not just a phrase—it's a commitment to prioritize the well-being of those I care for above all else.

Instead of focusing on what divides us, let's remember that we all share the *same* goal. Parents, doctors, you and I—*we all* want our children to be healthy. So in the words of my five-year-old, "Get ready to prepare!" We're about to embark on an exhilarating and, at times, uncomfortable odyssey into the world of vaccines. Hopefully, by the end of this book, we will all agree: Our collective health and the health of our children are worth a conversation—no matter how controversial the topic.

2

VACCINE EVOLUTION

THE PAST, PRESENT, AND FUTURE OF VACCINES

The science of medicine is ever progressive;
a physician who stops his labor becomes a common man.

—EDWARD JENNER,
"FATHER OF VACCINES AND IMMUNOLOGY"
AND CREATOR OF THE SMALLPOX VACCINE

VARIOLATION

Before we delve into the "good stuff," we should understand the history of vaccines. As far as I am aware, vaccination originated around the tenth century AD in China, where variolation was first used to protect against smallpox—a deadly viral disease that, at that time, caused severe illness and death on a global scale. Through this process, tiny amounts of the smallpox virus were introduced into healthy individuals, causing mild infection. In the earliest documented use of variolation practiced in China, smallpox scabs were blown into the nostrils of the healthy individual. (Yes, this sounds nauseating, but when death was the likely consequence of infection, snorting scabs proved a desirable alternative.)

By the early eighteenth century, variolation reached Europe. In 1717, Lady Mary Wortley Montagu, wife of the British ambassador to the Ottoman Empire, observed variolation performed in Constantinople. Having witnessed the high mortality rate from smallpox, Montagu introduced the technique in England. She also had her own children variolated. Montagu campaigned to perform the procedure across Europe, as a result of which variolation became a widely used method to prevent smallpox in England and other European countries. Utilizing modalities similar to those employed in the Ottoman Empire, a cut was inflicted on the patient. Next, material from the smallpox pustule of an infected person—ideally, someone with a mild case, was rubbed into the cut. The variolated individual typically developed a mild form of smallpox, with a much lower mortality rate than those who contracted the disease naturally, along with immunity against future smallpox infections.

While variolation resulted in more controlled infection, it was not entirely without risk. The procedure carried a mortality rate of around 1–2%, which is significantly lower than the 20–30% mortality rate of naturally occurring smallpox—though by modern standards, a 1-2% risk is still considered dangerous. Additionally, variolated individuals could transmit smallpox to others, increasing the risk of outbreaks.

In the early eighteenth century, variolation was introduced to the American colonies. During a smallpox outbreak in Boston in 1721, Puritan minister Cotton Mather and Dr. Zabdiel Boylston promoted the practice after learning of its success from African slaves. Initially, variolation faced significant opposition due to religious objections and fears over the risks it posed. Eventually, the procedure became widely used, marking the first known pervasive use of variolation in the Americas.

Variolation was a revolutionary step in the fight against infectious diseases. It shaped the modern understanding of immunology by demonstrating that controlled exposure to a pathogen could generate immunity—a principle that underpins today's vaccination programs.

THE INTRODUCTION OF MODERN VACCINES

Variolation laid the groundwork for modern inoculation. Ultimately, it was replaced by vaccination. In the late eighteenth century, Edward Jenner, who is frequently referred to as the father of vaccines and immunology, discovered the cowpox-based smallpox vaccine. Jenner observed that milkmaids that contracted cowpox were immune to smallpox. In 1796, Jenner inoculated a boy with cowpox from a cow named Blossom. When the boy was later exposed to smallpox, he did not contract it. Jenner termed this new process "vaccination" after the Latin word *vacca*, meaning "cow." Unlike variolation, vaccination used the much safer cowpox virus. It obviated the risk of infecting the patient with smallpox, significantly decreasing the possibility of adverse side effects. By 1980, Jenner's vaccine led to the eradication of smallpox. Smallpox remains one of the only human diseases to be completely eliminated through vaccination.

By the nineteenth century, Jenner's smallpox vaccine led to widespread adoption of vaccination, starting first in England and then spreading globally. In the 1800s, smallpox vaccination was mandatory in some countries. This was one of the first known widespread immunization campaigns.

In the 1880s, Louis Pasteur expanded upon Jenner's work, developing vaccines for rabies and anthrax. Pasteur discovered that weakening or killing a virus could create immunity, further laying the foundation for modern vaccines.

Several other notable vaccines were developed in the early twentieth century: In 1923, the diphtheria, in 1924, the tetanus, and in 1926, the pertussis (whooping cough) vaccines were discovered. In 1940, the combined DTP vaccine, which inoculated against diphtheria, tetanus, and pertussis, was introduced.

In 1955, Jonas Salk developed the first successful polio vaccine using an inactivated virus. In 1961, Albert Sabin introduced the oral polio vaccine, which has been widely used globally in an effort to eradicate the disease.

SANITATION VS. VACCINATION: UNDERSTANDING THE DRIVERS BEHIND DECLINES IN INFECTIOUS DISEASES

Although vaccines did reduce the rates and spread of disease, many infections were already on a sharp decline *before* vaccines were introduced. Advances in public health, including clean water supplies, improved sewage and sanitation systems, better housing, antibiotic innovations, and improved hospitals and medical care, were instrumental in controlling disease transmission through contaminated food, water, and crowded living conditions. Vaccine skeptics often argue that historical data shows a direct correlation between the decrease in mortality and incidences of infectious diseases, and significant medical and public health advancements in the nineteenth and early to mid-twentieth centuries.

British naturalist and biologist Alfred Russel Wallace was one of the first vaccine skeptics. Wallace is the lesser-known co-architect of the theory of evolution. In fact, Wallace independently conceived of the theory of evolution by natural selection. Alongside Charles Darwin, his insights played a central role in shaping the development of evolutionary theory. Initially, Wallace was a proponent of the smallpox vaccine—the primary vaccine used in his lifetime. He acknowledged its effect on mortality rates. But as he examined data and engaged in debates, he became a prominent critic of mandatory vaccination programs. In his 1889 book entitled *Vaccination: Proved Useless & Dangerous*, Wallace posited that vaccination was not as effective as public health authorities claimed. In analyzing government data, Wallace argued that improved sanitation, hygiene, and living conditions, *not* vaccination, were responsible for the decline in smallpox-related deaths.

Close to a century later, in their 1977 article, "The Questionable Contribution of Medical Measures to the Decline of Mortality in the United States in the Twentieth Century," John and Sonja McKinlay wrote: "Medical measures appear to have contributed little to the overall decline in mortality in the United States since about 1900." They contended that the significant reductions in mortality were primarily due to improvements in social and environmental factors, such as enhanced nutrition and sanitation, rather than medical interventions like vaccines and antibiotics.

Advocates of this view point to the significant decrease in the rates of infection and death from tuberculosis, cholera, scarlet fever, and typhoid that followed advances in sanitation and public health—citing the inescapable fact that no vaccines existed or were consistently used for any of these diseases at that time. Contemporaneous improvements to nutrition also enhanced individual immune resilience, which resulted in lower fatality from various infectious diseases.

Prior to 1940, sanitation and public health breakthroughs had a tremendous impact on overall health improvements and mortality rates. However, we cannot ignore the instrumental role vaccines played in the reduction and near elimination of many diseases. Vaccines mitigated the severity of illness and interrupted transmission. The precipitous and immediate decline in diseases has often followed the introduction of certain vaccines—an outcome that sanitation alone could not explain. For instance, sanitation had a minimal impact on the transmission of measles. Before the measles vaccine was introduced in 1963, nearly all children contracted measles by age fifteen. After the vaccine was introduced, the number of measles cases dramatically decreased. By the early 1980s, the instances of measles had declined by 99% in the United States, signifying an unequivocal correlation between vaccination and reduced incidence.

The smallpox vaccine is another notable example of the relationship between vaccination and disease elimination. Sanitation did not substantially influence smallpox transmission. The smallpox vaccine led to the eventual eradication of the disease.

Notably, much of the frequently cited decline in prevaccine mortality pertains to disease *severity*, as opposed to the actual incidence of disease. In other words, fewer people may have died from diseases like measles or whooping cough due to better health care and nutrition, but the number of infections, though lower than in decades past, remained high. Vaccines, in contrast, targeted disease *incidence* by stopping transmission within communities, reducing the number of new cases, and mitigating potential outbreaks.

While diseases and mortality rates were already on the natural downturn, the introduction of vaccines resulted in the staggering reduction of diseases that were once extremely common and even debilitating. In my opinion, this fact, which is supported by epidemiological graphs, is quite apparent. Still, we should not overlook the counterpoint: Modern advances in medicine, nutrition, sanitation, and technology inherently led to a sharp drop in diseases that were once prevalent and for which no vaccines are routinely used in the United States, such as tuberculosis and cholera. If in the 1960s, vaccines for tuberculosis and cholera were introduced and widely administered, we would now laud vaccines for the significant decline in these diseases. Because vaccines for these diseases are not commonly used in the United States, we can confidently say that other factors were responsible for the decline in tuberculosis and cholera. Would the same be true for other diseases, like diphtheria or mumps?

At the same time, chicken pox provides a perfect, real-world example of the efficacy of vaccines. As kids, many of us had chicken pox. Today children are unlikely to come into contact with the disease, largely due to the widespread use of the varicella vaccine. Most of us have witnessed this phenomenon in our lifetime, highlighting the role vaccines can play in controlling cases of certain diseases.

The impact of vaccines is not exclusively endemic to the United States. The 1960s and 1970s saw an uptick in global vaccination campaigns. In 1966, the smallpox eradication campaign marked a monumental achievement in global health, entirely eliminating smallpox. The last case of naturally transmitted smallpox occurred in Somalia in 1977. Building on this success, in 1974, the World Health Organization (WHO) launched the Expanded Program on Immunization (EPI), providing vaccines for tuberculosis (BCG), diphtheria, pertussis, tetanus, polio, and measles.

By 2000, the creation of the Global Alliance for Vaccines and Immunization (Gavi) further expanded vaccine access, particularly for diseases like Haemophilus influenzae type b (Hib), rotavirus, and pneumococcus. Supported by a 750-million-dollar contribution from the Gates Foundation, Gavi reduced vaccine costs and improved accessibility in low- and middle-income countries.

Between 2005 and 2015, these efforts majorly contributed to a decline in childhood mortality from vaccine-preventable diseases around the world. For instance, deaths from pneumococcal pneumonia fell by 38.8%; rotaviral enteritis, by 43.6%; measles, by 75.1%; and Haemophilus influenzae type b, by 60.7%. Pertussis-related deaths decreased by 41%; tetanus, by 57.2%; and diphtheria, by 61.3%. Overall, deaths of children under five years old declined by 27.2%, equating to 5.82 million lives saved worldwide.

Global collaboration played a pivotal role in these achievements. Gavi partnered with governments, pharmaceutical companies, and international organizations to develop new vaccines and increase coverage. The initiative also prioritized Millennium Development Goal 4 (MDG 4), focused on reducing child mortality.

Whether you choose to believe them or not, the CDC statistics illustrate just how impactful vaccination programs have been in the United States. Diseases such as smallpox and polio, which were once widespread and deadly, have been eradicated or nearly eliminated. Since vaccines became widely available, cases of other diseases, like measles and rubella, have dropped by more than 99%. Yes, sanitation and nutrition have played a role. And yes, much of the drop in morbidity and mortality occurred before vaccines were introduced. Nevertheless, this does not negate the profound effect vaccines have had on disease. The data overwhelmingly illustrates the role vaccines have played in transforming public health by preventing the resurgence of serious, and oftentimes life-threatening illnesses.

Disease	20th Century Annual Morbidity	2023 Reported Cases	Percent Decrease
Smallpox	29,005	0	100%
Polio	16,316	0	100%
Diphtheria	21,053	2	> 99%
Measles	530,217	47	> 99%
Mumps	162,344	429	> 99%
Haemophilus influenzae b	20,000	27	> 99%

Admittedly, I find it somewhat confounding that anyone could look at these statistics and still deny the impact vaccines have had on disease reduction. The below graph, adapted from the 2014 CDC Morbidity and Mortality Weekly Report (MMWR), shows a steep decline in Hib, corresponding to the introduction of the vaccine.

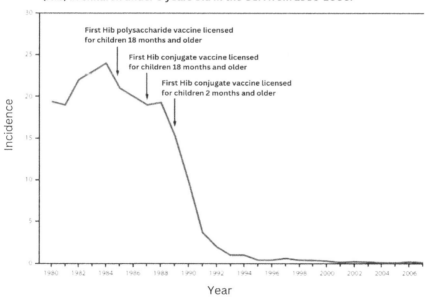

Estimated annual incidence per 100,000 of Haemophilus influenza type B (Hib) in children under 5 years old in the USA from 1980-2006.

To me, this graph illustrates the tremendous effect of the Hib vaccine. And if the sharp decline in Hib was not attributable to the vaccine, then this is quite the coincidence.

If the "sanitation versus vaccination" debate were a tennis match, your neck would hurt from watching the ball go back and forth over the net. Vaccines have played a crucial role in directly decreasing disease incidence, preventing transmission, and establishing community-wide immunity—something sanitation alone cannot achieve for all diseases. Yet advances in sanitation and public health have *also* greatly reduced exposure to pathogens and lowered mortality rates. The impacts of sanitation and vaccines are not mutually exclusive. This isn't as black-and-white as pro-vax versus anti-vax, or vaccination versus sanitation. Rather, both sanitation and vaccination have been, and remain pivotal, complementary strategies in combating infectious diseases.

MAJOR LEGAL CHANGES: NATIONAL VACCINE INJURY COMPENSATION PROGRAM

By construing §22(b)(1) to pre-empt all design defect claims against vaccine manufacturers for covered vaccines, the majority's decision leaves a regulatory vacuum in which no one—neither the FDA nor any other federal agency, nor state and federal juries—ensures that vaccine manufacturers adequately take account of scientific and technological advancements. This concern is especially acute with respect to vaccines that have already been released and marketed to the public. Manufacturers, given the lack of robust competition in the vaccine market, will often have little or no incentive to improve the designs of vaccines that are already generating significant profit margins. Nothing in the text, structure, or legislative history remotely suggests that Congress intended that result. I respectfully dissent.

—JUSTICE SONIA SOTOMAYOR, JOINED BY JUSTICE RUTH BADER GINSBURG IN DISSENTING FROM THE MAJORITY OPINION IN THE 2011 SUPREME COURT CASE, *BRUESEWITZ V. WYETH, LLC*

By the 1960s, the fight against infectious disease continued on a global scale. Vaccination programs expanded worldwide: In 1963, the measles, in 1967, the mumps, and in 1969, the rubella vaccines—among others—were developed. The 1960s marked a pivotal time in vaccine development. Over the course of the decade, new vaccines were introduced, and public health policies began to emphasize widespread immunization with the aim of preventing contagious disease outbreaks.

In the 1950s and early 1960s, the recommended vaccine schedule for children was far simpler and included DTP, polio, and smallpox. During the early 1960s, a child who received all recommended vaccines by the age of two would have been given only *four to five vaccines*, with several boosters throughout childhood.

Over the latter half of the twentieth century, the science of vaccinology continued to evolve. The early 1970s brought the measles, mumps, and rubella (MMR) combination vaccine. By the end of the 1970s, smallpox was eradicated worldwide, obviating the smallpox vaccine for general use. Over the course of the 1970s, the number of vaccines on the schedule remained relatively limited. In the mid-1980s, children were typically receiving about eight vaccines by the age of two, including three to four doses of the DTP, three doses of the OPV, and one dose of the MMR vaccines.

As the vaccine schedule expanded, major legal changes reshaped the landscape of vaccination in the United States. The broader use of vaccines was accompanied by growing claims of vaccine-related injuries. Consequently, vaccine manufacturers faced an increasing number of lawsuits—particularly related to the whole-cell DTP vaccine. The threat of liability prompted fears that companies would stop producing vaccines.

To address these concerns, in 1986, President Ronald Reagan signed into law the National Childhood Vaccine Injury Act (NCVIA). The NCVIA offered almost complete immunity (no pun intended) for vaccine manufacturers, shielding them from liability related to vaccine injuries—except in the case of fraud or willful misconduct. In addition, the NCVIA established the National Vaccine Injury Compensation Program (VICP) to compensate individuals injured by or experiencing serious side effects from vaccines. Compensation covers medical and legal expenses, loss of future earning capacity, and up to 250,000 dollars for pain and suffering; a death benefit of up to 250,000 dollars is also available. The program, which was established by the Department of Health and Human Services in 1988, is funded by an excise tax of seventy-five cents on every purchased dose of covered vaccine.

The NCVIA also established the Vaccine Adverse Event Reporting System (VAERS)—a national system for monitoring and reporting adverse events following vaccination. Jointly managed by the CDC and FDA,

VAERS serves as a warning system, monitoring potential safety concerns related to vaccines in the United States. VAERS is a passive surveillance system—meaning it relies on *voluntary* reporting of any adverse events after vaccination, regardless of whether these are thought to be linked directly to the vaccine. Over the past few years, especially following the COVID-19 vaccine rollout, VAERS saw a notable increase in reported events.

In 2020, prior to the COVID-19 vaccine rollout, the number of reports recorded by VAERS was in line with previous years—totaling approximately 50,000 reports across all vaccines. But by late 2021, COVID-19 vaccine-related entries made up over half of all reports submitted in VAERS's entire thirty-year history, reflecting both high vaccine administration and the heightened reporting requirements and awareness under Emergency Use Authorization (EUA). In stark contrast to typical annual totals from preceding years, in 2021, VAERS received approximately 752,660 reports in the United States. The high report volume was partly due to COVID-19 vaccine-specific reporting requirements that directed health-care providers to report adverse events after vaccination, regardless of causation or severity. Nonetheless, the significant increase in reporting led to some trepidation over the safety of the COVID-19 vaccine.

Despite heightened reporting specifically around COVID-19 vaccine-related injuries, the biggest problem with VAERS has historically been the under-reporting of vaccine-related concerns. Studies demonstrate that the system tends to capture just a small minority of actual adverse events that may be related to vaccines. A 2011 Harvard Pilgrim Health Care study analyzed data across 715,000 patients. It found that VAERS captures fewer than 1% of vaccine-related adverse events, attributing underreporting to the voluntary nature of VAERS and limited provider time.

Accordingly, VAERS is more of a preliminary signal detector than a comprehensive indicator of vaccine safety outcomes. When interpreting findings, understanding these structure and data limitations is crucial. While VAERS flags potential issues for further scientific scrutiny, it cannot independently confirm cause-and-effect relationships, rendering it merely one aspect of the broader vaccine safety evaluation process.

Many perceive the passage of the NCVIA a critical moment in vaccine history. The NCVIA stabilized vaccine production by shielding vaccine manufacturers from liability, except under very specific conditions, such as willful misconduct, inadequate warnings, instructions inconsistent with

FDA-approved labeling, or defectively designed vaccines that could have been made safer.

Proponents of this law champion it for its public and individual health implications. They aptly noted that the law paved the way for the further expansion of vaccine technology. However, opponents of the NCVIA consider it a slippery slope. They contend that limiting the liability of vaccine manufacturers also significantly limits accountability at the expense of safety and efficacy. Perhaps, there is some validity to *both* positions. One fact that remains unequivocally true: The NCVIA—and the billions of dollars awarded since its enactment to compensate individuals for injuries connected to vaccines—marked an *undeniable admission* that vaccines are *not entirely without side effects.*

To prevail under the VICP, (1) a claimant must prove that he or she experienced an injury, (2) the injury is one the law identifies as a possible vaccine injury, (3) the claim must be brought within the required time period, and (4) a causal connection between the vaccine and the injury exists. The claimant carries the burden of proof, which is the preponderance-of-the-evidence standard. This means the claimant must show that, more likely than not, his or her injury was caused by the vaccine. The VICP covers all vaccines listed on the Vaccine Injury Table maintained by the Secretary of Health and Human Services.

The most notable Vaccine Injury Compensation Program cases focused on vaccines and autism. In 2002, the Special Masters of the US Court of Federal Claims heard a set of cases known as the Omnibus Autism Proceeding (OAP). The OAP was a coordinated legal process established to address thousands of claims made through the VICP, alleging that vaccines, particularly the measles, mumps, rubella (MMR) vaccine, and vaccines containing the mercury-based preservative, thimerosal, could cause autism or autism-like symptoms in children. To streamline the legal process, the court grouped these 5,600 claims to ensure consistency in handling the common legal and scientific questions involved. After a thorough review of the evidence, testimony from medical experts, and extensive scientific studies, the court found no causal link between vaccines and autism in all six of the test cases heard. The court cited a lack of evidence that vaccines, including MMR and those containing thimerosal, caused or contributed to autism spectrum disorders (ASDs). The decisions in these test cases effectively set a precedent, leading to the dismissal of the majority of other autism-related claims under the Omnibus, which I will discuss in greater detail in a later chapter. (Stay tuned.)

Of the 2,865 non-autism-related VICP claims, 925 were compensated. The majority of the 925 compensated cases were awarded for recognized conditions listed on the Vaccine Injury Table or well-substantiated conditions known to have possible associations with vaccines, such as these:

1. *Anaphylaxis.* Severe allergic reactions that can occasionally occur after vaccination, often immediately after administration.

2. *Encephalopathy.* Neurological injuries, like encephalopathy (brain swelling or dysfunction), were among the compensated injuries, especially when associated with DTP (diphtheria, tetanus, pertussis) vaccines. Though relatively rare, this is a recognized risk and has been a common basis for compensation.

3. *Brachial Neuritis.* An injury to the nerve complex in the shoulder region that can cause arm weakness, often associated with the tetanus component of vaccines.

4. *Other Injuries.* Other conditions that are listed in the Vaccine Injury Table and associated with specific vaccines were also compensated, like Guillain-Barré Syndrome (GBS) with flu vaccines, thrombocytopenia (ITP) after MMR, and intussusception (bowel obstruction) related to the rotavirus vaccine.

Although no autism-related claims in the OAP were compensated on the grounds that vaccines caused autism, one unique case received compensation in connection with an autism-like developmental condition. The distinction cited by the court in *this* case is essential.

In 2007, the Hannah Poling case rose to prominence as the *only* instance in which the VICP awarded compensation for a vaccine-related injury that involved autism-like symptoms.

Hannah Poling had an underlying mitochondrial disorder—a rare genetic condition that affects cellular energy production. After receiving several vaccines, she experienced a marked regression in developmental milestones and subsequently exhibited autism-like symptoms. The VICP awarded compensation in Poling's case *not* on the basis that the vaccines caused autism but, rather, because the vaccines *may have exacerbated her preexisting mitochondrial disorder,* leading to a "regressive encephalopathy" with autism-like symptoms. This case, while frequently cited in discussions, did not establish a general link between vaccines and autism.

As of January 2025, $5.3 billion in compensation has been awarded under the VICP.

THE RAPID GROWTH OF THE VACCINE SCHEDULE IN THE 1990S

After the NCVIA conferred protection to vaccine manufacturers, vaccine technology continued to develop. The introduction of the Hib, varicella, hepatitis B, and pneumococcal vaccines in the 1990s and early 2000s further expanded the childhood vaccine schedule. In the late 1990s, children were receiving about *twelve to sixteen vaccines* by age two, including three doses of hepatitis B, four doses of DTaP, three to four doses of Hib, three doses of IPV, one dose of MMR, and one dose of varicella.

In the twenty-first century, new vaccines and combination shots were recommended including the rotavirus, HPV, meningococcal, influenza, COVID-19, and RSV vaccines.

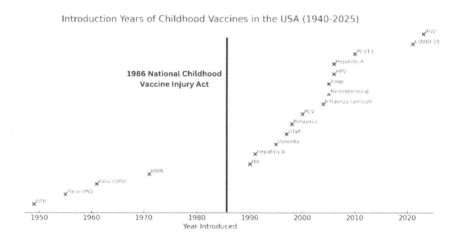

Introduction Years of Childhood Vaccines in the USA (1940-2025)

CHALLENGES AND TRENDS IN VACCINE ACCEPTANCE AND POLICY

Meanwhile, the seemingly accelerated development and administration of new vaccines fueled skepticism and concerns around vaccine recommendations. Marking a pivotal moment, the publication of a 1998 now-retracted study by Andrew Wakefield, which suggested a link between the MMR vaccine and autism, contributed to vaccine hesitancy. Wakefield's claim generated significant fear, precipitating the anti-vaccine movement.

Parents and advocacy groups primarily focused on the use of preservatives, such as thimerosal, and potential long-term side effects. Since then, vaccine hesitancy and the consequent decline in vaccine coverage has increased; children born in 2020 and 2021 have lower vaccination rates compared to those born in 2018 and 2019. According to a recent study in the *Journal of Human Vaccines and Immunotherapeutics*, one in three parents expressed concerns about vaccines to their pediatricians, and more than one in ten intended to follow an alternative immunization schedule. In the United States, parental hesitancy around vaccines is more prevalent than ever. In March 2020, data from the CDC's National Immunization Survey indicated that over one-third of children between nineteen and thirty-five months were not adhering to the recommended early childhood immunization schedule. In a 2024 journal article in *Vaccine*, the authors noted that, as of 2022, only 70.5% of US children between the ages of nineteen and thirty-five months were up-to-date on all recommended vaccines. As of 2022, the CDC's National Immunization Survey found that 1.3% of children between the ages of nineteen to thirty-five months did not receive any vaccinations at all. This marked an increase from previous years. Nearly every metric indicates a clear rise in vaccine hesitancy over the last decade—a trend that intensified in the aftermath of the COVID-19 pandemic.

The WHO has identified vaccine hesitancy as one of the top ten global health threats, emphasizing the importance of addressing these issues to maintain public health.

The rise in vaccine hesitancy can be attributed to several factors. Parents are worried about vaccine safety. They fear adverse reactions, autism, and other long-term side effects. Some parents believe natural infection is better for developing stronger immunity; others simply distrust public health recommendations and the pharmaceutical influence over regulatory agencies.

In recent years, in response to the growing anti-vaccine movement, the United States adjusted its vaccine policies. Several states, including California, passed laws eliminating religious and personal belief exemptions for school vaccinations, requiring all children to be fully vaccinated to attend public or private schools unless they have a medical exemption. For instance, in California, where I live, beginning January 1, 2021, under Senate Bills

(SB) 276 and 714, all new medical exemptions for school and childcare entry must be issued through the California Immunization Registry-Medical Exemption website (CAIR-ME). Medical exemptions can only be issued by medical doctors or doctors of osteopathic medicine who are licensed in California. The medical exemption must meet applicable CDC, Advisory Committee on Immunization Practices (ACIP), and American Academy of Pediatrics (AAP) criteria.

In California, when a doctor issues five or more medical exemptions in a given year, the California Department of Public Health (CDPH) is legally required to review those exemptions. This review ensures that exemptions align with the established medical standards and guidelines set by the CDC, ACIP, and AAP. Despite the technical legality of exemptions in the state, legislation such as SB 276 and SB 714 has significantly limited their issuance. If the CDPH finds that a doctor granted exemptions that are inconsistent with medical standards, the doctor may face severe consequences, like probation, license suspension or revocation, and public reprimand. These measures effectively deter many doctors from issuing exemptions, even in cases where an exemption might be appropriate and, arguably, medically indicated. Furthermore, these laws have shifted the decision-making process from the patient-provider relationship to an external authority that, while lacking personal familiarity with the patient, holds the power to revoke exemptions it deems unwarranted.

In 2023, more than five hundred California public schools were audited by the state after they reported that upward of 10% of their kindergarten or seventh-grade students were not fully vaccinated in the previous school year.

Meanwhile, the legal framework established by the NCVIA has remained largely intact, with vaccine manufacturers continuing to receive protection against liability through the VICP.

CURRENT VACCINE SCHEDULE AND NAVIGATING THE FUTURE OF VACCINATION

The current CDC/AAP recommended immunization schedule for children from birth through age six is concisely outlined below[1]:

1. *Vitamin K*: Birth.
2. *RSV*: Birth to eight months old, given during the winter.

---

1 For the most up-to-date schedule, please visit the CDC website.

3. *Hepatitis B (HepB)*: Birth, one to two months, and six to eighteen months.
4. *Rotavirus (RV)*: Two, four, and six months (series depends on the brand).
5. *Diphtheria, Tetanus, Pertussis (DTaP)*: Two, four, six, fifteen to eighteen months, and four to six years old.
6. *Haemophilus influenzae type b (Hib)*: Two, four, six, and twelve to fifteen months.
7. *Pneumococcal (PCV)*: Two, four, six, and twelve to fifteen months.
8. *Polio (IPV)*: Two, four, six to eighteen months, and four to six years.
9. *Influenza (flu)*: Annually from six months onward (with two doses given in the first flu season).
10. *Measles, Mumps, Rubella (MMR)*: Twelve to fifteen months and four to six years.
11. *Varicella (chicken pox)*: Twelve to fifteen months and four to six years.
12. *Hepatitis A (HepA)*: Twelve and eighteen months
13. *COVID-19*: Eligible at six months, dose timing varies by vaccine (with a two-to three-dose series depending on brand and annual boosters).

A number of these are combination vaccines, which reduce the total number of pokes. If children were to receive single vaccines (not including the COVID-19 and flu vaccines), then by the ages of four to six, they will have received over thirty pokes. If they were to also receive the COVID-19 and flu vaccines, then they would have received a total of more than forty pokes. This represents a marked increase from just a few decades earlier.

Yes, we have come a long way from inhaling infected scab particles. Since the 1960s, the United States childhood vaccine schedule has expanded considerably, with more vaccines regularly introduced to prevent a wider range of diseases. Although in many ways, this has proven a public health victory, resulting in the near elimination of diseases such as polio and measles in the United States, it has concurrently sparked debates over vaccine safety, bodily autonomy, choice, and policy.

The vaccine skeptic crowd often cites the number, "seventy-two vaccines." This does sound like a *lot* of vaccines. I believe this figure is not entirely transparent and intentionally alarmist. To be clear, this number is not indicative of the number of pokes received but, rather, the collective total sum of antigens across all shots. For instance, the DTaP (diphtheria, tetanus, pertussis) vaccine is a singular shot that contains three of these seventy-two vaccines. I'm going to get a little technical here, so bear with me. The number seventy-two is based on counting the letters *D, T,* and *P.* The DTaP vaccine actually contains four to five antigens—*more* antigens than its acronym suggests. It consists of diphtheria toxoid, tetanus toxoid, acellular pertussis components, plus a detoxified pertussis antigen, filamentous hemagglutinin, the adhesion protein Pertactin, and adhesion protein Fimbriae types 2 and 3 . . . Who wants to get this technical though?

Yes, the number of pokes a child endures is significantly lower than the big, scary total number of antigens received. The number of pokes *is* high though—and growing. With the addition of the RSV, COVID-19, and flu vaccines, many children will have received over one hundred antigens from immunizations by the age of eighteen. So if we really want to fearmonger, let's dispense with this "seventy-two" business and use a more accurate triple-digit figure.

Seemingly, Jenner and Pasteur were not financially motivated. These scientists strived to eradicate diseases that were decimating populations, and they succeeded. The concept of vaccines is undeniably good, and the protections vaccines offer are invaluable. Yet we must simultaneously weigh the cumulative impact a high number of vaccines has on developing immune systems. As we navigate the future of inoculations, the question remains: *Do we draw the line somewhere, or do we continue to give more vaccines ad infinitum?*

The ongoing expansion of the vaccine schedule spotlights several competing considerations: On the one hand, it marks a positive step in protecting children from a growing number of preventable, debilitating, and even fatal diseases. On the other, as the number of recommended vaccines increases, in perpetuity, a number of parents and health-care professionals are asking: "Is there such a thing as too much?" and "Who decides how much is too much?"

3

THE INFLUENCE ECONOMY

THE COST OF CONTROLLING THE MESSAGE

*I'm just scared that the tentacles of the pharmaceutical industry
are so deeply entrenched in politics and in media that you can't
just shake them off. You can't just say, "Hey, you can't advertise
on TV anymore," or "Hey, you no longer have exemption from
responsibility from the side effects of certain drugs."*

—JOE ROGAN

Years ago, I posted several interesting and thought-provoking articles to
one of my social media pages. One of these articles suggested that foods
containing dyes were linked to behavioral and other health issues and,
therefore, potentially harmful to children. I posted these articles without
comment and explicitly refrained from expressing an opinion one way or
another. In response, a prominent Allopathic physician who works with
children, reprimanded me for "perpetrating faux-scientific alarmism." He
claimed that by "spreading information that is not true," I was "endangering
kids." Many years later, I remain genuinely perplexed as to why or how an
article that links the consumption of dyes and refined sugars to behavioral
issues "endangers kids."

The second article presented research connecting certain pesticides
to cancer and behavioral diseases in children. Another physician chided:
"Provide evidence-based advice and medicine to people—not these
fearmongering conspiracy theories." No *reasonable* human being would
have classified these articles as "fearmongering conspiracy theories."
Furthermore, a rudimentary search would have yielded dozens of peer-
reviewed, evidence-based journal articles linking the chemicals cited in

each respective article to a slew of diseases—albeit even in the absence of any studies, common sense would dictate that consuming chemical-laden foods is an inherently unhealthy practice that endangers kids significantly more than did my posting these articles. Then again, Voltaire said, "Common sense is not so common." In reply to this physician's comment, I explained that a brief search generated a bevy of legitimate, peer-reviewed journal articles—published in top medical journals, no less. I shared a few of these peer-reviewed, evidence-based studies with this physician. He facetiously answered: "Happy you searched for 'a few minutes.' That's great." Blinded by a level of vitriol for anything that deviated from his dogmatic understanding of "science," this physician was unwilling to accept a viewpoint that was inconsistent with his own, *even after he was proven wrong.*

Despite the wealth of peer-reviewed studies that link certain pesticides to cancer and behavioral concerns, and artificial dyes to cancer and hyperactivity in children (so much so, in fact, that, in January 2025, red dye No. 3 and, in April 2025, eight other petroleum-based dyes were banned from food in the United States), I was branded a "faux-scientific alarmist" guilty of "spreading information that is not true." I'll bet those guys are going to just *love* this book!

The buzzwords "pseudoscience," "fearmongering," "misinformation," "disinformation," and "conspiracy theorist"—to name a select few—have been weaponized to automatically disqualify anyone who questions scientific "gospel." Science, by its very definition, requires us to question theories to advance our understanding of the physical and natural world. Yet we are told that *vaccine science* is settled, and we should trust it implicitly. This concept of science we are asked to indiscriminately accept contravenes with the word's very definition.

Notwithstanding the disproportionately aggressive responses I received to these relatively innocuous articles I posted, I don't blame these physicians or others like them. They genuinely felt it their sacred duty to police the internet for any information that may promulgate a distrust of science and the institutions that purport to uphold it.

So how did we get to the point where any information that deviates from the narrative is automatically pilloried and branded one of these derisive buzzwords? Why did it become our moral imperative to defend companies, products, and chemicals? When did we rob human beings of the right to think for themselves? When did physicians anoint themselves the gatekeepers of scientific dogma? Why do they perceive themselves as the masked crusaders of the internet tasked with fighting inquiry and dialogue? The answer may lie in the historic alliance between medicine and the pharmaceutical industry.

JOHN D. ROCKEFELLER AND THE MARRIAGE BETWEEN PHARMA AND MEDICINE

We will need to travel back to the late 1800s, when John D. Rockefeller had become extremely wealthy by extracting oil from the ground. By the twentieth century, through his ownership of the Standard Oil Corporation (which was subsequently split into Mobil, Chevron, Exxon, etc.), Rockefeller controlled 90% of all petroleum refineries in America. Around this time, the science world was getting excited about the newfound ability to create a variety of compounds, specifically petrochemicals, from oil. Rockefeller eventually learned that, by using the petroleum derivative coal tar, he could manufacture pharmaceuticals.

Also in the early 1900s, scientists were making groundbreaking discoveries in the field of health, including the discovery of essential vitamins, such as B1, B2, biotin, vitamin C, vitamin A, and vitamin D. By identifying these vitamins, scientists changed the landscape of disease treatment and prevention. Using simple vitamin remedies, doctors were now able to prevent and even cure conditions previously caused by vitamin deficiencies, like scurvy and rickets. Scientists were attempting to recreate synthetic versions of these vitamins in a laboratory.

As an interesting aside, vitamin B1 (also known as thiamine) was discovered by Polish scientist Casimir Funk in 1912. He named this miracle remedy *vitamine*—combining the word *vital* (due to the vitamin's integral role in health) with the word *amine*, referring to the vitamin's composition (as in thi-*amine*).

Now back to Rockefeller . . . Numerous reports suggest that Rockefeller recognized the threat these increasingly popular natural remedies posed to his bottom dollar. Not only were natural and herbal remedies regularly prescribed in the United States in the early 1900s, but they were actually proving effective against a number of previously incurable diseases. In the United States, many medical colleges and doctors were practicing holistic medicine, using extensive knowledge from Europe and Native American traditions.

Rockefeller took action. Using his vast oil wealth, he formed a "drug trust" alliance between the Rockefeller empire and the German chemical and pharmaceutical company IG Farben, which subsequently became Bayer. Rockefeller had his proverbial finger in both pies: he controlled a significant portion of the product needed to manufacture the petrochemicals that were used to make pharmaceuticals and simultaneously controlled or partially influenced the companies that manufactured them. Petrochemicals could be patented and sold for high profits, proving them to be highly lucrative.

Rockefeller hired educator and reformer Abraham Flexner to prepare a report, known as the Flexner Report, which, in 1910, was submitted to Congress. While there was undeniable validity to a number of Flexner's findings, Flexner (not surprisingly) concluded that colleges for the education of the various forms of alternative medicine should be closed and that modalities like homeopathy, osteopathy, physiomedicalism, and other alternative practices should be abandoned. He went so far as to classify them as "quackery" effusively throughout his report.

Flexner also praised several schools for excellent performance, including Western Reserve (now Case Western Reserve), Michigan, Wake Forest, McGill, and Toronto. Flexner touted Johns Hopkins as the model for medical education. In his report, Flexner issued the following recommendations:

1. Reduce the number of medical schools and the number of, what he deemed, poorly trained physicians.
2. Increase the prerequisites to enter medical training.
3. Train physicians to practice in a scientific manner and engage medical faculty in research.
4. Give medical schools control of clinical instruction in hospitals.
5. Hire trained, full-time staff for medical education.
6. Grant medical schools increased funding.
7. Strengthen state regulation of medical licensure.

Yes, on their face, these recommendations seem as though they would optimize patient care. At the same time, they conveniently eliminated integrative health-care modalities from medicine.

But wait! The plot thickens. In his report, Flexner proclaimed Johns Hopkins a "small but ideal medical school, embodying in a novel way, adapted to American conditions, the best features of medical education

42

in England, France, and Germany." Flexner further asserted that all the other medical schools were subordinate in relation to this "one bright spot." In 1916, Johns Hopkins University and William Henry Welch, MD (the founding dean of the Johns Hopkins School of Medicine and *key medical adviser to the Rockefeller Foundation*), received a 267,000-dollar donation from the Rockefeller Foundation to found the Johns Hopkins School of Hygiene and Public Health. (This is the modern equivalent to approximately 7,951,571 dollars). Through his financial contribution, Rockefeller secured his place as an influential voice in the "one bright spot" medical school that would ultimately train budding physicians to prescribe his pharmacological products. Moreover, Rockefeller ensured that the dean was indebted to him. What could possibly go wrong?

In addition to influencing a pharmaceutical company that manufactured drugs made from the petroleum product he also largely controlled, Rockefeller succeeded in reducing the number of medical schools, streamlining the curriculums taught at each, and financially entangling himself with the institution deemed most exemplary. These changes led to an amazing boon in science and medicine. However, at the risk of venturing too deep down the conspiracy theory rabbit hole, these changes also cleared a direct path for Rockefeller to cultivate practitioners beholden to him and his pharmacological products. Of course, this would equate to sizable profits. If he were alive today, Rockefeller would have likely labeled me a "fearmongering conspiracy theorist." Though a brilliant deflection from his diabolically genius, albeit transparent agenda, Rockefeller's conspicuous web of collusion and resulting conflicts of interest are *not* conspiracy theory; they are incontrovertible, historically accurate facts.

Universally recognized as the father of medicine and namesake of the Hippocratic oath, Hippocrates taught, "Let food be thy medicine and medicine be thy food." He also reminded physicians: "The greatest medicine of all is teaching people how not to need it." Of course, there is no profit in these principles. Neither Rockefeller nor Flexner were medical doctors, medical professors, or scientists. Yet they forever reshaped the paradigm of medicine, moving away from the pedagogy of the father of medicine himself and replacing it with a pharmaceutical-driven model. To this day, the Flexner Report remains the foundation for medical education in the United States. For over a century, physicians have been programmed to trust their training. And in large part, they should. They should also be taught to question, because not always (but *sometimes*), financial motives *may* supersede competing public health concerns.

PHARMA'S ENTANGLEMENT WITH DOCTORS, RESEARCH, AND MEDICAL LEARNING INSTITUTIONS

The groundwork had been laid. During the latter half of the twentieth century, pharmaceutical companies heavily influenced some doctors through lavish gifts, vacations, and perks. To address these conflicts of interest in medicine, laws were passed to ensure that clinical decisions were made based on the best interests of patients and not financial incentives. In 1972, the Anti-Kickback Statute and, in 1989, the Stark Law were enacted. Later in 2010, the Physician Payments Sunshine Act mandated transparency by requiring disclosure of all financial relationships between physicians and pharmaceutical companies. These measures did curb direct financial incentives for individual physicians, yet pharmaceutical companies continued (and still continue) to exert substantial influence over the medical field through large-scale institutional donations. According to a 2009 *Time Magazine* article, 1,600 of Harvard's 8,900 professors and lecturers admitted that either they or a family member had a business link to pharmaceutical companies—some worth hundreds of thousands of dollars—which could at least implicitly bias their teaching or research.

In 2010, Pfizer donated $85 million dollars to UCSF for medical research; In 2018, Novartis made a multimillion-dollar grant to Harvard Medical School. These are merely a select few among an endless number of such similar donations. It's a little-known fact that you can actually look up the financial relationships that drug and medical device companies have with health-care providers (including *me*) on the site OpenPaymentsData.cms. gov. Although sizable donations support education and foster innovation, the source of these donations raises questions about the potential indirect pharmaceutical influence on medical curriculum and research priorities.

Moreover, between 2020 and 2022, pharmaceutical companies paid over $1 billion to peer reviewers and top medical journals, such as *JAMA* and *The New England Journal of Medicine*—this according to a 2024 research letter that, funnily enough, was published in *JAMA*. The letter revealed that payments came in the form of consulting fees, travel, and speaking compensation, calling into question whether these financial ties may subtly influence scientific research and publications and further erode trust.

This systemic financial entanglement highlights the urgent need for greater transparency and independence in medical research, education, and decision-making so that public health remains the greatest priority.

POLITICAL CONTRIBUTIONS

It's no secret that in addition to donating to medical schools and research institutions, pharmaceutical companies routinely donate to political campaigns. The statistics are easily accessible to the general public. Frankly, the why should be fairly obvious. While there may be no "smoking gun" written contract, this Faustian bargain is, instead, sealed with a wink and a handshake. Pharmaceutical companies are not benevolent entities who indiscriminately donate large sums of money to starving orphans in third-world countries. Instead, they routinely donate millions of dollars to politicians running for election—presumably in the hope that, once elected, these politicians will curry favor.

In 2024, Politico reported that pharma lobbyists *increased* campaign spending as compared to previous years. According to Open Secrets, during the 2024 presidential election, presidential candidate Kamala Harris received nearly $11 million from the pharmaceutical and health product sector, while Donald Trump received approximately $1.6 million. In the first quarter of 2024, health lobbying continued to grow from previous years. Health lobbyist group PhRMA spent $9.6 million; Pfizer, $3.55 million; Novartis, $3.51 million; and Amgen, $3.33 million.

THE "REVOLVING DOOR" BETWEEN PHARMA AND THE FOOD AND DRUG ADMINISTRATION

Pharmaceutical enmeshment doesn't end there. In what is sometimes described as the "revolving door," Food and Drug Administration (FDA) employees often matriculate to positions at pharmaceutical companies.

In 2016, Dr. Vinay Prasad and Dr. Jeffrey Bien, both of whom are affiliated with Oregon Health and Science University, conducted a study on career trajectories of FDA medical reviewers specializing in hematology-oncology. Their research letter to the *British Medical Journal*, which tracked fifty-five reviewers from 2001 to 2010 using sources like LinkedIn and PubMed, revealed that 57% of those who left the FDA subsequently engaged with the pharmaceutical industry.

Prasad stated: "If you know in the back of your mind that your career goal may be to someday work on the other side of the table, I wonder whether that changes the way you regulate. Are you more likely to give [companies] the benefit of the doubt? Are you less likely to beat them up hard over [using bad comparisons in drug studies]?"

To me, this is analogous to the relationship between a contractor and a building inspector. When a homeowner hires a contractor to renovate a home, those renovations must first be approved by an independent inspector, whose job it is to ensure that the construction is properly performed. This arm's-length relationship is, of course, necessary to ensure the safety of the homeowner who does not possess the requisite expertise to evaluate the contractor's work. If, due to some self-serving arrangement between the building inspector and the contractor, the building inspector turns a blind eye to work improperly performed by the contractor, the safety of the homeowner may be jeopardized.

These statistics are not in and of themselves definitive proof of collusion. However, these findings, along with the apparent "revolving door" between the FDA and the pharmaceutical industry, do beg the inescapable question as to whether securing a lucrative position with a pharmaceutical company incentivizes at least some FDA employees to turn a blind eye to otherwise questionable data.

ADVERTISING AND THE MEDIA

Only two countries in the *entire world* allow pharmaceutical companies to advertise on television: the United States and New Zealand. The history of pharmaceutical advertising in the United States is fascinating but lengthy. At the risk of deviating too far off course, I won't go into it in tremendous depth. Rather, I have isolated a few key points germane to our understanding of pharmaceutical advertising and the potential conflicts of interest it poses in the modern day.

In 1938, the federal government passed the Wheeler-Lea Act, which, in part, prohibited unfair and deceptive practices in commerce. In the committee report, the chairman of the House Committee emphasized that the public should be protected against the "abuses of advertising; the imposition upon the unsuspecting; and the downright criminality of preying upon the sick as well as the consuming public through fraudulent, false or subtle misleading advertisements." The Wheeler-Lea Act effectively handed over to the Federal Trade Commission (FTC) significant authority to regulate drug advertising.

Since ads in medical journals were exempted from the FTC's regulatory authority, drug manufacturers focused their efforts on advertising to physicians through these medical journals. Included among such ads was one for Diabinese (chlorpropamide)—an oral antidiabetic introduced by Chas. Pfizer & Co. Inc. in 1958. Despite a report prepared for the company showing a 27% incidence of serious side effects, like jaundice, the ad claimed an "almost complete absence of unfavorable side effects." A pharmaceutical company would *never* mislead or outright lie, right? In response to such misleading and even patently false advertisements—which targeted physicians and made safety claims rarely backed by actual evidence— Congress began to focus more intently on pharmaceutical marketing practices.

In 1962, after serious birth defects resulted from the use of thalidomide in Europe, Congress passed the Kefauver-Harris Amendments to the Federal Food, Drugs, and Cosmetics Act (FDCA), which dramatically expanded the FDA's authority over prescription drugs. It required pharmaceutical companies to prove a drug was safe and effective before marketing it—perhaps marking the origin of these ubiquitous buzzwords. These amendments transferred the regulatory authority over the advertising of prescription drugs from the FTC to the FDA and additionally required that drugs meet a high standard of scientific evidence in order to receive FDA approval.

By 1969, the FDA mandated that drug advertisements proffer a "true statement of information in brief summary relating to side effects, contraindications, and effectiveness." Among other stringent prerequisites, it was now compulsory that prescription drug advertisements strike a fair balance—meaning, they present information on the drug's side effects and contraindications together with information regarding its efficacy.

In the early 1980s, several savvy pharmaceutical marketers deviated from advertising directly to physicians. Instead of paid advertising, they experimented with public relations strategies. For instance, soon after Syntex, an analgesic, was introduced in the United Kingdom in 1978, the drug became a topic of discussion on talk shows, as a result of which its use increased. In the early 1980s, Pfizer followed suit by launching a public relations campaign called Partners in Health Care to increase awareness of what it touted as underdiagnosed conditions, such as diabetes, angina, arthritis, and hypertension. Pfizer's ads made no mention of any particular drugs, yet they prominently displayed Pfizer's name in the hope that patients suffering from one of these conditions might ask their physicians to prescribe a Pfizer product.

Between the 1950s and the early 1980s, no pharmaceutical companies were running product-specific ads in the mass media. In 1981, Boots pharmaceuticals used print and television ads to promote Rufen, a prescription pain reliever. Rufen was marketed as a more cost-effective alternative to the leading brand. In 1982, after market research demonstrated that a small percentage of patients who could benefit from the pneumonia vaccine Pneumovax were receiving it, Merck and Dohme advertised the vaccine to people over the age of sixty-five.

In 1982, Eli Lilly and Company launched an antiarthritic drug called Oraflex. Eli Lilly distributed 6,500 press kits to television networks and radio stations. While the company did furnish some cautionary information, the campaign focused on the claim that Oraflex might prevent the progression of arthritis. This representation went beyond the approved product label. The use of Oraflex, which may have been more pervasive due to the marketing campaign, resulted in a number of adverse drug events. Ultimately, Eli Lilly voluntarily pulled the drug from the market a mere five months after it was introduced.

Because pharmaceuticals were not directly marketed to consumers prior to the early 1980s, the FDA had little need to regulate direct-to-consumer advertising. In 1983, FDA commissioner Arthur Hull Hayes requested that the pharmaceutical industry cease advertising drugs to the public. Hayes believed that direct-to-consumer advertising would lead patients to pressure physicians to prescribe unnecessary or unindicated drugs, increase the price of drugs, confuse patients, potentiate the use of brand-name products rather than cheaper but equivalent generic drugs, and foster increased drug taking in an already overmedicated society.

Despite the unassailable correlation between direct-to-consumer marketing of pharmaceuticals and an increase in their prescription and use, in September 1985, *the FDA inexplicably rescinded the moratorium on direct-to-consumer advertising*, mandating *only* that the ads meet the same legal requirements as those directed at physicians. Notwithstanding the compelling evidence to the contrary, the FDA commissioner at the time, Frank E. Young, proclaimed that the FDA did not believe the advertisement of pharmaceuticals on television would result in increased use. This decision ran contrary to the findings made by every other public health authority around the world, including the FDA itself in the 1950s, 1960s, and early 1980s.

Notably in 2013, many years after his term as FDA commissioner ended, Young joined Braeburn Pharmaceuticals as executive vice president of clinical and regulatory affairs, where he contributed to the development of new drug applications to the FDA for evaluation of Braeburn's Probuphine (buprenorphine) implant, which—not surprisingly—was approved on May 26, 2016. Probuphine is the first buprenorphine implant for the maintenance treatment of opioid dependence. Young's subsequent employment by a pharmaceutical company—and one that would ultimately profit from advertising its product directly to consumers—calls into question the impetus for the 1985 legislation.

Today in the United States, television commercials make up a significant portion of pharma's advertising budget. Some reports indicate that up to three-quarters of pharma's total advertising budget is allocated to television ads. In 2020, pharma advertisement accounted for 75% of *all* television ads collectively.

According to Kantar Media, pharmaceutical companies are among, if not *the* largest advertisers on US television, *expending approximately $6.88 billion* in 2021 on direct-to-consumer advertising for drugs. The fact that pharmaceutical companies profit from direct-to-consumer advertising is not, in and of itself, nearly as disconcerting as the fact that pharmaceutical ad spending provides significant revenue for the networks and media companies, potentially incentivizing these outlets to avoid unfavorable reporting on pharmaceutical practices.

Major media companies—upon which the public relies for objective and transparent journalism—have indirect or even direct financial ties with pharmaceutical companies through advertising or investments. This results in an invariable conflict of interest, whereby these media organizations may hesitate to report critically on the companies on which they rely for substantial revenue.

Some journalists have shared anecdotal accounts of pressure to avoid content that could jeopardize pharmaceutical sponsorships. In some cases, investigative reports on controversial pharmaceutical issues (such as opioid advertising and prescription practices) faced delays or rejections by editors concerned about alienating major advertisers.

Moreover, media coverage of health topics frequently emphasizes pharmaceutical solutions, often without so much as first suggesting less invasive lifestyle changes or alternative interventions. Some critics argue that this creates a bias toward medicalizing health issues and suppresses viable nonpharmaceutical approaches.

Sure, common sense dictates that media outlets would be reluctant to alienate their most significant revenue streams. But for those unwilling to rely on common sense alone, studies show that articles backed by pharmaceutical funding are less likely to report adverse outcomes of medications. In fact, they tend to present drugs more favorably . . . obviously. A 2010 analysis, published in *PLOS Medicine*, found that studies conducted by pharmaceutical companies tended to be more favorable toward pharmaceutical products than studies that were not conducted by pharmaceutical companies. If networks received the bulk of their advertising revenue from regenerative organic farmers, would our news cycle look different?

Because the financial influence over the media, medical, and research institutions isn't enough, pharmaceutical companies also fund patient advocacy groups, which, in turn, provide information to the media. A 2017 study in *The New England Journal of Medicine* found that 83% of US-based patient advocacy groups reported receiving funding from pharmaceutical companies, and 36% disclosed that drug, device, or biotech companies had representatives on their boards.

THE "TENTACLES" OF THE PHARMACEUTICAL INDUSTRY

I share this admittedly lengthy history of profit-driven pharmaceutical enmeshment *not* to invite allegations that I am a conspiracy theorist. (Those will inevitably follow *without* my solicitation.) Rather, I offer it to show pharma's protracted entanglement in virtually every significant sphere—the training of physicians, the regulation of advertisements, the media, politics, and advocacy groups, to name just a few. One would be hard-pressed to chew on this information without simultaneously digesting the difficult truth: Pharma's tentacles are indeed so deeply entrenched that it stands in the optimal position to shape the narrative—such that even highly intelligent physicians illogically consider it their sworn duty to defend artificial dyes over the health of our children.

It's not surprising though. Author Jop Helm said: "When the powerful control the narrative, they hold the reins of perception. In the era of corporate western media, the masses must question what they're being fed, lest they become unwitting pawns in the game of power."

These well-intentioned professionals—who protect pharmaceuticals from the so-called "misinformation"—are all too often the unsuspecting minions whose strings are pulled by pharma Svengalis. I humbly admit I was one of them and, to some degree, I still am. I did not question. I did not ever think to.

Taking a page from Rockefeller's seminal playbook, pharmaceutical companies routinely make large donations to medical schools. Eager for future donations, these medical schools are unlikely to require "Should You Trust Big Pharma?" 101 as part of their core curriculums. Instead, from day one, would-be physicians are programmed to implicitly trust and defend their school's benefactors. Pharma knows that by funding biased studies that, in turn, are published in the most reputable medical journals, top doctors from the top universities can and will parrot the research for years to come.

Media outlets derive a majority of their advertising revenue from pharma ads, thereby disincentivizing, if not outright silencing reporting that would prove unfavorable to the pharmaceutical companies. This ensures that the public and the medical community maintain their pristine perceptions of pharma.

Politicians who receive massive donations from pharmaceutical companies feel a compunction to reciprocate once elected. They enact legislation that shields pharma from liability and allows pharma to run direct-to-consumer television and radio ads.

Pharma's reach is so deliberately pervasive that consumers and the medical community trust pharma because pharma spends tremendous sums of money on making certain that consumers and the medical community trust it. These "you scratch my back, I'll scratch yours" alliances allow pharma to skew research and favorably present data, with little to no accountability, at the ultimate expense of the consumer.

It, thus, stands to reason that—just maybe—pharma *might* deliberately withhold or even conceal the potential risks associated with its highly profitable products (vaccines included) from physicians and consumers alike. This is not to say that all pharmaceutical products are bad or that all studies funded by pharma are biased. Many medications and pharmaceutical interventions are truly miraculous. We are fortunate to live in a time when such tremendous medical advances exist. But when pharma massively profits from controlling seemingly every aspect of the narrative, we must at least wonder whether the science presented to us is, in fact, as they say, settled.

LISTENING TO PARENTS: NAVIGATING VACCINE CONCERNS WITH COMPASSION AND OPENNESS

As a pediatrician, I trust parents. In particular, I trust moms. I believe them when they look me in the eye and tell me that, upon receiving a vaccine, their child went from totally developmentally typical to displaying a gamut of uncharacteristic behavior like noticeable speech regression, inability to make eye contact, rocking back and forth, and inconsolable screaming, among others. We cannot, in the same breath, say vaccines are "*completely* safe and effective" and yet award billions of dollars for injuries proven in a court of law to be causally related to vaccines. These stories are far too numerous to ignore. Sadly, not only are these parents marginalized — they are actually vilified by all the players who should be sounding the alarm.

When perfectly pro-vax parents voice concerns over their child's adverse reaction to a vaccine, we owe it to those parents, that child, and *all* children to listen. These parents have no ulterior motives. These are not anti-vax conspiracy theorists. They are moms and dads who meticulously follow the schedules recommended by the CDC and AAP. They want their children to receive the protections vaccines offer. They do not, however, expect to have their lives altered by the adverse events that sometimes follow. Unlike the pharmaceutical companies—who are beholden to their shareholders and unabashedly driven by profit—these parents care *solely* about the health and safety of their children—so much so that they eagerly run to get their children vaccinated. When we take a step back and examine the potential respective motives at play, moms and dads have no fathomable incentive to fabricate adverse reactions.

As physicians, we owe it to our young and vulnerable patients to approach this uncomfortable conversation with an open mind—to lift the blindfold from our eyes, planted there from years of indoctrination. And this is no easy task. When a physician takes an oath to *first and foremost* do no harm, he or she cannot reconcile the fact that he or she may have inadvertently harmed a patient. It is far too bitter a pill to swallow. Instead, we physicians lean deeper into the mantra "safe and effective" to assuage our guilt. If we refuse to question whether vaccines *may*, at least on occasion, cause serious adverse side effects, we can mollify our conscience.

Likewise, it may be that physicians are afraid to draw attention to themselves and jeopardize their livelihoods. I don't blame them. I was. Hell, I still am. For many years, we worked tirelessly and diligently for the privilege to practice our chosen profession. Our families financially rely on us. We have watched medical boards eagerly make examples of physicians who voiced concerns—which, for many, were rooted in reasonable scientific hypotheses.

We stand at a crossroads. Who do we choose to believe? Why do we choose to believe corporations over moms or dads? I in no way purport to abolish vaccines or promote vaccine hesitancy. I want children to be protected against debilitating diseases. At the same time, I do not want that protection to come with other health consequences. I do believe that consumers and the doctors who stand in the middleman position deserve complete transparency, particularly when it comes to products that are injected into children's bodies. Silencing conversation serves only to raise inexorable suspicion. The increasing distrust of pharma and medicine is not misinformation promulgated by a contingent of misanthropes. Rather, it is the unfortunate result of a culture that has somehow accepted suppressing reasonable inquiry—even when those silencing the conversation massively profit from doing so.

Going forward, the moral and existential debates that the medical community and parents must grapple with are whether the information we are being provided (or not provided) is truly accurate or whether bigger self-interests are shaping the information in a way that may not be entirely in our best interest. We must carefully contemplate future additions to the schedule through independent, objective research and by performing long-term studies on the cumulative impact of the ever-expanding schedule.

In the introduction to this book, I vowed to bridge the gap. Understanding each side of the debate—even if you disagree with it—is rudimentary to respectful discourse. The verifiable facts are inescapable. Tens, if not hundreds, of thousands of *pro-vax* parents cannot all be saying the same thing without at least some merit. Children's health must *always* supersede corporate gain. Acknowledging these truths does not earn you the title "anti-vax conspiracy theorist." Instead, it renders you an open-minded, compassionate, intelligent, and solution-oriented human being. The goal is not to do away with vaccines but for consumers and the medical establishment to join forces and demand transparency from the companies manufacturing them and to make those products as safe as possible. This starts with the fundamental agreement that we just *might* be misplacing our trust in the corporations whose tentacles are strategically, pervasively, and yes, deeply entrenched.

4

BETWEEN SCYLLA AND CHARYBDIS

WEIGHING THE OPTIONS

That's the problem with vaccines. When they work, absolutely nothing happens. Nothing. Parents go on with their lives, not once thinking that their child was saved from meningitis caused by Hib or from liver cancer caused by hepatitis B or from fatal pneumonia caused by pneumococcus or from paralysis caused by polio. We live in a state of blissful denial.

—PAUL OFFIT, MD
PEDIATRIC INFECTIOUS DISEASE SPECIALIST, VACCINE EXPERT
PROFESSOR OF PEDIATRICS AT THE UNIVERSITY OF PENNSYLVANIA
DIRECTOR OF THE VACCINE EDUCATION CENTER AT CHILDREN'S HOSPITAL OF
PHILADELPHIA (CHOP), COINVENTOR OF THE ROTATEQ VACCINE

Throughout this book, I will share my thoughts; I will never tell you what to do. The purpose of this book is to arm you with critical information essential to make the best decisions for *your* family. Those decisions are reserved for *you*, not me.

Of course, I must urge you to follow the vaccine schedule recommended by the CDC and AAP. Deemed optimal by scientists far smarter than I, the current schedule was carefully crafted by health-care professionals over the course of many years. It is continually adjusted based on what is believed to be best and safest for your child. (I swear, no scary men in black suits pulled me into an unmarked van and coerced me to say this!) Because you likely glossed over the disclaimer at the beginning of this book, it bears repeating: The CDC and AAP recommendation is that your child obtain *all* vaccines on the schedule at the ages recommended by the CDC, AAP, or your local health authority, consistent with the standard of care. Let me be abundantly clear: I am *not* advising that you deviate from the recommended schedule. I am not advising you of anything.

Phew! Now that we've gotten that out of the way, many of you reading this book may be inherently curious about the alternatives. You might be disappointed when I don't expressly validate your contrarian beliefs. You may hope I suggest a vaccine schedule that deviates from the standard of care so you can proudly wield these pages on the treacherous vaccine battlefield, a.k.a. the social media comments section. If so, you have come to the wrong place. The only schedule a physician can recommend is the standard of care, which, in the United States, is the CDC schedule. Should you choose to follow a different schedule or altogether opt your child out, these are serious medical decisions that you should make after conferring with your child's doctor. This book is solely intended for educational purposes and is not a substitute for medical advice. If the men in black suits are reading this (assuming they've made it past the sensationalistic media headlines referring to me as a "tinfoil-hat-wearing, anti-science crackpot"), there you have it. Here's the part where you insert the joke about beating a dead horse.

If you are one of those parents struggling with whether to follow the recommended schedule or a slow schedule or entirely eschew vaccinations, how do you make such a difficult and potentially life-altering decision? Sure, if your almighty crystal ball revealed your child would contract the measles or end up in the Pediatric Intensive Care Unit for two weeks after developing Hib meningitis, you would (most likely) eagerly rush to vaccinate. On the other hand, if your crystal ball prognosticated that your child would experience a severe reaction to the DTaP vaccine, you may choose not to give it.

In Homer's *Odyssey*, the protagonist, Odysseus, is faced with the existential challenge of sailing between two inescapable threats: Scylla, a rock shoal described as a six-headed sea monster, and Charybdis, a formidable whirlpool. Whereas avoiding the monster would mean sailing too close to the whirlpool, avoiding the whirlpool would mean sailing too close to the monster. Ultimately, Odysseus is advised to choose the six-headed sea monster and lose only a few sailors, rather than risk losing his entire ship in the whirlpool. Despite two very difficult options, one poses a greater risk than the other. In choosing whether to vaccinate or not, it may often seem as though we parents literally stand between Scylla and Charybdis—or, put yet another way, *between a shot and a hard place.*

Conflicted parents should contemplate a risk-benefit analysis—one rooted in actual data. Although I will strive to address the known theoretical benefits of each vaccine along with the known theoretical risks posed by the diseases against which they are designed to protect, the conclusion may not always be readily apparent. You will choose to take the path of the six-headed monster—whatever that may mean to you. For some, that might be the recommended CDC schedule. For others, it could mean choosing not to vaccinate.

This delicate balancing act is ultimately designed to select the path we deem safest . . . or least risky. Whereas one parent may be utterly horrified by the prospect of giving a vaccine, another parent may be similarly horrified by the prospect of not giving it. No matter how minor the risks may or may not be, the undeniable risk inherent to either decision is a gamble. The difficulty in what feels like "betting it all on black or on red" is highlighted by two equally tragic didactic stories.

The first is the story of AR, a vibrant four-month-old baby girl, giggling at her parents' funny faces and cooing at the family dog. Concerned about potential vaccine side effects, AR's parents decided to delay vaccination. "She's healthy, and we're breastfeeding," they reasoned. "Her immune system will be fine."

One night, AR developed a high fever and struggled to breathe. Her parents rushed her to the emergency room, where she was later diagnosed with Hib meningitis. The doctors worked tirelessly, administering antibiotics and fluids, but the infection had already taken hold. Over the next two days, AR's condition deteriorated. The swelling in her brain caused seizures. Despite their best efforts, the medical team informed AR's devastated parents that AR had suffered irreversible brain damage.

AR survived. Yet her life was forever altered. She was left with profound hearing loss, cognitive impairments, and motor difficulties. Her parents were haunted by the knowledge that a simple vaccine might have prevented the ordeal.

The second (and slightly different) story involves another four-month-old baby girl, JR. This bright-eyed child was growing, curious, and developmentally on track. At her four-month checkup, JR received the Hib vaccine.

For a day or two after, JR seemed fussier than usual. Her parents chalked it up to the common postvaccine crankiness. A week later, JR started to display alarming symptoms. Her legs were weak, and she wasn't kicking like before. Within days, she was struggling to lift her head. Panicked, her parents rushed her to the hospital, where she was later diagnosed with Guillain-Barré Syndrome (GBS) — a rare, albeit known, vaccine complication.

The doctors explained that GBS occurs when the body's immune system mistakenly attacks the peripheral nerves, sometimes triggered by an infection or, in rare cases, a vaccine. JR was admitted to the pediatric ICU. There, JR received immunoglobulin therapy and intensive care. After weeks of treatment and months of physical therapy, JR slowly regained some of her strength. By her first birthday, she was crawling but had lingering partial paralysis in her legs.

Her parents remain haunted by the fact that, in their perception, a vaccine they gave their child may have caused a lifelong disability.

These examples may make it feel a little bit like "You're damned if you do, and you're damned if you don't." So how do you make the right decision for your child? Of course, you may follow the CDC guidelines. Yet if you fall into the undecided camp, consider the following: What is the risk your child will contract the disease? Is there currently a threat of contracting this disease in your area? What are the chances your child will be exposed? If your child is exposed, how likely is he or she to get infected? How dangerous is the disease? What are the chances your child will get extremely ill or even die from it? What are the odds your child will end up in hospital? Which treatment options are available?

Once you answer these questions, you must weigh them against all available prophylactic measures. What vaccine is available? How effective is it? What are the recommendations from the major public health organizations? What are the short- and long-term risks of the vaccine? What are the odds your child will experience a minor reaction versus a severe one? Are the possible severe reactions, even if rare, worse than the risks posed by the disease? Are the odds of a severe vaccine reaction higher or lower than the odds that your child will die from the disease?

The answers better position you to weigh the risks and make educated decisions. The difficulty lies primarily in the fact that the information may not always be at our disposal, rendering a risk-benefit analysis complicated. Often, we have few alternatives but to, as we are told, "trust the science." Further muddying the waters are added considerations, such as (1) as vaccination rates decline, the risk of outbreaks correspondingly increases and (2) the public health implications of not vaccinating. For instance, measles may not be an immediate concern in your area *this* week. In the past five years, there may have been zero cases in your community. However, if everyone in your area stops vaccinating and one person contracts measles, the disease could rapidly spread without sufficient time to administer the vaccine.

As the 2019 GlaxoSmithKline PRIORIX study and measles outbreak in Samoa that same year reveal, the decision to vaccinate or not vaccinate is not always simple. Anyone who claims that it is, is downplaying the six-headed monster and the whirlpool.

In 2022, as an alternative to the only measles, mumps rubella vaccine used in the United States—the MMR II, manufactured by Merck—the FDA-approved PRIORIX for individuals, twelve months and older to protect against measles, mumps, and rubella. One of the studies that led to its approval was published in a highly regarded journal *The Journal of Pediatric Infectious Disease Society*. The findings were based on the type of exemplary randomized, double-blind, controlled placebo testing that is deemed top-level science.

Although we will discuss the significance of placebos in greater detail later in this book, for the purpose of this example, you need to know that placebos are used to help researchers determine the effectiveness of a new treatment by comparing the results of the placebo group to the results of the group that receives the active treatment. The placebo is ideally inactive and has no real effect. Since the placebo group should not experience any reactions, any effect observed in the treatment group can be attributed to the experimental compound.

Except in the PRIORIX study, the placebo group received the MMR II vaccine. "What the f@*k!" you so eloquently blurt out. In this study, PRIORIX wasn't tested against an *inactive* substance that has no real effect. It was tested against *another vaccine*. When researchers compared PRIORIX with the MMR II placebo group, they found PRIORIX elicited robust immunoresponses. They concluded that the vaccine *raised no safety concerns* and that *no safety concerns were detected*.

No safety concerns? How can researchers truly evaluate safety concerns when two MMR vaccines are compared to each other? What if the MMR II and PRIORIX vaccines both caused seizures? If PRIORIX did not cause *more* seizures than the MMR II vaccine, then researchers could correctly state that PRIORIX raised no safety concerns—even though many parents would agree that seizures are, in fact, a safety concern. If PRIORIX had been tested against an inert substance that did not cause seizures, then researchers might have been unable to conclude that PRIORIX raised no safety concerns. The fact that the side effects from two different vaccines are similar does not automatically prove either vaccine safe; it simply renders them comparable.

To truly make a claim that a vaccine is safe, it would need to be tested against an inert placebo—a substance, like saline, that is devoid of therapeutic value. While PRIORIX may be safe, this study is misleading, at best. The more accurate claim regarding the safety of PRIORIX would have been "We did not find any specific safety concerns with PRIORIX compared to MMR II." Moreover, adverse events were monitored for just 180 days. Were there any potential side effects beyond that timeframe? We don't know because they weren't studied.

Notably, as is the case with *most* vaccine studies, *the vaccine manufacturer and its paid partners performed the study*. I know what you're thinking: Wait, that's a conflict of interest. *Ding, ding, ding!* You get a gold star. Yes, GlaxoSmithKline had every incentive to test PRIORIX in a way that would optimize the outcome. Of course, this does not, in and of itself, equate to foul play. By proving PRIORIX is safe, GlaxoSmithKline not only secured FDA approval but ensured a stream of revenue that accompanies its sale. This, ladies and gentlemen, is the very definition of conflict of interest. GlaxoSmithKline wasn't hiding it though. The paragraphs-long list of potential conflicts of interest from this study are disclosed . . . if anyone bothers to actually look. I've taken the liberty of pasting these paragraphs below for your perusal. (Shock and awe ensue . . . or maybe don't.) It is difficult to ignore that this study was funded by GlaxoSmithKline, conducted by GlaxoSmithKline teams using GlaxoSmithKline grants, and involved paid vaccine speakers:

> *Acknowledgments. We thank SR, PhD, and UM, PhD (both XPE Pharma & Science, Wavre, Belgium, care of GSK), for providing medical writing services and AK, PhD (XPE Pharma & Science, care of GSK), for publication management.*

Financial support. This work was supported by GlaxoSmithKline Biologicals SA (GSK), which was the funding source and was involved in all stages of study conduct and analysis. GlaxoSmithKline Biologicals SA also took responsibility for all costs associated with the development and publishing of this article.

Potential conflicts of interest from this study. N. P. K., L. W., J. A. F., M. C., and C. P. report receiving grants from the GSK group of companies. N. P. K. also reports receiving grants from Merck & Co, Pfizer, Inc, Sanofi Pasteur, Novartis (now in the GSK group of companies), Protein Science (now Sanofi Pasteur), and MedImmune. L. W. also reports receiving grants from Merck & Co and Novartis and personal fees from Sanofi Pasteur for consulting services. M. C. also reports receiving a grant from the National Institute of Allergy and Infectious Diseases for clinical study. C. P. also reports receiving grants from Sanofi Pasteur and Regeneron. R. A.-E., M. P., P. G., S. C., and O. H. are employees of the GSK group of companies. R. A.-E., P. G., S. C., and O. H. hold shares in the GSK group of companies as part of their employee remuneration. M. M. P. reports receiving a grant, speaker's honorarium, and consulting fee from Novartis and Sanofi Pasteur. J. D.-D. reports receiving grants, a speaker's honorarium, and a consulting fee from the GSK group of companies, MSD, and SPMSD. G. S. M. is a scientific advisor and investigator for the GSK group of companies, Merck & Co, Novartis, Pfizer, Inc, Sanofi Pasteur, and Seqirus and reports receiving speaker's honoraria from Pfizer, Inc, and Sanofi Pasteur. K. P. R. reports receiving research support from Novartis and research support from the GSK group of companies. I. M. served as a site investigator for the GSK group of companies and received funding as part of her involvement in the trial; she is an employee of Pfizer, Inc. T. V. declares receiving payment for lectures in the past from the GSK group of companies. C. B. and A. C. were employees of the GSK group of companies at the time the study was conducted.

All other authors: No reported conflicts of interest. All authors have submitted the ICMJE Form for Disclosure of Potential Conflicts of Interest. Conflicts that the editors consider relevant to the content of the manuscript have been disclosed.

I am not saying the results of this study are wrong or that PRIORIX is unsafe. What I am saying is, I don't know. Based on this study alone, we can conclude merely that the MMR II vaccine and PRIORIX appear to share comparable safety profiles—whether that's good or bad. The length of the disclosure list, which is so long that you likely stopped reading it after the first several sentences, speaks for itself.

Reading this gives you pause. Now you're not so sure you should give your child the measles vaccine. You have pored over the vaccine inserts. You've mulled it over with your friends and consulted with your child's pediatrician. You're still reluctant to give your child the measles vaccine. You've heard that, at one time in the United States, roughly five hundred children died from measles each year and that predated many of today's medical advances. You're fairly certain the risk to your child is slim to none. You're not alone.

In 2018, parents in Samoa thought the same thing. Samoa's measles vaccination coverage dropped to approximately 31–34%, a significant decrease from 74% in 2017. This decline was partly due to a tragic incident. After receiving improperly prepared MMR vaccines, two infants died, leading to public mistrust and suspension of the vaccination program.

In September 2019 (the same year GlaxoSmithKline was conducting PRIORIX trials), Samoa experienced a measles outbreak. By January 2020, over *5,700 cases had been reported, resulting in eighty-three deaths*, predominantly among children under five years old. This devastating story underscores the implications herd immunity has on public health and serves as a stark reminder that measles can be deadly.

Although conflicting and varying data around the measles vaccines may lead to understandable skepticism, real-world examples may offer invaluable guidance. If someone tells you measles poses no threat to your child, that is untrue. If someone tells you the vaccine science is settled—meaning, we know *all* potential risks associated with the MMR vaccine—that, too, to the best of my knowledge, is untrue. Both sides of this debate offer valid arguments. Safety and efficacy are not mutually exclusive propositions. The fact that it works does not automatically render it safe. Perhaps it is. However, the bias inherent to the research casts sufficiently reasonable doubt on the findings. Seemingly, PRIORIX is no more dangerous than the MMR II vaccine. This does not mean PRIORIX or, for that matter, the MMR II vaccine are entirely without risk. When you stand between a shot and a hard place, there are indeed so many shades of gray. You must weigh the risks against the benefits and ultimately choose the safest path.

In the next chapter, we will examine vaccine terminology and look closely at each individual vaccine on the schedule. Fair warning: It will perhaps be the most monotonous part of this book. This chapter is necessary to lay the foundation for the salacious, page-turning content that follows. (Teaser: For one particular chronic condition, there is basically no evidence to make the statement "the science is settled." Seriously, get the popcorn ready—*extra grass-fed, organic* butter.) We cannot speak the language of vaccines until we understand the terminology. For each disease, we will examine the various vaccines available for children and the ingredients in each. We will explore efficacy claims for each vaccine along with the dangers associated with the diseases they are designed to protect against. This conversation will be data -driven and, to the extent possible, objective.

5

SPEAKING THE LANGUAGE OF VACCINES

Joel "Gator" Warsh seems to be the next in a growing list of fringe, wayward pediatricians who peddle poorly-supported opinions upon unsuspecting patients and families. Such practices put patients at risk, and erode the credibility of the field of Pediatrics. In the era of "fake news," it is important for credible pediatricians and public-at-large to spotlight the unfortunate tendencies of some physicians to market themselves instead of championing science, however well-intentioned they may appear to be.

—LOCAL PEDIATRICIAN, 2019

I am unsubscribing from your emails Dr. Gator . . . you should be telling EVERYONE to NOT consider vaccinating their children . . . Very dangerous, and children hardly ever get these so-called diseases . . . NO more emails from you thank you . . .

—EMAIL FROM RC, A (FORMER) EMAIL SUBSCRIBER, 2022

We've made it to the boring part I hyped up in the last chapter—the one where you'll learn some cool science jargon. So that it's not a total snooze-fest, I prefaced this chapter with a few (of many) amusing messages I received over the years, fondly saved for posterity in a folder titled "Troll Joel." No matter how objectively I attempt to present the information, my mere existence seems to offend someone. Even my basic definition of the common vaccine vernacular will, with absolute certainty, invite vitriol. There is truly no pleasing everyone.

Without further ado, let's dive in, because we cannot participate in intelligent discourse and, accordingly, make informed decisions until we familiarize ourselves with rudimentary vaccine terminology. This is the less sexy—but no less important—part of the book where we learn to speak the language of vaccines.

TERMINOLOGY

Vaccines are biological preparations designed to stimulate an immune response, providing protection against infectious diseases. Childhood vaccines are formulated to protect children from a range of potentially severe diseases that could have significant health consequences. To appreciate the way vaccines work, we need to comprehend the different types of vaccines, their components, and their unique roles in immunity. Vaccines typically consist of the following:

1. *Antigens.* The primary component of vaccines, antigens are the specific parts of a pathogen (an organism that causes disease). Injecting these antigens triggers an immune response. Simply put, the antigen may be a virus, bacteria, chemical, toxin, or other substance that signals the body to produce antibodies, which are proteins produced by the body's immune system to identify, neutralize, and kill antigens. The immune system learns to recognize these antigens so that in the future, it can respond quickly when it encounters that particular pathogen.

2. *Adjuvants.* Added to some vaccines to boost the body's immune response to the antigen, adjuvants are substances, like aluminum salts, that increase the effectiveness of the vaccine, particularly during the initial dose.

3. *Stabilizers.* These components prevent vaccines from losing potency during storage and transport. Common stabilizers include sugars and proteins, which help maintain vaccine efficacy until administration.

4. *Preservatives.* Used to prevent contamination, preservatives, like thimerosal, prevent the growth of bacteria or fungi in vaccine vials.

5. *Inactivators.* These are chemicals, like formaldehyde, used to inactivate bacteria, toxins, or viruses in some vaccines.

6. *Trace residuals.* Trace amounts of substances, like antibiotics, might be present from the production process, usually in minute amounts.

7. *Buffers.* These substances maintain the vaccine's pH, ensuring stability and comfort during administration. Some of the most common buffers are phosphate, histidine, and citrate buffers.

TYPES OF IMMUNIZATIONS

Vaccines are categorized by the way they present the antigen to the immune system. Each type comes with its unique advantages, with some better suited for specific pathogens or age groups.

1. *Live attenuated vaccines.* These vaccines contain live, weakened forms of the pathogen. Live attenuated vaccines are unable to cause disease in healthy individuals. Because they closely mimic natural infections, they typically provide strong, lasting immunity. Examples of live attenuated vaccines are the MMR and varicella vaccines. Benefits to live attenuated vaccines include long-term immunity, often with fewer doses. However, they are not recommended for immunocompromised and pregnant individuals due to the live pathogen, even though it is weakened.

2. *Inactivated (killed) vaccines.* Unlike live attenuated vaccines, inactivated vaccines contain pathogens that have been killed so they cannot cause disease. The immune system responds to the dead pathogen, generating immunity. The inactivated polio vaccine (IPV) is a common example.

3. *Subunit, recombinant, polysaccharide, and conjugate vaccines.* These vaccines use specific pieces of the pathogen—such as proteins, sugars, or the capsid—as opposed to the entire organism. By focusing on essential parts, they effectively stimulate immunity. Examples include the hepatitis B, HPV, and Hib vaccines. They generally require multiple doses to achieve immunity.

4. *Toxoid vaccines.* Toxoid vaccines target bacterial toxins rather than the bacteria itself. They contain inactivated toxins, known as toxoids, which train the immune system to recognize the harmful effects of the toxin without exposure to active toxins. The diphtheria and tetanus vaccines are examples. Toxoid vaccines are effective at preventing disease symptoms caused by bacterial toxins but also often require booster doses.

5. *mRNA vaccines.* Using a copy of the messenger RNA molecule, these vaccines provide genetic instructions for cells to produce a protein associated with the pathogen, sparking an immune response.

6. *Immunoglobulin-based prevention (monoclonal antibody).* Using monoclonal antibodies, these types of immunizations provide passive immunity and are specifically designed to protect against a pathogen

like RSV. Rather than stimulating the body's own immune response to build memory, this immunization instead offers immediate, short-term protection. Monoclonal-based immunizations are not technically vaccines as they do not stimulate an immune response.

7. *Passive prophylaxis.* The vitamin K shot is also not a vaccine but provides a substance the body uses rather than stimulating an immune response. It aids newborns by preventing vitamin K deficiency bleeding (VKDB).

Simply put, a vaccine stimulates the immune system to create its own long-term protection. This is known as active immunity. In contrast, passive monoclonal antibody therapy like the RSV and vitamin K shots are often referred to as "vaccines" because they are injected in a similar manner, though they are not technically vaccines.

INGREDIENTS

The most common ingredients found in vaccines, along with a brief description of each, are as follows:

1. *Aluminum salts.* Aluminum salts, such as aluminum hydroxide and aluminum phosphate, are adjuvants that boost the immune response. They make the vaccine more effective, especially initial doses.
2. *Formaldehyde.* Used to inactivate bacterial toxins and viruses during the vaccine production process, formaldehyde may be present in residual amounts that are considered safe, trace levels.
3. *Thimerosal.* A mercury-based preservative, thimerosal is used to prevent contamination by bacteria and fungi in some multidose vials.
4. *Gelatin.* A stabilizer used to protect vaccines from temperature changes during storage and transport, the gelatin in vaccines is usually derived from porcine (pork) sources.
5. *Sucrose or lactose.* These are sugars used as stabilizers to maintain vaccine effectiveness during storage.
6. *Sorbitol.* Another sugar alcohol stabilizer, sorbitol, is often used in combination with gelatin or sucrose.

7. *Polysorbate 80.* This is an emulsifier that helps vaccine ingredients blend together and stabilize, especially in vaccines with lipid or fat-based components.

8. *Monosodium glutamate.* A stabilizer in some vaccines, monosodium glutamate protects against degradation from heat, light, or acidity during storage. Yes, monosodium glutamate—commonly known as MSG—is not exclusive to Chinese food or unhealthy snacks. It is also used as a stabilizer and preservative in many vaccines.

9. *Antibiotics.* Antibiotics, such as neomycin and polymyxin B, are used to prevent bacterial contamination during production.

10. *Human serum albumin.* A protein derived from human blood, human serum albumin is sometimes used as a stabilizer, particularly in vaccines produced using cell cultures.

11. *Egg protein.* Used as a growth medium for certain viruses, like the influenza virus, this ingredient is present in trace amounts in some vaccines.

12. *Lipid nanoparticles.* In mRNA vaccines, like the COVID-19 vaccines, lipid nanoparticles are used to encase and protect the mRNA, allowing it to enter cells more effectively.

13. *Yeast proteins.* In vaccines, such as the hepatitis B vaccine, yeast cells are used to produce antigens. Some trace amounts of yeast proteins may be present in the final product.

14. *2 Phenoxyethanol.* This is a preservative that is sometimes used as an alternative to thimerosal.

15. *Potassium or sodium chloride.* These are salts that help balance the pH and maintain stability in the vaccine solution.

KEY VACCINE CONCEPTS

1. *Herd immunity*: Also known as community immunity, herd immunity is a form of indirect protection from infectious diseases that occurs when a significant portion of a population becomes resistant to an infection. Consequently, the spread of infection diminishes. Herd immunity is achieved either through vaccination or when a sufficient number of naturally infected individuals recover from the disease, thereby decreasing the likelihood of infection for individuals who are

not immune. Herd immunity thresholds vary by disease based on their contagiousness. For instance, to attain herd immunity from measles, which is highly infectious, approximately 95% of the population must have immunity against the disease.

2. *Vaccine schedule.* The recommended timeline for administration of vaccines, according to various age groups and health conditions, to ensure optimal immunity.

3. *Booster shot.* An additional dose of a vaccine given periodically to boost the immune system's memory of the antigen and maintain sufficient immunity over time.

4. *Vaccine adverse events.* Any medical event that follows vaccination that may but does not necessarily have a causal relationship to the administration of the vaccine. Adverse events can range from minor side effects, like pain at the injection site, to more serious outcomes.

COMMON RISKS ACROSS VACCINES

Common minor side effects of most vaccines are typically mild and transient, indicating the body's immune response to the vaccine. Among them are the following:

- *Local reactions.* Pain, redness, or swelling at the injection site are frequent, occurring in up to 80% of vaccine recipients.
- *Systemic reactions.* Symptoms such as fever, fatigue, headache, muscle or joint pain, and chills are also common.
- *Gastrointestinal symptoms.* Nausea, vomiting, or diarrhea can occur—though these are less common.

These side effects usually resolve on their own within a few days. Whereas serious side effects are less common, the following more severe side effects may occur in certain individuals, depending on the vaccine:

- *Allergic reactions.* Among other allergic reactions, anaphylaxis is a severe, potentially life-threatening allergic reaction that can cause difficulty breathing, hives, swelling, and a drop in blood pressure.
- *Neurological reactions.* Guillain-Barré Syndrome (GBS) is a rare autoimmune disorder in which the body's immune system attacks the nerves, potentially causing muscle weakness or paralysis.

- *Seizures.* Seizures can occur and are often triggered by fever after vaccination—namely, in children. Febrile seizures occur in 1 per 3,000 doses of vaccines like MMR or DTaP.
- *Encephalopathy.* A very rare inflammation of the brain, encephalopathy potentially leads to seizures or altered mental states.
- *Bell's palsy.* Temporary facial paralysis, where one side of the face may become weak or droop.
- *Cardiovascular and blood disorders.* Included among such disorders are myocarditis and pericarditis—an inflammation of the heart muscle or lining, primarily noted after mRNA COVID-19 vaccines in young males. Myocarditis and pericarditis were noted in 1 to 4 patients per 100,000 doses. Thrombosis with thrombocytopenia syndrome (TTS) is a condition involving blood clots combined with low platelets.
- *Autoimmune reactions.* Immune thrombocytopenic purpura (ITP) is a condition causing low platelet counts, leading to easy bruising or bleeding. ITP has been seen in 1 per 40,000 doses after MMR vaccination.
- *Severe skin reactions.* Stevens-Johnson syndrome (SJS) is a rare but serious skin reaction that can cause peeling, blisters, and severe rash.
- *Respiratory reactions.* Bronchospasm is a sudden constriction of the muscles in the walls of the bronchi, leading to difficulty breathing. While rare, it may occur after vaccination, especially in individuals with asthma or severe allergies.
- *Severe gastrointestinal reactions.* Gastroenteritis and intussusception are severe inflammation and blockage of the stomach and intestines, sometimes associated with the rotavirus vaccine.
- *Hypotonic-hyporesponsive episode (HHE).* HHE is a condition where a child may become pale, limp, and unresponsive for a short period after vaccination, typically within forty-eight hours of receiving vaccines, such as DTP. This occurs in approximately 1 per 1,750 doses of DTP vaccine.
- *Arthralgia.* Otherwise known as temporary joint pain or swelling, arthralgia is particularly noted with MMR or rubella-containing vaccines. It occurs approximately 1 per 10,000 to 1 per 100,000 doses.

- *Ocular reactions.* Optic neuritis is the inflammation of the optic nerve, potentially leading to visual disturbances or vision loss. Although rare, optic neuritis has been reported with the influenza and hepatitis B vaccines.

In summary, *serious* side effects from vaccines are stated to be extremely rare, with most occurring at documented rates of 1 per 10,000 to 1 per 1,000,000.

Nearly *all* vaccine inserts also state: "Carcinogenesis, mutagenesis, impairment of fertility has not been evaluated," which means that the vaccine was not specifically tested in long-term studies to determine whether it causes cancer, genetic mutations, or fertility issues.

THE IMMUNE SYSTEM

A discussion of vaccines would be incomplete without simultaneously addressing the system they are designed to protect.

The immune system is the body's incredible defense network—a powerful army tirelessly working to defend the body against harmful invaders such as bacteria, viruses, and toxins. It consists of *innate immunity* and *adaptive immunity.* Whereas innate immunity provides immediate but nonspecific defense, such as skin, mucus, and white blood cells, adaptive immunity recalls past infections to respond more effectively in the future.

(For those of you in the Super Nintendo generation, adaptive immunity is kind of like that moment when you finally defeated Bowser in the last level of Super Mario World. Once you achieved this Herculean feat, you knew how to beat him again the next time you played the game.)

The adaptive immune system relies on antibodies, which are proteins produced by B cells that recognize and neutralize pathogens. Another key player, T cells, help coordinate the immune response and destroy infected cells.

Immunity can be active or passive. As memory cells are created, active immunity develops when the immune system is directly exposed to a pathogen, either through infection or vaccination, leading to long-term protection. Passive immunity occurs when antibodies are transferred from another source, such as from mother to baby through the placenta or breast milk, or through immune globulin therapy or monoclonal antibody, like the RSV immunization—providing temporary protection using premade antibodies. While active immunity lasts far longer, passive immunity offers immediate but short-lived defense and is typically used for emergency protection against diseases such as rabies or hepatitis exposure. Both types of immunity play essential roles in keeping us protected from infections.

6

INSIDE THE SYRINGE
A CLOSER LOOK AT INDIVIDUAL VACCINES

Our greatest responsibility is to be good ancestors.
—JONAS SALK, DEVELOPER OF THE INACTIVATED POLIO VACCINE

Now that you are familiar with the terminology, we are in a position to discuss the individual childhood vaccines recommended by the CDC. This chapter will provide you with the foundational science lesson necessary to understand the more exciting stuff to come. Specifically, for each vaccine, we will explore the underlying disease against which the vaccine is designed to protect. We will also list the vaccine's ingredients and discuss its efficacy and dosing.

For those expecting a debate about the good, the bad, the ugly, and everything in between, be patient. I promise, we will most definitely get there. In subsequent chapters, we will dissect the common concerns and controversies. I will answer your burning questions. To start, though, a rudimentary grasp of the vaccines and diseases is indispensable to our impending conversation. We will begin by addressing the first three shots administered shortly after birth—hepatitis B, RSV, and vitamin K. Next, we will cover the vaccines given in infancy and childhood, along with the available combination shots, followed by those given to older children. We will round out our discussion of individual vaccines with the flu and COVID-19 vaccines before diving into the tantalizing content you came for.

HEPATITIS B

Because hepatitis B is one of the very first vaccines parents are asked to administer to their newborn baby, it is a good place to start. Hepatitis B, caused by the hepatitis B virus (HBV), is a serious viral infection that leads to inflammation of the liver. It can result in both acute (short-term) and chronic (long-term) illness. Acute hepatitis B often presents with flu-like symptoms such as fever, fatigue, loss of appetite, nausea, and vomiting. Some individuals may also experience abdominal pain, particularly in the upper right side where the liver is located. As the infection progresses, more specific symptoms, like dark urine, pale stools, joint pain, and jaundice (yellowing of the skin and eyes), may occur. These symptoms typically appear within one to four months after exposure to the hepatitis B virus.

Some people may experience mild or no symptoms; others can have more severe manifestations. Most individuals with acute hepatitis B recover fully, though in rare cases hepatitis B can lead to fulminant liver failure (a rapid and severe form of liver damage that leads to life-threatening complications). On the other hand, if left untreated, chronic hepatitis B can lead to long-term issues such as cirrhosis (scarring of the liver), liver failure, liver cancer, and death.

Hepatitis B is primarily spread through contact with infectious body fluids, like blood, semen, and vaginal fluids. Common means of transmission include:

- mother to child during childbirth (vertical transmission),
- unprotected sexual contact with an infected person,
- sharing needles or syringes (i.e., in IV drug use),
- direct contact with open sores or blood from an infected person, and
- needlestick injuries in health-care settings.

In 2020, a total of ten cases of perinatal hepatitis B (meaning, it was transmitted from mom to baby) were reported to the CDC. Hepatitis B is not transmitted by casual contact. For example, unless they have contact with blood, blood products, or blood-contaminated fluids, hospital employees are at no greater risk than the general public. In 2020, only nine total cases of transmission in adults came from nonsexual household contact.

The risk of developing chronic hepatitis B depends largely on the age at which the infection occurs. Approximately 90% of infants who contract hepatitis B at birth or in the first year of life will develop chronic hepatitis B. This is because their immune systems are not fully developed to clear the virus effectively. Around 25–50% of children infected between ages one and five will develop chronic hepatitis B. In contrast, fewer than 5% of adults who contract hepatitis B will develop a chronic infection. Most adults are able to mount an effective immune response that clears the virus from their system.

The primary risk for children, especially newborns, is contracting hepatitis B during birth if the mother is infected with the virus. Illustrating this risk is the devastating story of a three-month-old baby girl, Rashida. On December 13, 2000, Rashida was brought to a local Michigan hospital emergency department following a five-day history of fever, diarrhea, and jaundice. Rashida was diagnosed with hepatic (liver) failure due to hepatitis B virus infection. On December 16, Rashida was transferred to another hospital for possible liver transplantation. After the transfer, she developed seizures. Her condition deteriorated rapidly. On December 17, Rashida passed away.

Investigation revealed that Rashida's mother had tested positive for the hepatitis B Surface Antigen (HBsAg) during her pregnancy but that the test result was communicated incorrectly as "hepatitis negative" to the hospital where Rashida was born. Neither the laboratory nor the prenatal care provider reported the HBsAg-positive test results to the local health department as required by state law. The infant received no hepatitis B vaccine and no hepatitis B immune globulin (HBIG) at the time of birth.

The hospital where Rashida was born had suspended administration of the hepatitis B vaccine to all newborns during the summer of 1999 due to the concern about the presence of thimerosal used as a preservative in hepatitis B vaccine. The first dose of hepatitis B vaccine wasn't administered to Rashida until two months of age. Had it been administered upon Rashida's birth, this tragedy could and probably would have been averted.

In 2020, 11,635 new cases of chronic hepatitis B were identified and reported in the United States, which equates to a rate of 5.0 cases per 100,000 people. In 2021, 2,045 acute cases of hepatitis B were reported across all age groups, with the majority of new cases occurring in adults. Cases in children, especially newborns, remain very low. According to CDC data, acute cases in the 0–19 age group were 0.1 per 100,000 between 2006 and 2010, and 0.0 per 100,000 between 2011 and 2020.

There are several hepatitis B vaccines: ENGERIX-B, by GlaxoSmithKline, and RECOMBIVAX HB, by Merck.

The active ingredient in ENGERIX-B is the recombinant hepatitis B surface antigen (HBsAg) produced in yeast cells. Other ingredients include aluminum hydroxide, sodium dihydrogen phosphate dihydrate, disodium phosphate dihydrate, sodium chloride, and water for injection.

The active ingredient in the RECOMBIVAX HB vaccine is recombinant hepatitis B surface antigen (HBsAg), which is also produced in yeast cells. Other ingredients include aluminum hydroxyphosphate, formaldehyde, sulfate, amino acids, dextrose, mineral salts, and water.

Both ENGERIX-B and RECOMBIVAX HB contain 0.25 mg of aluminum per 0.5 mL dose.

According to the CDC guidelines, recommended dosing for infants and children for the hepatitis B vaccine typically includes three doses, with the first given within twenty-four hours of birth; the second, at one to two months of age; and the third, between six and eighteen months of age.

Some wonder whether all three doses are necessary. After the first dose, approximately 30–50% of recipients develop some protective antibodies against the hepatitis B virus (HBsAg-specific antibodies). After the full series, meaning all three doses, is administered, the vaccine provides 95% protection against hepatitis B. The vaccine elicits strong immunogenicity in infants and young children, particularly when given in the first twenty-four hours after birth.

Hepatitis B vaccines are highly effective, providing long-lasting protection for at least twenty to thirty years after the full series is completed.

VITAMIN K

Like the hepatitis B vaccine, the vitamin K immunization is administered shortly after birth. In the 1930s, scientists first identified the role vitamin K plays in blood clotting. Researchers noticed that newborns were at a higher risk of bleeding disorders. This was attributed to the low levels of vitamin K at birth.

By the 1940s, early research showed that giving vitamin K to newborns could prevent life-threatening bleeding, leading to the development of the vitamin K immunization as a standard preventive measure.

Vitamin K is a fat-soluble vitamin essential for blood clotting. It exists in two main forms: vitamin K1 (phylloquinone), found in leafy green vegetables, and vitamin K2 (menaquinone), found in fermented foods and animal products. Certain types of bacteria produce vitamin K in the gut, mostly in the large intestine. These bacteria synthesize vitamin K2, which, to some extent, is absorbed—though the efficiency of this process can vary based on an individual's gut health and microbiome composition.

While the body can produce some vitamin K2 through gut bacteria, dietary sources of both K1 and K2 are generally needed to maintain adequate levels, especially since vitamin K plays critical roles in bone health, cardiovascular health, and coagulation. Vitamin K deficiency is rare in adults but can be more common in newborns, who lack a well-developed gut microbiome and, therefore, do not produce sufficient vitamin K at birth. Moreover, vitamin K transfer through the mother's placenta during pregnancy is limited, and breast milk contains low vitamin K stores—even breastfed infants do not receive a more significant amount of vitamin K. Accordingly, the vitamin K shot is recommended at birth to help the infant's body produce the proteins needed for blood clotting and prevent excessive bleeding.

Why is blood clotting such a big deal? Vitamin K deficiency bleeding (VKDB) is a condition whereby newborns or infants experience severe bleeding due to insufficient vitamin K. Prior to the introduction of routine vitamin K administration, VKDB was a major concern for newborns. The mortality rate for infants with late VKDB (two weeks to six months after birth) was around 20%, and survivors often suffered from long-term neurological damage due to bleeding in the brain.

Although more rare, early VKDB (within twenty-four hours of birth) occurs primarily in infants whose mothers were on certain medications during pregnancy that interfere with vitamin K. Without prophylaxis, this risk is approximately 1 in 60 to 1 in 250 newborns. The risk of classic VKDB (two to seven days after birth) is approximately 0.25–1.5% (1 in 100 to 1 in 400 newborns) without the vitamin K shot. Late VKDB is the most dangerous because it frequently involves intracranial hemorrhage (brain bleed). The risk is 1 in 14,000 to 1 in 25,000 for infants who do not receive the vitamin K shot, especially in exclusively breastfed babies. Additionally, infants who do not receive the vitamin K shot are eighty-one times more likely to develop late VKDB than those who do.

Whereas statistics show that 4.4 to 7.2 infants out of 100,000 who do not receive any vitamin K at birth will develop late VKDB, they also show that 0 to 0.4 out of 100,000 infants who receive the vitamin K shot at birth get late VKDB. For infants who receive a 1 to 3 mg dose of oral vitamin K 1.4 to 6.4 of them out of 100,000 will develop late VKDB. For infants who receive 1 mg of oral vitamin K at least three times during infancy (typically one week and four weeks), 2.6 out of 100,000 will develop late VKDB. Statistics from Germany, Switzerland, and Denmark show that somewhere between 0 and 0.9 infants out of 100,000 will develop late VKDB when they receive a 2 mg dose of oral vitamin K at least three times during infancy (administered either four to six days, and again, at four to six weeks *or*, alternatively, 2 mg of oral vitamin K given after birth, followed by 1 mg of oral vitamin K every week for three months).

In the United States, it is common practice to administer vitamin K injections to newborns shortly after birth to prevent VKDB. The shot, phytonadione (Vitamin K1), is manufactured by several companies, such as Pfizer, Amphastar Pharmaceuticals, and International Medication Systems Ltd. (IMS) (generic). The active ingredient is phytonadione. Other ingredients typically include polysorbate 80, which helps dissolve the vitamin K in a liquid solution; propylene glycol, which acts as a solvent and stabilizer; and benzyl alcohol, which is used as a preservative in some formulations. The inactive ingredients vary slightly by manufacturer but typically contain buffering agents to maintain pH stability.

The primary difference between formulations lies in the preservative content. Preservative-free formulations are recommended for newborns and those at risk of allergic reactions or sensitivities to benzyl alcohol—although from a practical standpoint, I'm not sure how anyone would know if a one- to two-hour-old baby has these sensitivities. In infants, benzyl alcohol can cause gasping syndrome when given in large amounts. The preservative-free version still contains the following inactive ingredients: polysorbate 80 NF, propylene glycol USP, sodium acetate anhydrous USP, acetic acid, glacial USP, and water for injection USP.

The initial 1 mg dose of vitamin K1 is administered via intramuscular injection in the thigh, within one to two hours after birth.

In 1961, the AAP started recommending that all newborns receive a single dose of vitamin K to prevent VKDB. After the widespread adoption of the vitamin K shot, cases of VKDB dramatically decreased. Today, the vitamin K shot is considered the standard of care in many countries, and its routine administration has virtually eliminated VKDB in most developed nations.

Some parents prefer to administer oral vitamin K. When oral vitamin K is given in lieu of the vitamin K shot, the risk of VKDB is reduced although not altogether obviated. Oral vitamin K is not as effective as the injection. While oral doses can help prevent early and classic VKDB, multiple doses are required (typically three doses over several weeks or a dose per week for three months). Adherence can prove challenging for parents during what are arguably the most difficult months of parenthood.

In summary, the introduction of vitamin K support in the mid-twentieth century revolutionized newborn care, significantly reducing the rates of severe bleeding and preventing the life-threatening complications of VKDB. Prior to this intervention, newborn bleeding disorders were much more common and carried high rates of mortality and neurological damage.

RSV

Next in line in our discussion of individual vaccines is the RSV immunization. Respiratory syncytial virus (RSV) is a common respiratory infection that typically causes mild coldlike symptoms in healthy children and adults but can be more severe in infants, young children, and the elderly, most notably those with weakened immune systems or underlying health conditions. RSV can lead to bronchiolitis (inflammation of the small airways in the lung) and pneumonia, which may require hospitalization, chiefly in infants under one year of age.

RSV is a significant cause of respiratory infections in infants, and approximately 90% of children will have been infected with the virus by age two. Though most recover without any complications, RSV is one of the leading causes of hospitalizations in infants and, in some, can result in long-term respiratory complications.

Each year in the United States, RSV is responsible for approximately 58,000 to 80,000 hospitalizations among children under five years old, and tragically, between 100 and 300 of these children die each year from the virus.

Currently, two options exist for the RSV immunization. Each uses different formulations and mechanisms to target the virus.

One RSV immunization, known as Beyfortus (nirsevimab), is manufactured by AstraZeneca and Sanofi and comes in 0.5 mL and 1 mL forms. The 0.5 mL contains 50 mg nirsevimab-alip, arginine hydrochloride (8 mg), histidine (1.1 mg), L-histidine hydrochloride monohydrate (1.6 mg), polysorbate 80 (0.1 mg), sucrose (21 mg), and water for injection (USP). The 1 mL contains 100 mg nirsevimab-alip, arginine hydrochloride (17 mg), histidine (2.2 mg), L-histidine hydrochloride monohydrate (3.3 mg), polysorbate 80 (0.2 mg), sucrose (41 mg), and water for injection (USP).

Unlike traditional vaccines, which stimulate the body's immune system to produce antibodies over time, nirsevimab provides preformed antibodies directly to offer immediate protection. It acts against the F protein of the RSV virus, preventing it from entering host cells.

It is suggested for all infants under eight months old entering their first fall/winter RSV season to provide protection for the duration of the season and for older infants who are at high risk. The vaccine may be given as early as the first week of life. The recommended dosage for neonates and infants born during or entering their first RSV season is 50 mg if under 5 kg (11 lb) in body weight, or 100 mg if greater than or equal to 5 kg in body weight.

Manufactured by Pfizer, RSVPreF (ABRYSVO) is another available RSV vaccine. A more traditional vaccine, it is recommended for pregnant women. Given during pregnancy, this vaccine prompts the mother's immune system to produce antibodies against RSV, which are then passed to the fetus through the placenta, offering protection to the newborn. A single-dose vaccine given to the mother between weeks thirty-two and thirty-six of pregnancy is designed to protect infants during the first six months of life.

According to the insert, Beyfortus carries with it the potential for hypersensitivity reactions, such as anaphylaxis. Serious hypersensitivity reactions have been reported after the administration of Beyfortus. These reactions included hives, shortness of breath, cyanosis, and hypotonia.

Pre-licensure testing of Beyfortus demonstrated a 74.5% reduction in the relative risk of medically attended RSV lower respiratory tract infections compared to placebo. A study conducted in Galicia, Spain, during the 2022–2023 RSV season, reported an 82% effectiveness of Beyfortus in reducing RSV hospitalizations among infants. A CDC study revealed that early data from the New Vaccine Surveillance Network indicated that nirsevimab was 90% effective in preventing RSV-related hospitalizations in infants. Among the infants who received Beyfortus in clinical trials, no deaths were attributed to RSV.

Immunizing against RSV is a fairly recent development. The vaccines are new. Death from RSV is very rare, so much so that no children died in the trials. In the United States, it is reported that approximately one hundred to three hundred children die annually from RSV.

For those who subscribe to "the more the merrier" school of thought, adding another vaccine to the battery of newborn vaccines may prove . . . well . . . all the merrier. However, many parents may be reluctant to give another vaccine to their newborn baby, particularly when that vaccine is new and doesn't come with any long-term data. Yet studies show that the RSV vaccine is extremely effective in protecting children from a disease that roughly 90% of them will have contracted by the time they are two years old and that, for some, can result in serious complications, hospitalization, and even death. A close family member of mine was hospitalized in the intensive care unit (ICU) with RSV. Babies don't come with crystal balls. There is no way for parents to predict whether their child will be one of the unlucky few that end up in the pediatric ICU, strapped to a breathing machine. Of the existing vaccines available, the RSV immunization appears to merit serious consideration.

DTAP

Any discussion around early childhood vaccines would be incomplete without the DTaP (diphtheria, tetanus, acellular pertussis) vaccine. A combination shot, the DTaP vaccine provides protection against several serious diseases, the first of which is diphtheria. Diphtheria is caused by the pathogenic bacterium, corynebacterium diphtheriae, and spreads through respiratory droplets or direct contact with infected individuals or carriers. The symptoms of diphtheria—which I share cautiously and with the keen knowledge that some of you will swear you've come down with it the next time you experience the slightest throat tickle—include sore throat, low-grade fever, and a thick gray membrane covering the throat and tonsils, which can cause breathing difficulties. In severe cases, it can lead to heart, kidney, and nerve damage due to a toxin produced by the bacteria. In all likelihood, your sore throat isn't *this*.

Diphtheria. It sounds so antiquated—like the type of disease that plagued humanity back when men rocked sartorial jabots and those funny colonial-era buckle shoes. No, diphtheria isn't as prevalent as it may have been when men's fashion was undeniably more interesting (or some might even say "cooler"). This is not because diphtheria simply went by the wayside along with double-breasted waistcoats. Rather, vaccination played a significant role in obviating what was once a common and deadly disease. In the 1920s, the United States reported around 100,000 to 200,000 cases of diphtheria annually, with approximately 13,000 to 15,000 deaths each year. Diphtheria is now extremely rare in the United States, with a mere handful of cases reported in the last few decades. Between 1996 and 2018, the United States reported only fourteen cases of diphtheria and one death. These numbers, although a testament to the efficacy of vaccination and public health, in no way render diphtheria any less serious or deadly.

The second disease against which the DTaP combination shot protects, tetanus is a serious infection caused by *Clostridium tetani* bacteria found in soil, dust, and manure. Tetanus is contracted when the bacteria enters the body through cuts, punctures, or wounds. Symptoms include muscle stiffness, principally in the jaw (lockjaw), followed by stiffness throughout the body, painful muscle spasms, and in severe cases, respiratory failure or cardiac arrest, which can lead to death.

In the 1940s, around five to six hundred cases of tetanus were reported annually. Since then, tetanus cases have significantly decreased. The CDC reported that between 2009 and 2019, there was an average of approximately thirty cases annually in the United States, with a case-fatality rate of about 10–20%, mainly in unvaccinated or under-vaccinated individuals. Once infected, Tetanus Immune Globulin (TIG) may help with symptoms.

Most of us have heard that if we step on a rusty nail, we must immediately receive a tetanus shot. Whoever ran the smear campaign against rusty nails deserves some sort of PR award. Rust does not cause tetanus. Rather, tetanus is caused by a bacterium called *Clostridium tetani* that can live in soil, dust, and animal feces sometimes harbored in the rusty nail. The rust itself is not the source of tetanus, and there is no general need to worry about contracting tetanus from a rusty nail, *except* under very specific circumstances.

The association between rusty nails and tetanus originated from the understanding that rusty objects are often found outdoors—where the *Clostridium tetani* bacterium is prevalent in the soil. If a rusty nail punctures the skin, it can create an anaerobic (low oxygen) environment in the wound that is ideal for the bacterium to multiply and release its toxin, causing tetanus. The deeper and more anaerobic the wound, the higher the risk of tetanus infection. Tetanus is more likely to occur on farms compared to urban or suburban areas. *Clostridium tetani* thrives in environments commonly found on farms because *Clostridium tetani* spores are naturally present in soil and animal feces. Farms, with their abundance of livestock and outdoor activities, frequently have higher levels of these spores. Thus, wounds contaminated with soil or manure are at greater risk for tetanus.

Farmwork typically involves handling sharp tools, heavy equipment, and materials like barbed wire or nails, as a result of which injuries and puncture wounds are more prevalent, especially for those working barefoot or without proper protective gear. Moreover, injuries may not be immediately treated on a farm, thereby increasing the chance of infection. Prompt cleaning and care of wounds are crucial in preventing tetanus.

The AAP *Red Book* does recommend giving the Tdap vaccine within forty-eight to seventy-two hours of injury, including from a rusty nail. It is biologically plausible that Tdap, when administered immediately after injury, may offer some protection, albeit not everyone agrees with this statement. If a person is already infected with tetanus, the Tdap or DTaP vaccines are not the first-line treatment for an active tetanus infection. Vaccines are designed to prevent infections by helping the immune system recognize and fight pathogens before they can cause illness. This process can take anywhere from several days to weeks—not fast enough to counteract an active tetanus infection, which progresses rapidly.

Standard recommendations are that after sustaining a wound that is dirty and severe, but before any symptoms of tetanus present, a person who has had fewer than three prior doses of tetanus toxoid or an unknown history of prior doses should receive TIG *as well as* the tetanus toxoid vaccine.

Once symptoms present, the DTaP or other tetanus vaccines are no longer helpful and TIG is the appropriate medical intervention. TIG provides immediate passive immunity by neutralizing the tetanus toxin that has not yet bound to nerve endings. TIG is typically given as an injection at the time of diagnosis. TIG provides temporary immunity by directly providing antitoxin. This ensures that protective levels of antitoxin are achieved even if an immune response has not occurred.

Turning now to the third and final disease against which the DTaP vaccine is designed to protect is pertussis, otherwise known as whooping cough. Caused by the bacterium *Bordetella* pertussis, pertussis is transmitted through airborne droplets from coughing or sneezing. Pertussis begins with coldlike symptoms and is often followed by severe coughing fits that might end with a "whoop" sound upon inhalation—hence the name whooping cough. Pertussis is most dangerous for infants under six months old, who run the greatest risk of developing pertussis-related complications (i.e., pneumonia, seizures, brain damage, or death). Roughly one out of twenty pertussis patients develop pneumonia. In fact, the most common complication and cause of death from pertussis in infants is a secondary infection from pneumonia. About one-third of infants with pertussis require hospitalization. Apnea—a condition characterized by pauses in breathing—occurs in approximately 68% of infants under twelve months old. Less serious complications include otitis media (middle ear infection), anorexia, and dehydration.

Adolescents and adults may also develop complications of pertussis such as difficulty sleeping, urinary incontinence, pneumonia, rib fracture resulting from coughing fits, syncope, and weight loss. For older children and adults, the symptoms of pertussis are typically milder. Severe complications, like pneumonia and neurologic issues, are less common in these age groups. Still, infected individuals can spread the disease.

Before the pertussis vaccine was introduced in the 1940s, pertussis was a leading cause of childhood illness and death in the United States, with more than 200,000 cases and about 9,000 deaths annually. Between 2000 and 2017, the United States reported 307 deaths from pertussis. Children under two months old sadly accounted for 84% of these deaths.

Although pertussis cases undeniably decreased, the disease has resurged in recent years, with fluctuating case numbers. In 2012, the United States experienced a significant pertussis outbreak, with over 48,000 reported cases and twenty deaths. In 2019, the United States reported 18,617 cases, and in 2023, it reported 2,815 cases of pertussis across all age groups. While many attribute the resurgence of pertussis to the unvaccinated, multiple more recent outbreaks have also occurred in vaccinated individuals.

The DTaP vaccines offered in the United States are DAPTACEL, manufactured by Sanofi Pasteur, and INFANRIX, manufactured by GlaxoSmithKline. DAPTACEL contains the active ingredients: diphtheria and tetanus toxoids and acellular pertussis antigens, filamentous hemagglutinin, pertactin, and fimbriae types 2 and 3. The inactive ingredients are aluminum phosphate, as an adjuvant; formaldehyde, as a preservative; 2-phenoxyethanol, as a preservative; polysorbate 80; and water for injection.

The active ingredients in INFANRIX are diphtheria and tetanus toxoids and acellular pertussis antigens, filamentous hemagglutinin, and pertactin. The inactive ingredients are aluminum hydroxide, as an adjuvant; polysorbate 80; formaldehyde; sodium chloride; and water for injection.

Doses are recommended at two months, four months, six months, fifteen to eighteen months, and again, at four to six years. DAPTACEL contains 0.33 mg of aluminum per dose, in the form of aluminum phosphate. INFANRIX contains 0.5 mg of aluminum per dose, as aluminum hydroxide.

The DTaP vaccine has proven successful in protecting against diphtheria, tetanus, and pertussis, though efficacy can vary somewhat for each disease component. The efficacy of the DTaP vaccine against diphtheria and tetanus is estimated to be over 95% after the complete series of doses. The efficacy of the DTaP vaccine against pertussis is roughly 85% after the full series in infancy. However, immunity for pertussis tends to wane over time, leading to reduced efficacy in older children and adolescents. Studies have found that DTaP protection against pertussis decreases by about 10% per year after the last dose, making booster doses important. The series of the first five doses offers robust initial protection. The waning immunity against pertussis has led to recommendations for booster doses, such as the Tdap booster given at eleven to twelve years. The Tdap booster is also given to pregnant women during *each* pregnancy to provide immunity from mother to infant.

HIB

The next in our long list of childhood vaccines is the Haemophilus influenzae type b (Hib) vaccine. Haemophilus influenzae is a bacterium consisting of several different types, categorized from type a to type f based on distinct surface antigens. Among these, Hib has historically been the most disconcerting due to its ability to cause severe invasive diseases, including meningitis, pneumonia, and epiglottitis, particularly in children under five years of age.

Transmission occurs through respiratory droplets, making it easy for Hib to spread in close-contact environments like day care centers. Given that Hib primarily affects young children under the age of five and individuals with weakened immune systems, the contagious nature of this pathogen renders it all the more dangerous. In fact, for young children, Hib was once a leading cause of bacterial meningitis—an infection of the membranes surrounding the brain and spinal cord, and epiglottitis that can lead to fatal swelling of the windpipe and block the airway. The advent of the Hib vaccine has dramatically reduced the incidence of Hib infections in countries with high vaccination rates.

Prior to the initiation of a vaccine program, Hib was estimated to account for nearly twenty thousand cases of invasive infections annually in the United States, approximately twelve thousand of which were meningitis. Infants younger than six months old accounted for roughly 17% of all Hib infections, with the peak incidence of Hib meningitis occurring between six and eleven months of age. About 47% of all cases of Hib occur by one year of age, with the remaining 53% of cases occurring over the next four years.

The mortality rate from Hib meningitis is roughly 5%. In addition, up to 35% of survivors develop neurologic sequelae, including seizures, deafness, and neurodevelopmental concerns. Other invasive diseases caused by this bacterium are cellulitis, epiglottitis, sepsis, pneumonia, septic arthritis, osteomyelitis, and pericarditis.

In a 2020 article entitled "Vaccine's Safety, Morality Hit Home for Girl's Parents," published in *The Tennessean*, author Bill Snyder tells the story of Suzanne and Leonard Walther, who had such serious concerns about the safety and morality of vaccination that they decided to delay vaccinating their infant daughter while they sought answers to their questions. In the meantime, their daughter contracted Hib. Although, fortunately, she recovered, Suzanne Walther later said, "I don't want my child to be the one in three million children who suffers a potentially fatal reaction to a vaccine, but I also don't want mine to be the one in ten that dies if they get the disease."

Since the introduction of the Hib vaccine in the United States in the 1980s, cases of invasive Hib disease among children under five have decreased by over 99%. In 2018, the CDC reported only thirty-eight cases of Hib in young children, a stark contrast to the tens of thousands of cases seen annually in the prevaccine era.

In 2022, in the European Union, over 2,300 invasive Haemophilus influenzae cases were reported, though most were caused by nontypeable strains—those not covered by the Hib vaccine. About 211 cases were attributed to type b, primarily in young children. Additionally, Hib disease is still estimated to cause significant illness and mortality in regions with limited vaccine access.

In the United States, there are several available Hib vaccines: ActHIB, by Sanofi Pasteur; PedvaxHIB, by Merck; and HIBERIX, by GlaxoSmithKline. The formulations and schedules vary from vaccine to vaccine.

The ActHIB vaccine contains the Hib polysaccharide linked to tetanus toxoid protein. The Hib polysaccharide is linked to tetanus toxoid protein to enhance immune response. Polysaccharides alone are poorly immunogenic in young children. Conjugating them to a protein carrier helps stimulate a stronger, longer-lasting immune memory by engaging T cells. The ActHIB vaccine also contains sodium chloride and aluminum and may contain traces of residual formaldehyde from the manufacturing process.

The PedvaxHIB vaccine contains the Hib polysaccharide linked to a meningococcal protein carrier. It contains sodium chloride and aluminum hydroxyphosphate sulfate and may include trace amounts of formaldehyde.

The HIBERIX vaccine contains Hib polysaccharide conjugated (fused) with tetanus toxoid protein. It also contains aluminum phosphate and sodium chloride and may also include residual formaldehyde. Unlike ActHIB and PedvaxHIB, HIBERIX contains lactose as a stabilizer.

PedvaxHIB contains 0.225 mg of aluminum hydroxyphosphate sulfate. ActHIB and HIBERIX do not contain aluminum.

The Hib vaccine is typically given as a series, with doses spaced out over the first few years of life. Whereas the primary series of ActHIB and HIBERIX, which consists of three doses, is given at two, four, and six months of age, the primary series of PedvaxHIB consists of only two doses and is given at two and four months of age. All Hib vaccines require a booster dose at twelve to fifteen months of age.

Studies show the tetanus-conjugated vaccines provide excellent immunity when the full four-dose series is completed. Clinical trials report over 95% efficacy in preventing Hib disease in fully vaccinated children. The tetanus-conjugated design is effective but typically requires the full series to reach optimal immunity levels.

PedvaxHIB uses an outer membrane protein (OMP) from *Neisseria meningitidis* as the conjugate. This formulation triggers a faster and robust immune response compared to tetanus toxoid-conjugated vaccines. As a result, PedvaxHIB can provide significant immunity with a three-dose schedule. This may prove beneficial in settings with higher disease risk or vaccine access challenges. Studies indicate that PedvaxHIB offers over 98% efficacy after the completion of the three-dose series.

POLIO

Next on our list of vaccines administered in early childhood is the polio vaccine. For most parents, the polio vaccine is, simply put, a no-brainer—as the very word "polio" conjures terrifying imagery of debilitating paralysis. Polio, or poliomyelitis, is an infectious viral disease. It is primarily spread by the fecal-oral route of transmission. It may also be spread by the pharyngeal route or, in layman's terms, the throat. Poliomyelitis is derived from the Greek words *polios*, meaning "gray," and *myelós*, meaning "marrow" (referring to the spinal cord). Coupled with the suffix "-itis"—meaning, inflammation—poliomyelitis literally translates to "inflammation of the gray matter of the spinal cord."

Polio primarily affects young children. In severe cases, it can lead to irreversible paralysis and sometimes death. The disease is thought to date back thousands of years, with evidence of polio-like symptoms depicted in ancient Egyptian art. As far as medical science is concerned, though, polio did not become a widespread epidemic until the late nineteenth and early twentieth centuries. Until the late 1800s, polio was relatively rare. In the early twentieth century, major polio epidemics affected the United States and parts of Europe, terrifying communities as the virus spread rapidly and often left children paralyzed. In 1916, one of the worst polio outbreaks in the United States led to twenty-seven thousand cases and over six thousand deaths.

In the early twentieth century, the diagnostic resources available to identify and study diseases were relatively limited. They didn't have swabs, bloodwork analysis technology, or those rapid tests that, for a cool ten bucks, you can pick up from your local drugstore—or, for us entitled millennials, have delivered directly through our favorite on-demand delivery services. Back then, the lack of advanced laboratory capabilities meant that diagnosis was determined by the clinical symptoms. Because polio was characterized by paralysis, muscle weakness, and stiffness, these symptoms alone defined the disease—regardless of whether polio virus actually caused them. This approach has led to considerable debate among modern researchers regarding the accuracy of these early polio diagnoses.

In fact, historical records reveal that some cases labeled as polio may not have been caused by the poliovirus as understood today. Alternative causes have been proposed, including, among them, exposure to toxic substances like mercury and arsenic. During this era, many medications contained high doses of mercury or arsenic, which are known to cause neurological symptoms similar to those of polio. Furthermore, the early twentieth century saw a significant increase in the use of pesticides for crop spraying, introducing additional neurotoxic substances into the environment.

These confounding factors suggest that, in some cases, acute pesticide exposure or poisoning from heavy metals may have been misdiagnosed as polio. Delving into historical data, researchers continue to uncover the true causes of these neurological symptoms in the context of the medical and environmental conditions of the time.

Despite this, the poliovirus is, sadly, very real; it is unpredictable, crippling, and potentially devastating. Iconic figures, such as President Franklin D. Roosevelt, who suffered paralysis as a result of polio, brought public attention to the disease, fueling the establishment of organizations, like the March of Dimes, that have played a key role in funding research.

In 1955, Dr. Jonas Salk developed the groundbreaking inactivated polio vaccine (IPV). Marking a turning point, in the 1960s, Dr. Albert Sabin developed the oral polio vaccine (OPV). Widespread immunization campaigns in the 1950s and 1960s drastically reduced polio incidence in developed countries. In 1988, the WHO launched the Global Polio Eradication Initiative, which has since eliminated polio from much of the world, although a few areas still face challenges with endemic transmission.

The IPV currently given to children differs significantly from the original Salk IPV. As the demand for IPV grew, so, too, did the demand for the monkey kidney cells needed for the original version of the vaccine. In the late 1970s, a group of researchers at the National Institute for Public Health in the Netherlands created a new product called enhanced potency IPV (eIPV), in which the vaccine was made from purified virus grown in large bioreactors as opposed to monkey kidney cells. The pharmaceutical company Pasteur Mérieux (now Sanofi Pasteur) made further improvements to the vaccine. Pasteur Mérieux replaced monkey kidney cells with Vero cells. The vaccine contained more protective D-antigen and could be combined with other vaccines such as DTP, improving its cost-efficiency.

The original Salk vaccine also used strains of poliovirus that were selected based on their availability and growth characteristics in cell culture at the time. Over the years, the strains in IPV have been optimized for improved immunogenicity. The current IPV formulations often use the Sabin strains—derived from the live attenuated OPV developed by Albert Sabin.

Prior to the introduction of the IPV in 1955, large outbreaks of poliomyelitis occurred each year in the United States. By the time the OPV was introduced in 1961, the annual incidence of paralytic disease of 11.4 cases per 100,000 population declined to 0.5 cases. Incidence continued to decline thereafter to a rate of 0.002 to 0.005 cases per 100,000 population.

Of the 127 cases of paralytic poliomyelitis reported in the United States between 1980 and 1994, six were imported (caused by wild polioviruses), two were indeterminate, and 119 were vaccine-associated paralytic poliomyelitis (VAPP)—resulting from the use of live, attenuated OPV. Yes, you read that correctly. In what can be described only as tragic irony, people were contracting polio *from the vaccine*. Consequently, in 1999, an all-IPV schedule was adopted to eliminate VAPP cases.

Even though polio sounds scary, and of course it can be for the unlucky few, approximately 90–95% of poliovirus infections are asymptomatic. Minor, nonspecific illness, consisting of low-grade fever and sore throat, occurs in 4–8% of infections. Meningitis occurs in 1–5% of patients a few days after the minor illness has resolved. Rapid onset of asymmetric acute flaccid paralysis occurs in 0.1–2% of infections, and residual paralytic disease involving motor neurons (paralytic poliomyelitis) occurs in about 1 per 1,000 infections.

Since the WHO launched the Global Polio Eradication Initiative in 1988, polio cases have decreased by over 99% worldwide. At that time, polio paralyzed or killed approximately 350,000 people annually across 125 countries. By 2023, fewer than thirty cases of wild poliovirus were reported globally, and most cases were confined to just a few countries—namely, Afghanistan and Pakistan. Polio no longer poses the threat it once did. However, vaccine-derived polio cases still materialize in some areas.

In the United States, the last known case of naturally occurring wild poliovirus was reported in 1979. Since then, polio has been eliminated in the United States, although in 2022, a case of paralytic polio was reported in New York state. This case was *vaccine-derived*, meaning it was contracted through a mutation in the weakened virus used in the OPV. The United States now exclusively uses the IPV, which does not contain the live virus. But some countries still use OPV due to its ease of administration.

In recent years, vaccine-derived outbreaks have been documented in multiple countries, including regions in Africa (specifically, Nigeria, the Democratic Republic of Congo, and Somalia) and in parts of Asia and the Middle East.

Of the available polio vaccines, one routinely used in the United States for children is IPOL, manufactured by Sanofi Pasteur. It provides immunization against all three poliovirus types.

The active ingredients in the current iteration of IPOL are inactivated poliovirus types 1, 2, and 3. The inactive ingredients are 2-phenoxyethanol, as a preservative, formaldehyde, which is used to inactivate the virus, and trace amounts of calf serum albumin, and antibiotics, such as neomycin, streptomycin, and polymyxin B. Aluminum is not used as an adjuvant in IPV.

The four-dose series of IPOL is administered, respectively, at two, four, six to eighteen months, and four to six years.

In addition to the live, attenuated poliovirus strains, the OPV contains the inactive ingredient magnesium chloride, a stabilizer designed to preserve the virus during storage and transportation.

The OPV is successful in inducing strong immunity in the intestines, helping to stop person-to-person transmission of the virus. As the weakened poliovirus can spread, OPV also provides community-level protection, boosting immunity in populations where vaccination coverage is low.

In countries with active polio transmission, the WHO recommends OPV doses at birth, six, ten, and fourteen weeks, sometimes supplemented by IPV to boost immunity.

The IPV has demonstrated high efficacy in preventing polio and is widely used in countries where the wild poliovirus has been eliminated. It provides over 90% immunity to all three types of poliovirus after two doses and at least 99% immunity after three doses. While IPV induces strong immunity in the bloodstream—protecting individuals from paralytic polio—it does not create the same level of intestinal immunity as OPV. This means IPV-vaccinated individuals are less likely to get polio but may still carry and shed the virus if exposed. For this reason, the IPV is often combined with OPV in areas with active poliovirus transmission.

PCV

Perhaps paling in notoriety to polio, pneumococcus is, nonetheless, equally precarious. Pneumococcus, caused by the bacterium *Streptococcus pneumoniae*, is a leading cause of bacterial infections worldwide and remains a significant public health concern globally. Responsible for a range of illnesses that are notably severe in young children, older adults, and immunocompromised individuals, this bacterium is a primary agent behind several diseases, such as pneumonia, meningitis, and bacteremia (bacteria in the blood), as well as less severe infections like otitis media (middle ear infection).

Leonardo DaVinci was considered a "Renaissance man" because he was so proficient and educated in a wide range of fields. To put things in perspective, if DaVinci was a bacterium, he'd probably be pneumococcus. The cause of *so many* horrific maladies, pneumococcus is the insidious "Renaissance man" of the infectious disease world.

One of the most common and dangerous forms of pneumococcal disease is pneumococcal pneumonia—an infection of the lungs. Symptoms include high fever, chills, productive cough, chest pain, and difficulty breathing. Pneumococcal pneumonia can even lead to serious complications such as respiratory failure or sepsis.

Highlighting the gravity of pneumococcal pneumonia is a true story—tragically, one of many of its kind. In 1996 (four years before the pneumococcal conjugate vaccine [PCV] was licensed in the United States), a three-year-old little boy, Leo, underwent two days of emergency room visits and was admitted to the hospital for four days, where he was treated for pneumococcal pneumonia, sepsis, and pleural effusions (fluid in the lungs). On his return home, he faced weeks of illness and months of recovery. His parents agonized as they anxiously monitored their little boy's breathing quality and watched him struggle to breathe. Fortunately, Leo made a full recovery.

Pneumococcus isn't a one-trick pony. Another disease it causes is pneumococcal meningitis. When pneumococcus infects the membranes surrounding the brain and spinal cord, it leads to meningitis, a life-threatening condition. Symptoms include severe headache, stiff neck, sensitivity to light, fever, and altered mental status. It can result in complications like hearing loss, neurological damage, and in severe cases, death. Children under five are more vulnerable to this form of meningitis.

However, that isn't all pneumococcus can do. Bacteremia occurs when pneumococcus enters the bloodstream and leads to systemic infection. It can cause sepsis—an overwhelming immune response that can result in organ failure and death. Bacteremia often occurs in conjunction with pneumonia or meningitis and requires prompt treatment.

Pneumococcus doesn't stop there though. Oh no, the list goes on. It is also a common cause of otitis media, an infection of the middle ear in young children, leading to ear pain, fever, and hearing difficulties. Recurrent ear infections can sometimes lead to hearing loss and speech or developmental delays, rendering prevention important in children.

Pneumococcus can also infect the sinuses, causing sinusitis. Symptoms include facial pain, nasal congestion, and headache. Though generally less severe, sinusitis can still be uncomfortable and, if untreated, lead to more serious complications.

Yes, so proficient at harming humans in so many different ways, pneumococcus may just win the award for the most versatile bacterium. It also secures the nomination in the highly contagious category. Spread through respiratory droplets, pneumococcus is easily communicable, especially in crowded or close-contact settings. Children may carry the bacteria asymptomatically in their nose and throat, increasing transmission risks in households and communities. My wife and I recently took our five-year-old son roller-skating. At one point, she turned to me and, with a disgusted look on her face, said, "Yuck! Pneumococcus everywhere." I've ruined her. Alas, she wasn't wrong—albeit, in California, where we live, most children have been vaccinated against it.

In 2021, lower respiratory infections, including pneumococcal pneumonia, were responsible for approximately 2.2 million deaths worldwide. Pneumococcal disease is a leading cause of vaccine-preventable deaths among children under five, particularly in low- and middle-income countries.

In the United States, approximately 30,000 cases of invasive pneumococcal disease (IPD) are reported annually in all age ranges, along with severe infections that lead to approximately 150,000 hospitalizations each year.

Vaccines, such as Prevnar 13 (PCV13), Vaxneuvance (PCV15), and PCV20, are highly effective in preventing severe pneumococcal disease. In 2019, the incidence of IPD among children under five years old was approximately 8.8 cases per 100,000. This reflects a substantial decline from the prevaccine introduction rates in the 1990s, which were around 100 cases per 100,000.

Before widespread vaccination, pneumococcal pneumonia was a leading cause of hospitalization among US children; each year, approximately 100,000 to 175,000 children under five were hospitalized with pneumonia. After the introduction of the vaccine, hospitalizations have declined by 66–69%. Vaccination has also led to a significant decrease in cases of pneumococcal meningitis among children and resulted in a 41% reduction in otitis media visits, from 78 to 46 visits per 100 children annually.

The two main pneumococcal vaccines currently given to children in the United States are Prevnar (PCV13 or PCV20), manufactured by Pfizer, and Vaxneuvance (PCV15), manufactured by Merck.

As the number in its name suggests, Prevnar 13 is a 13-valent PCV and Prevnar 20 is a 20-valent pneumococcal conjugate vaccine. In plain English, this means that the main ingredients are polysaccharide antigens that cover multiple serotypes of *Streptococcus pneumoniae*. (Okay, maybe that wasn't such plain English.) More simply put, this vaccine protects against either thirteen or twenty different strains of pneumococcus. I know, why don't they just say that? Prevnar contains the carrier protein Diphtheria CRM197, which helps the immune system recognize and respond to the polysaccharides. It also contains aluminum phosphate as an adjuvant, as well as sucrose, sodium chloride, polysorbate 80, and water for injection. The aluminum content is approximately 0.125 mg per dose. Dosing is recommended at two, four, and six months and, again, between twelve and fifteen months old, for a total of four doses in children.

PCV 15, as the name also suggests, is a 15-valent pneumococcal conjugate vaccine consisting of polysaccharide antigens that cover fifteen serotypes. It includes the same thirteen *Streptococcus pneumoniae* serotypes covered by Prevnar 13 but also protects against two additional serotypes—22F and 33F—and, thus, may offer broader protection. Like Prevnar 13, PCV 15 contains the carrier protein Diphtheria CRM197 and uses aluminum phosphate as an adjuvant, with an aluminum content of 0.125 mg per dose. And like Prevnar 13, PCV 15 contains sodium chloride, polysorbate 80, and water for injection. Doses are similarly recommended at two, four, and six months and, again, between twelve and fifteen months old.

Studies show that Prevnar is highly effective in preventing IPD caused by the serotypes included in the vaccine. The vaccine has been shown to reduce the rate of IPD by approximately 90% among vaccinated children for those specific strains. Widespread use of Prevnar has significantly reduced cases of pneumococcal meningitis, bacteremia, and pneumonia in children. By reducing nasopharyngeal carriage of pneumococcus, Prevnar has been shown to provide indirect protection, in the form of herd immunity, thereby decreasing transmission within communities.

In clinical trials, PCV 15, too, has been shown to elicit a strong immune response comparable to PCV13 for the thirteen shared serotypes, with additional immunity against the two extra serotypes. These two serotypes have been implicated in a small but increasing number of cases of IPD, so their inclusion may improve protection.

While no long-term data exists on the indirect benefits of PCV15 on herd immunity, the vaccine's immune response profile indicates it should offer similar community protection as Prevnar.

ROTAVIRUS

Next on our list of early childhood vaccines is the rotavirus vaccine. A contagious virus that primarily affects infants and young children, rotavirus causes gastroenteritis, which is characterized by diarrhea, vomiting, fever, and abdominal pain. Before the introduction of vaccines, rotavirus was one of the most common causes of severe diarrhea in young children globally, leading to significant morbidity and mortality, especially in developing countries.

Rotavirus spreads easily through the fecal-oral route, either directly, from person-to-person contact, or indirectly, through contaminated surfaces (known as fomites), food, and water. Able to survive on surfaces for days, rotavirus is notably resilient, proving it difficult to control.

The virus itself belongs to the *Reoviridae* family. Possessing a unique structure, rotavirus consists of a double-stranded RNA genome enclosed in a triple-layered protein coat. This isn't all that significant, though you should understand that the particular chemical structure of rotavirus allows it to evade parts of the immune response, which is the reason it is so highly infectious. Although several strains of rotavirus exist, group A is the most common and is responsible for the majority of infections in humans.

Symptoms of rotavirus infection typically appear one to three days after exposure and generally last about a week. For many children, especially in high-income countries, rotavirus may present as a mild illness. Yet for the malnourished or those who have limited access to medical care, rotavirus can result in severe dehydration and complications requiring hospitalization. Because immunity to rotavirus develops gradually, repeated infections are common. The symptoms tend to grow milder with subsequent infections.

Prior to the introduction of the vaccine in 2006, nearly all children were infected with rotavirus by age five. Before the vaccine existed, rotavirus was responsible for more than 400,000 doctor visits and over 200,000 emergency room visits in the United States each year, and twenty to sixty children under five died from rotavirus or complications from it annually. In 2016, rotavirus was responsible for approximately 128,500 deaths among children under five years old globally. That same year, an estimated 258 million episodes of rotavirus-induced diarrhea occurred in this age group.

After widespread vaccination, the United States has seen a 58–90% decline in laboratory-confirmed rotavirus cases, along with a significant reduction in rotavirus-related hospitalizations and emergency room visits. The latest available data shows that the United States continues to experience low rates of rotavirus-related hospitalizations and deaths.

In the United States, the two available rotavirus vaccines are ROTARIX, by GlaxoSmithKline, and RotaTeq, by Merck.

ROTARIX is a monovalent vaccine containing a single strain of live, attenuated human rotavirus. While the main ingredient is the live, attenuated rotavirus strain, it additionally includes the stabilizers sucrose, salts, and amino acids. It also contains Dulbecco's Modified Eagle Medium—a medium used to support the growth of cells. ROTARIX does not contain aluminum. Two doses are recommended, with the first at two months and the second at four months. All dosing should be completed by twenty-four weeks of age.

RotaTeq is a pentavalent vaccine containing, as the root "pent" suggests, five live, attenuated human-bovine reassortant rotavirus strains (G1, G2, G3, G4, and G6), which are main ingredients in the vaccine. RotaTeq similarly contains the stabilizers, sucrose, salts, and buffer solutions, along with cultured Vero cells, derived from African green monkey kidney cells. Like ROTARIX, RotaTeq does not contain aluminum. RotaTeq requires three doses, respectively at two, four, and six months, with the series to be completed by thirty-two weeks of age.

Studies generally show that both ROTARIX and RotaTeq provide strong protection against severe rotavirus infections. In clinical trials, ROTARIX has demonstrated approximately 85–96% efficacy against severe rotavirus disease in the first year postvaccination. It maintained around 79–88% efficacy against hospitalizations and severe cases of rotavirus in the second year of life. RotaTeq showed about 74–98% efficacy against severe rotavirus gastroenteritis in the first year after vaccination and around 85–98% efficacy in preventing hospitalizations and severe cases in children under two years old.

These vaccines have significantly reduced rotavirus hospitalizations and severe cases of rotavirus, particularly in countries with routine vaccination.

MMR

The next early childhood vaccine on our list, the MMR, is a combination vaccine that protects against three highly contagious viral diseases: measles, mumps, and rubella. Each of these diseases poses significant health risks and can lead to severe complications, especially in children and vulnerable populations. Prior to widespread vaccination, these diseases were prevalent worldwide, causing high rates of illness, hospitalization, and even death.

The first *M* in MMR, measles is, without a doubt, the illustrious star of this combination vaccine and the one on which the bulk of our discussion will focus. Caused by the *measles virus*, measles is known for its high transmission rate and characteristic red rash. The virus spreads through respiratory droplets, with symptoms like high fever, cough, runny nose, and conjunctivitis, followed by the appearance of a rash. Measles can lead to serious complications, including pneumonia, encephalitis, and death.

Prior to the introduction of the measles vaccine in 1963, measles was historically one of the most common and deadly diseases affecting children worldwide. The United States saw an average of three to four million cases per year, resulting in approximately 48,000 hospitalizations. Between 400 and 500 deaths were attributed to measles annually. Globally, measles was one of the leading causes of childhood mortality, and in the 1950s and early 1960s, millions of deaths were reported annually from measles. After the widespread use of the vaccine in the United States, measles cases precipitously dropped by over 99%; worldwide, measles cases have declined by 75%.

Among the common serious complications associated with measles, pneumonia is the leading cause of measles-related deaths. It affects approximately 6% of infected children. Encephalitis occurs in about 1 per 1,000 cases and can result in permanent brain damage or death. Subacute sclerosing panencephalitis (SSPE)—a rare but fatal condition affecting the central nervous system—can develop years after measles infection, occurring in 4 to 11 out of 100,000 cases. Measles may also cause something known as immune amnesia. As the name suggests, immune amnesia occurs when memory B cells (the immune system's means of remembering past pathogens) are infected, effectively erasing that memory. This results in a higher susceptibility to other infections for months or even years after recovering from measles. Research suggests that immune amnesia can occur in a significant portion of those affected, potentially impacting up to 50% of those infected with measles.

While such complications are more rare and the survival rate is fairly high, measles can prove fatal. Roald Dahl—prolific and beloved author of the books *Charlie and the Chocolate Factory*, *Matilda*, and *BFG*, to name a very select few—lost his eldest daughter, Olivia, to measles when she was seven years old. In a personal essay written in Olivia's memory and aimed at parents who refused to vaccinate their children against measles in the United Kingdom, Dahl recounted: "As the illness took its usual course I can remember reading to her often in bed and not feeling particularly alarmed about it. Then one morning, when she was well on the road to recovery, I was sitting on her bed showing her how to fashion little animals out of colored pipe cleaners, and when it came to her turn to make one herself, I noticed that her fingers and her mind were not working together and she couldn't do anything. 'Are you feeling alright?' I asked her. 'I feel all sleepy,' she said. In an hour, she was unconscious. In 12 hours she was dead." Dahl noted, "It really is almost a crime to allow your child to go unimmunized."

Perhaps measles is so dangerous because it is highly contagious. In fact, it is one of the most infectious diseases known to exist, with an R_0 (basic reproduction number) between 12 and 18. This means a single infected person can spread measles to twelve to eighteen others in a susceptible population. This is among the highest R_0 for any infectious disease. For comparison, the R_0 for influenza is 1 to 2. The steep transmission rate, principally in crowded or unvaccinated communities, proves measles containment challenging. The virus can remain airborne or survive on surfaces for up to two hours, which further contributes to its spread.

If one person infected with measles is in a room with a group of unvaccinated individuals, almost everyone in the room is likely to become infected. The CDC and WHO emphasize that with such high contagion, maintaining high vaccination rates (around 95%) is crucial to achieve herd immunity and prevent outbreaks.

The success of vaccination programs has nearly eradicated measles in many areas. In 2000, measles was declared "eliminated" in the United States. While many incorrectly construe this to mean that there were zero cases of measles, in reality, it means that there had been no continuous disease transmission for more than twelve months within any particular geographic area. In fact, that very year, the United States reported eighty-six cases of measles and ten outbreaks involving three or more cases across nine states.

The distinction between eliminated and eradicated is significant. Elimination refers to the interruption of endemic transmission, not a complete absence of cases. Even as measles was declared "eliminated," outbreaks continued to occur and were primarily attributed to travelers from regions where measles had not been eliminated, underscoring the importance of exercising ongoing precaution.

In 2024, the United States reported a total of 284 measles cases across thirty-two jurisdictions, including California, Florida, and New York City. Given the highly transmissible nature of measles, this number is relatively low. Still, outbreaks continue to occur, even in countries with high overall vaccination rates.

Turning now to the second *M* in MMR, mumps is caused by the mumps virus. Also spread through respiratory droplets or direct contact with an infected person, mumps is classically characterized by fever, headache, and swelling of the salivary glands, namely, the parotid glands, resulting in swollen cheeks and jaw. Complications can include orchitis (testicular inflammation), which can cause infertility, as well as pancreatitis, encephalitis, and hearing loss. In 2024, the United States reported 357 cases of mumps.

The lone *R* in MMR stands for rubella—otherwise known as German measles. Although a typically milder disease, rubella may have serious implications for pregnant women as it can cause congenital rubella syndrome (CRS) in the fetus. CRS may result in miscarriage, stillbirth, or severe birth defects, like hearing loss, heart defects, and intellectual disabilities. Rubella symptoms are typically mild and include fever, rash, and swollen lymph nodes. Rubella remains very rare in the United States. However, the risk to fetuses underscores the importance of vaccination.

The MMR II vaccine, produced by Merck, is most exclusively used in the United States. The active components are the live attenuated (weakened) viruses for measles, mumps, and rubella. It employs the stabilizers, sorbitol, and hydrolyzed gelatin to protect the viruses in the vaccine. MMR II additionally contains sodium phosphate, sucrose, and recombinant human albumin, as preservatives, along with trace amounts of neomycin—an antibiotic that prevents bacterial contamination. The MMR vaccine is produced by culturing the measles and mumps viruses in chick embryo cell culture and growing the rubella virus in human diploid cell cultures (WI-38). The MMR II vaccine does not use aluminum as an adjuvant. The first dose of MMR II is given between twelve and fifteen months of age. The second dose is given between four and six years of age (or, if given earlier, then at least twenty-eight days after the first dose).

After the full two-dose series, the MMR II vaccine has high efficacy rates for each of its components, with approximately 97% efficacy against measles, roughly 88% efficacy against mumps, and about 97% efficacy against rubella.

In 2022, PRIORIX—an MMR vaccine—was approved for use in the United States, though it is not yet commonly administered. Manufactured by GlaxoSmithKline, PRIORIX is used in several countries, namely, parts of Europe and Canada.

The CDC and several studies report that the efficacy rates for both vaccines generally provide lifelong immunity against measles and rubella. Mumps immunity can occasionally decrease over time, though outbreaks remain relatively low among vaccinated populations.

VARICELLA

The varicella vaccine is a relative newcomer to the cohort of early childhood vaccines. Varicella, commonly known as chicken pox, is a highly contagious viral illness that, for many of us, conjures memories of red itchy spots, oatmeal baths, and calamine lotion. Before the vaccine became widely available in 1995, chicken pox was nearly universal in childhood. While chicken pox is generally considered a mild illness, it is not without risks. Each year, thousands of children are hospitalized, and a small percentage experience severe complications, like bacterial infections, pneumonia, and in rare cases, encephalitis. Adults, pregnant women, and immunocompromised individuals are at higher risk for severe disease.

The chicken pox vaccine fundamentally changed the way we think about varicella. With routine immunization, cases have drastically decreased, sparing many children from infection. Prior to the introduction of the varicella vaccine, the United States reported approximately four million cases of chicken pox annually, leading to about 10,500 to 13,500 hospitalizations and 100 to 150 deaths each year.

The implementation of the varicella vaccination program has resulted in a significant decline in cases. By 2019, varicella incidence had decreased by over 97% among individuals under twenty years old, effectively rendering hospitalizations and deaths in this group rare occurrences. Despite the success of the vaccination program, varicella outbreaks still occur, particularly in settings with close contact, such as schools and childcare centers. These outbreaks are more common in communities with lower vaccination coverage.

The varicella vaccine given in the United States is VARIVAX, manufactured by Merck. The active ingredient in VARIVAX is the live attenuated varicella-zoster virus. Inactive ingredients include sucrose, hydrolyzed gelatin, sodium chloride, monosodium L-glutamate, sodium phosphate monobasic, potassium chloride, and other residual components from manufacturing, like trace amounts of the antibiotic neomycin and fetal bovine serum used during virus cultivation. Varicella is cultured in MRC-5 human diploid cells, which are derived from lung fibroblast cells. VARIVAX does not contain aluminum.

The first dose of VARIVAX is administered between twelve and fifteen months of age. The second dose is administered between four and six years of age.

The efficacy of the VARIVAX vaccine against varicella has been studied extensively, showing high levels of protection, especially when given as a two-dose series. After two doses, VARIVAX is 98–99% effective at preventing all cases of varicella. Studies further indicate that immunity from VARIVAX is long-lasting, with protection sustained for at least ten to twenty years postvaccination.

HEPATITIS A

Rounding out the list of early childhood vaccines is the hepatitis A vaccine. Hepatitis A—a non-enveloped RNA virus belonging to the *Picornaviridae* family—is a highly contagious liver infection caused by the hepatitis A virus (HAV). Unlike other forms of viral hepatitis, hepatitis A does not cause chronic liver disease but can lead to significant illness and, in rare cases, acute liver failure.

Hepatitis A is a global health concern; it is most prevalent in areas with poor sanitation and limited access to clean water. Due to improved hygiene and widespread vaccination programs, infection rates have decreased in high-income countries. Yet the disease remains endemic in many low and middle-income regions.

The virus spreads primarily through the fecal-oral route, often via contaminated food or water. (This is your polite reminder to wash your hands after using the bathroom!) Close person-to-person contact (i.e., within households or childcare settings) can also facilitate transmission. Individuals at higher risk include travelers to endemic areas, people experiencing homelessness, and those with underlying liver disease.

For hepatitis A, the incubation period—meaning, the amount of time it takes for symptoms to appear after exposure to the disease is approximately two to six weeks, which is relatively lengthy in the realm of infectious disease. Symptoms can vary in severity and run the gamut, from fever, fatigue, nausea, vomiting, abdominal pain, jaundice (a yellowing of the skin and eyes), dark urine and pale stools, and loss of appetite.

Children under six typically experience mild symptoms or asymptomatic infections; adults are more likely to experience severe symptoms. Hepatitis

A is generally self-limiting—meaning, most individuals recover fully within a few weeks to months. However, severe complications such as fulminant hepatitis (acute liver failure) can occur, particularly in older adults or individuals with preexisting liver conditions.

The WHO estimates that in 2016, approximately 7,134 deaths globally were attributable to hepatitis A, accounting for 0.5% of the mortality from viral hepatitis. Between November 2022 and September 2023, a foodborne hepatitis A outbreak in the United States affected individuals in California, Hawaii, Oregon, and Washington. The outbreak was linked to frozen strawberries imported from Mexico. Since 2016, widespread hepatitis A outbreaks have been reported in thirty-seven US states, primarily among persons who use drugs and those experiencing homelessness.

In the United States, two primary vaccines are approved for pediatric use: HAVRIX, manufactured by GlaxoSmithKline, and Vaqta, manufactured by Merck.

HAVRIX contains the inactivated hepatitis A virus antigen, which is propagated in MRC-5 human diploid cells. Aluminum hydroxide is added as an adjuvant. Other components include amino acid supplement in a phosphate-buffered saline solution and polysorbate 20. From the manufacturing process, HAVRIX also contains residual MRC-5 cellular proteins (not more than 5 mcg/mL), formalin (not more than 0.1 mg/mL), and neomycin sulfate. Each 0.5 mL pediatric dose of HAVRIX contains 0.25 mg of aluminum.

Vaqta, too, contains the inactivated hepatitis A virus antigen, but it uses aluminum hydroxyphosphate sulfate as an adjuvant. It is propagated in MRC-5 human diploid cells. Other components include sodium borate, sodium chloride, and water for injection. It may also contain residual formaldehyde, nonviral protein, DNA, Bovine Albumin, and neomycin. Each 0.5 mL pediatric dose contains approximately 0.225 mg of aluminum as aluminum hydroxyphosphate sulfate.

COMBINATION SHOTS

You've heard the adages "Kill two birds with one stone," "Everything but the kitchen sink" and "The more the merrier." Apparently, so have vaccine manufacturers. In fact, these aphorisms seem more like a pervasive ethos—except, instead of two birds, vaccine manufacturers aim for four or five because, after all, "the more the merrier." It's all about efficiency. In the vaccine world, combination shots are growing increasingly in vogue—a shot that protects against *more* diseases seems to be exceedingly desirable.

For some, this "kill [five] birds with one stone" approach may prove preferable. Combination shots not only translate to fewer tear-inducing pokes; they also mean that over the course of routine vaccination, a child will be injected with a reduced level of additives while simultaneously receiving the same protection.

Though we will weigh the pros and cons in later chapters, for now, we will simply examine the combination shots that are available and widely used. These shots—as their name suggests—combine various medleys of the individual, early childhood vaccines. The first of these combination shots is ProQuad, manufactured by Merk. ProQuad is a combination shot that inoculates against measles, mumps, rubella, *and* varicella (MMRV). The active ingredients include live attenuated measles, mumps, rubella, and varicella viruses. ProQuad also contains sucrose, hydrolyzed gelatin, sodium phosphate, monosodium glutamate, potassium chloride, potassium phosphate monobasic, trace neomycin, fetal bovine serum, sorbitol, and human albumin.

The MMRV vaccine carries a slightly higher risk of fever and febrile seizures in younger children, specifically between the ages of twelve and twenty-three months, than do the MMR II and varicella vaccines when each respective vaccine is administered separately. Similar to the MMR II, the MMRV vaccine does not contain aluminum. The MMRV vaccine requires two doses, the first of which is not actually the MMRV vaccine but a single dose of the MMR II vaccine and a single dose of the varicella vaccine. The second dose consists of the MMRV vaccine, and it is given between four and six years of age.

Another commonly used combination vaccine is Pentacel (DTaP-IPV-Hib), manufactured by Sanofi Pasteur. The active ingredients include diphtheria toxoid, tetanus toxoid, acellular pertussis, inactivated poliovirus (types 1, 2, 3), and Hib. Pentacel also contains aluminum phosphate, formaldehyde, glutaraldehyde, 2-phenoxyethanol, and polysorbate 80. Studies show that there is no significant difference in the safety profile of Pentacel when compared to separate DTaP, IPV, and Hib shots.

Pentacel is given at two, four, and six months and between fifteen and eighteen months, for a total of four doses.

The aluminum content in a single dose of Pentacel is 0.33 mg per dose. The aluminum content in the DTaP vaccine is around 0.33 to 0.625 mg per dose, depending on the brand; the aluminum content in Hib vaccines, such as PedvaxHIB, is 0.225 mg per dose (albeit, some Hib vaccines, like ActHIB, do not contain aluminum); the IPV vaccines do not contain aluminum. Thus, if a child receives the DTaP, IPV, and Hib vaccines separately, at the recommended doses, he or she will be injected with a combined total of approximately 0.33 mg to 0.85 mg of aluminum per dose, depending on the vaccine administered.

Yet another combination vaccine that takes this "the more [antigens] the merrier" approach is the relatively new kid on the block, VAXELIS (DTaP-IPV-Hib-HepB), manufactured by Merck and Sanofi Pasteur. Active ingredients include diphtheria toxoid, tetanus toxoid, acellular pertussis, inactivated poliovirus (types 1, 2, 3), Hib, and hepatitis B (HBsAg). VAXELIS is an army in a syringe; indeed, it is "everything but the kitchen sink." VAXELIS is the vaccine equivalent of the Battle of Winterfell in *Game of Thrones*, in which several houses unite to fight off the White Walkers. (Heck, VAXELIS even sounds similar to the name of one of the show's characters.)

Like Pentacel, VAXELIS provides protection against diphtheria, tetanus, pertussis, polio, and Hib. However, VAXELIS additionally protects against hepatitis B. The shot contains the inactive ingredients aluminum phosphate, polysorbate 80, formaldehyde, neomycin, and polymyxin B. Studies show that the safety profile for VAXELIS is comparable to the separate vaccines DTaP, IPV, Hib, and hepatitis B.

The aluminum content per dose of VAXELIS is 0.319 mg. If combining hepatitis B, at 0.25 mg, DTaP, at 0.33 to 0.625 mg, Hib, at 0-0.225 mg, and IPV, at 0 mg, the total aluminum content ranges from 0.58 mg to 1.1 mg per dose, depending on the brands used. For those keeping an aluminum scorecard, a single dose of VAXELIS will inoculate against the same diseases while delivering considerably less aluminum per dose. VAXELIS is given at two, four, and six months, for a total of three doses.

The last of the combination vaccines is PEDIARIX (DTaP-HepB-IPV), manufactured by GlaxoSmithKline. PEDIARIX provides protection against several diseases—diphtheria, tetanus, pertussis, hepatitis B, and polio. PEDIARIX is given at two, four, and six months of age and contains the active ingredients diphtheria toxoid, tetanus toxoid, acellular pertussis, hepatitis B (HBsAg), and inactivated poliovirus (types 1, 2, 3). The inactive ingredients in PEDIARIX are aluminum hydroxide, polysorbate 80, formaldehyde, neomycin sulfate, and polymyxin B.

Studies show that PEDIARIX demonstrates no significant safety concerns as compared to the individual components. This combination shot contains similar preservatives and stabilizers as the single vaccines, with an aluminum content of 0.85 mg per dose, largely due to the combined DTaP and HepB components. DTaP contains between 0.33 and 0.625 mg of aluminum, hepatitis B contains 0.25 mg of aluminum, and IPV does not contain any aluminum. If a child were to receive each of these three vaccines individually, he or she would receive a combined total of 0.58 mg to 0.875 mg per dose, depending on the DTaP brand used. Therefore, even though PEDIARIX results in fewer injections, the aluminum content is roughly the same per dose as receiving the DTaP, hepatitis B, and IPV vaccines individually.

For those concerned with aluminum content (and we will discuss aluminum in much greater detail in a later chapter), combination shots, such as Pentacel and VAXELIS, offer lower levels of aluminum per dose than giving each component individually.

HPV

As we leave the electrifying world of combination vaccines, we turn now to vaccines administered in later childhood. The first of these is the human papillomavirus (HPV) vaccine. HPV is a highly prevalent virus. Of the two hundred various strains of HPV, approximately forty can infect the genital tract. HPV is primarily transmitted through skin-to-skin contact, most often via sexual intercourse, making it one of the most common sexually transmitted infections worldwide. The CDC estimates that nearly all sexually active people will be exposed to HPV at some point in their lives.

HPV is typically divided into two categories: low-risk types and high-risk types. Low-risk HPV strains are generally benign, potentially causing warts on various parts of the body, including the hands, feet, and genital area. They are not associated with cancer. In contrast, roughly fourteen strains of HPV are considered high-risk (i.e., they can lead to cancer). The most notable types, HPV-16 and HPV-18, account for about 70% of cervical cancers. Besides cervical cancer, high-risk HPV can contribute to cancers of the throat, mouth, anus, and genitals in both men and women.

For many individuals, HPV infections are transient and resolve spontaneously without intervention. But some high-risk infections persist and can lead to cellular changes that, over time, may evolve into cancer. HPV infections are incredibly common, with millions of new cases each year in the United States alone. Most infections are asymptomatic and self-limiting. Yet due to the link between high-risk HPV strains and certain cancers, HPV remains a significant public health concern. The CDC reports that HPV is responsible for nearly all cases of cervical cancer, contributing to approximately 12,000 cases and over 4,000 deaths annually in the United States. In addition to cervical cancer, HPV is also responsible for increasing rates of oropharyngeal and anal cancers, particularly in men.

To address HPV's impact, vaccines were developed to prevent infection with the most harmful strains. The HPV vaccine targets specific high-risk types, including HPV-16 and HPV-18—associated with the highest risk of cancer. Vaccination is most effective when administered before individuals are exposed to the virus, which is the reason it is generally recommended for preteens, both boys and girls, between ages eleven and twelve. The vaccine is also recommended for older adolescents and young adults who may not have completed the series or were previously unvaccinated.

Since its introduction, the HPV vaccine has shown promising results in reducing the prevalence of HPV infections, precancerous lesions, and associated cancers—in particular, cervical cancer. In fact, studies have demonstrated a significant decrease in cervical precancers among vaccinated populations. A meta-analysis of studies from fourteen high-income countries found that within a decade of vaccine introduction, cervical precancers had declined, with an 83% decrease in HPV-16 and HPV-18 among girls between the ages of thirteen and nineteen, and a 66% decrease among women between the ages of twenty and twenty-four. In a study conducted in the United States, Australia, and several European countries, cases of CIN2+ (a high-grade precancerous lesion) dropped by 51% among vaccinated women between the ages of fifteen and twenty-four. These calculable reductions reveal just how instrumental the HPV vaccine has been in preventing HPV infections and subsequent cancer development.

Gardasil 9, manufactured by Merck, is the HPV vaccine predominantly administered in the United States. Previously, HPV vaccines such as Cervarix, manufactured by GlaxoSmithKline, and the original Gardasil, also manufactured by Merck, were available. In more recent years, Gardasil 9 is the only HPV vaccine distributed in the United States. It contains the active components: recombinant L1 proteins of HPV types 6, 11, 16, 18, 31, 33, 45, 52, and 58. Gardasil 9 employs amorphous aluminum hydroxyphosphate sulfate as an adjuvant. Each 0.5 mL dose contains 0.5 mg of aluminum. Other inactive ingredients in Gardasil 9 are sodium chloride, L-histidine, polysorbate 80, sodium borate, and residual yeast protein. Gardasil 9 offers broader protection compared to its predecessors by covering additional HPV types associated with cancers and genital warts.

The dosing schedule varies by age to optimize immunogenicity and protection. If given between the ages of nine and fourteen, Gardasil 9 is administered in a two-dose series, with the second dose administered six to twelve months after the first. If given between the ages of fifteen and forty-five, Gardasil 9 is administered in a three-dose series, with the second dose given one to two months after the first, and the third dose administered six months after the first.

It has been shown to be 97–99% effective in preventing infections with HPV-16 and HPV-18, as well as five other cancer-causing types (31, 33, 45, 52, and 58). It also prevents types 6 and 11, which cause most cases of genital warts. Studies also demonstrate that Gardasil 9 reduces the risk of cervical, vulvar, vaginal, and anal cancers significantly by preventing the initial HPV infections that lead to these cancers. The vaccine offers long-lasting protection, with studies showing immunity lasting at least ten years or more.

MCV

Another vaccine administered to older children—with the first dose typically given between eleven and twelve years of age—is the meningococcal vaccine. Meningococcus, or *Neisseria meningitidis*, is a bacterium responsible for causing meningococcal disease, a serious infection that can lead to meningitis (inflammation of the protective membranes covering the brain and spinal cord) and septicemia (bloodstream infection). Meningococcal disease can be devastating, with rapid progression that can result in severe complications, such as brain damage, hearing loss, or even death within hours of the first symptoms. Meningococcal disease primarily affects infants, adolescents, and young adults—specifically, in crowded settings like college dorms and military barracks. Meningococcal outbreaks are uncommon and predominantly impact communities where close contact is frequent, facilitating the spread of the bacteria through respiratory and throat secretions—often with life-altering outcomes.

Among the several serogroups of *Neisseria meningitidis,* serogroups A, B, C, W, and Y are the most common causes of disease worldwide. In the United States, serogroups B, C, and Y are most prevalent. According to the CDC, in 2023, approximately 438 cases of meningococcal disease were reported in the United States. Even with appropriate antibiotic treatment, the fatality rate is about 10–15%. Survivors can face long-term disabilities, including limb loss, deafness, and neurological impairment.

In the United States, the three meningococcal vaccines given are Menactra and MenQuadfi, manufactured by Sanofi Pasteur, and MENVEO, manufactured by GlaxoSmithKline. The active components in Menactra are polysaccharides from meningococcal bacteria groups A, C, W, and Y conjugated to diphtheria toxoid protein. In MenQuadfi, these bacteria groups are conjugated to tetanus toxoid. Inactive ingredients include sodium phosphate, sodium chloride, and residual formaldehyde.

The active components in MENVEO are meningococcal polysaccharides from groups A, C, W, and Y, conjugated to CRM197, a nontoxic mutant of diphtheria toxin. Inactive ingredients include sucrose, potassium dihydrogen phosphate, disodium phosphate, and residual formaldehyde. MENVEO does not contain any aluminum.

One dose is given between ages eleven and twelve, with a booster recommended at age sixteen to extend protection during the highest risk years, which are considered to be between the ages of sixteen and twenty-one. None of these three meningococcal vaccines contain aluminum.

Meningococcal conjugate vaccines, like Menactra, MenQuadfi, and MENVEO, are highly effective in protecting against the targeted meningococcal strains A, C, W, and Y. Studies show that in adolescents and young adults, meningococcal vaccines are 85–90% effective at preventing meningococcal disease caused by serogroups A, C, W, and Y. Because immunity wanes after five years, a booster dose is recommended. The vaccines also help reduce asymptomatic carriage of the bacteria in the nose and throat, contributing to herd immunity by reducing transmission.

There are also separate vaccines available for just the meningococcal B (MenB) strain, which is not included in the Menactra, MenQuadfi, and MENVEO vaccines. Men B is a rare but serious bacterial infection caused by *Neisseria meningitidis* serogroup B. In the United States, there are two

MenB vaccines available: BEXSERO (a two-dose series) and TRUMENBA (a two- or three-dose series, depending on risk factors). Unlike the routine meningococcal vaccines, which cover the meningococcal strains A, C, W, and Y, MenB vaccination is optional for healthy adolescents in the United States, though it is recommended for those aged sixteen to twenty-three, based on shared clinical decision-making. In the United States, MenB accounts for about 40% of meningococcal disease cases among young adults, with an estimated 300 cases per year—albeit incidence has declined due to improved vaccination and awareness.

INFLUENZA

While the final two vaccines—influenza and COVID-19—are not specific to early or late childhood, they nonetheless warrant mention in this chapter as they are recommended by the CDC. Turning first to influenza—commonly known as the flu—this disease is a contagious respiratory illness caused by influenza viruses. Influenza infects the nose, throat, and sometimes the lungs, leading to mild to severe illness and, in some cases, death. The flu spreads primarily through respiratory droplets when an infected person coughs, sneezes, or talks. It can also spread by touching surfaces contaminated with the virus and then touching the face.

Influenza viruses are classified into four main types: A, B, C, and D. However, only types A and B are responsible for the seasonal flu epidemics seen each winter in many parts of the world. Influenza A viruses are particularly intriguing because they can infect both animals and humans. They are known for their ability to mutate, leading to new virus strains and even pandemics. The twentieth and early twenty-first centuries saw several significant flu pandemics; among them is the 1918 Spanish flu, which claimed millions of lives worldwide, and the 2009 H1N1 pandemic, caused by a novel strain of influenza A.

Typically less severe than influenza A, influenza B can still cause significant illness and contribute to annual flu seasons. In contrast, influenza C causes mild respiratory illness and is not typically associated with epidemics. Influenza D primarily affects cattle.

The seasonal flu impacts millions each year. The CDC estimates that between nine million and forty-one million people in the United States alone contract influenza annually. Hospitalization numbers vary from year to year, ranging from 140,000 to 710,000. In the United States, an average of 12,000 to 52,000 influenza-related complications and deaths are reported each year. Young children, pregnant women, and those with certain chronic conditions are at increased risk of severe flu complications, like pneumonia, respiratory failure, and exacerbation of underlying health conditions.

The flu vaccines available in the United States include the standard-dose inactivated influenza vaccine (IIV), the high-dose vaccine for older adults, the live attenuated influenza vaccine (LAIV) administered via nasal spray, and the adjuvanted and recombinant vaccines designed to improve immune responses in those over sixty-five.

The influenza vaccines available for young children in the United States are FluLaval Quadrivalent, manufactured by GlaxoSmithKline; Fluzone Quadrivalent, manufactured by Sanofi Pasteur; and FluMist Quadrivalent (nasal spray), manufactured by AstraZeneca. The active components in FluLaval Quadrivalent are inactivated (killed) influenza viruses. It consists of two A strains and two B strains and contains the inactive ingredients sodium chloride, potassium chloride, magnesium chloride, sodium phosphate, monobasic potassium phosphate, egg protein, polysorbate 80, octylphenol ethoxylate (a stabilizer), and trace amounts of formaldehyde. It does not contain aluminum.

The active component in Fluzone Quadrivalent is also the inactivated (killed) influenza viruses—two A strains and two B strains. The inactive ingredients are sodium phosphate, sodium chloride, polysorbate 80, egg protein, trace amounts of formaldehyde, and gelatin; it does not contain aluminum.

Unlike the other flu vaccines, FluMist Quadrivalent (nasal spray) contains the live attenuated (weakened) influenza viruses—two A strains and two B strains. The inactive ingredients in FluMist Quadrivalent are gelatin hydrolysate, sucrose, arginine hydrochloride, monosodium glutamate, gentamicin (an antibiotic), and egg protein. It, too, does not contain aluminum.

Whereas Fluzone and FluLaval both contain inactivated viruses and are injected, FluMist contains live attenuated viruses and is sprayed into the nasal passages. For many parents, FluMist is, therefore, preferable, although FluMist is not recommended for children under two years of age or those with certain health conditions, like asthma.

To achieve full immunity against the flu, children under nine years old who are receiving the flu vaccine for the first time are recommended to take two doses of the flu vaccine, spaced four weeks apart. Thereafter, it is recommended that they be given one dose of the flu vaccine annually, before or during flu season.

In addition to single-dose influenza vaccines, multidose vial formulations of flu vaccines are available. These are typically used in large vaccination settings (i.e., public health clinics or hospitals), where multiple doses can be drawn from a single vial. As a single vial is used multiple times, these multidose vials contain thimerosal—a preservative used to prevent bacterial and fungal contamination. Thimerosal contains ethylmercury, which has been a source of concern due to associations with mercury exposure. (For those of you jumping up and down in your seats, rest assured, we will most definitely explore thimerosal in greater depth in later chapters.)

For parents who prefer to avoid thimerosal, single-dose flu vaccines, such as Fluzone or FluLaval single-dose formulations, do not contain thimerosal. These thimerosal-free options are widely available and predominantly used for children.

Each year, the flu vaccine is designed to protect against the influenza viruses, which research suggests will be most common. By analyzing global influenza surveillance data, tracking circulating strains, and using epidemiological modeling to forecast which variants are most likely to dominate in the upcoming flu season, vaccine makers predict which flu strains to include in the annual flu vaccine. Consequently, annual vaccination is considered crucial for protection. In years when the vaccine matches the circulating strains well, efficacy is higher, often reaching up to 60%. In years when there is a significant mismatch between the vaccine strains and circulating viruses, the efficacy may drop, sometimes below 30%.

In the United States, the CDC provides vaccine efficacy data for each flu season. During the 2019–2020 season, the flu vaccine was about 39% effective overall. The results varied slightly during the 2018–2019 influenza season, when, due to a mismatch with circulating strains, vaccine effectiveness ranged from 9% against A(H3N2) to 44% against A(H1N1).

Overall, the percentage of children receiving one or more doses of the flu vaccine during the 2023–2024 season was 55.4%. This was a decrease of 2.0 percentage points from 57.4% during the 2022–2023 season and a decrease of 8.3 percentage points compared with 63.7% who received one or more doses during the 2019–2020 prepandemic season.

CORONAVIRUS DISEASE 19 (COVID-19)

We've made it to the grand finale—the last and perhaps most infamous vaccine on the list, coronavirus disease 19 (COVID-19). The source of significant controversy, social media wars, lost friendships, and the subject of countless conspiracy theories, the COVID-19 vaccine is both literally and figuratively a sore spot for many. Whereas some laud—nay, deify—the vaccine, others revile it. With a level of passion and hatred befitting of a soap opera or Joan Collins novel, people feel strongly about the COVID-19 vaccine because it emerged from a devastating global pandemic that posed existential challenges. For many, the memory is so recent that it still carries a palpable sting and is triggering.

Whatever your personal feelings about it, the COVID-19 vaccine has undeniably reshaped the global health landscape. Because during the COVID-19 pandemic nearly every layperson suddenly became an epidemiologist, you likely already know that COVID-19 is a complex and evolving infectious disease caused by the novel coronavirus SARS-CoV-2. A thorough exploration of COVID-19's implications, from public health responses to vaccine development, would warrant an entire book unto itself. The narrative around COVID-19 continuously shifts; therefore, I cannot cover the disease or the vaccine comprehensively in *this* book—though to the extent the COVID-19 vaccine is now part of the recommended schedule, I will touch upon it briefly.

Coronaviruses (not specifically COVID-19) are a common class of viral illnesses that account for approximately 15–30% of minor colds in children each year. These viruses are part of a large family known to cause a spectrum of respiratory illnesses. Before the global awareness brought by COVID-19, coronaviruses were one of the routine causes of common coughs, runny noses, and colds. While the COVID-19 virus is in the same family as other coronaviruses, COVID-19's high transmissibility and potential for severe complications, especially among vulnerable populations, have made it uniquely challenging to control and manage.

COVID-19 impacts all age groups, albeit older adults, individuals with underlying health conditions, and those with compromised immune systems are particularly at risk for severe disease. Symptoms range widely, from asymptomatic cases to severe respiratory failure, and can include fever, cough, loss of taste or smell, fatigue, and shortness of breath. The virus is primarily transmitted through respiratory droplets, though it can also spread through aerosols in enclosed spaces, leading to large outbreaks, notably in settings where people are in close proximity for extended periods.

Unless you live in a cave with no internet or telephone access, completely cut off from the rest of the world, you lived through the COVID-19 pandemic. You experienced firsthand the unprecedented response by political leaders, scientists, public health experts, and pharmaceutical companies—all working tirelessly to formulate and deliver COVID-19 vaccines on a mass scale. This effort was expedited by previous research on similar viruses, such as SARS and MERS, and by the leveraging of newer vaccine technologies. Within a year of the virus's identification, several vaccines became available and were widely administered in the United States under the Emergency Use Authorization (EUA).

The primary vaccines developed for COVID-19 are the mRNA vaccines—with one manufactured by Pfizer and the other by Moderna. These vaccines use mRNA technology to instruct cells in the body to produce a protein resembling a part of the virus, triggering an immune response. Johnson & Johnson developed a viral vector vaccine, which used a modified virus to deliver genetic material that teaches the body to recognize and fight SARS-CoV-2. And though less common, protein subunit vaccines, which contain harmless pieces of the virus to stimulate an immune response, were also used.

The mRNA vaccines represent a significant change in vaccine technology, marking the first time such vaccines have been distributed on a large scale. These vaccines have been celebrated as monumental achievements in modern medicine; they have also sparked ongoing debates. Among the key concerns are the durability of the immunity the mRNA vaccines confer and the necessity of booster doses, along with the short- and long-term impacts of this new technology. Additionally, the COVID-19 vaccines have spurred discussions about potential adverse reactions, such as myocarditis, predominantly in young males, and other possible side effects.

Whereas the scientific community was excited by the rollout of this new vaccine technology, others were skeptical. Many individuals were concerned about the rapid development timeline, the lack of long-term safety data, and the emergency use authorization process. As vaccine mandates were introduced in certain sectors and boosters became recommended for specific populations, disagreements intensified over personal freedoms, public health, and vaccine efficacy against emerging variants like delta and omicron.

Despite the fact that ongoing research and adjustments are a natural part of science, the fast pace of updates has caused confusion and contributed to mistrust. The shifting guidance on booster doses, changing eligibility criteria, and the mixed messaging regarding immunity and efficacy duration have been sources of public frustration and discourse.

Given that the mRNA vaccine technology is relatively new, the data and information around the mRNA COVID-19 vaccine are constantly emerging. According to the Commonwealth Fund, the COVID-19 vaccine saved the United States $1.15 trillion and 3 million lives. Other sources state the vaccine killed more people than it saved.

Perhaps unlike any other vaccine, the COVID-19 vaccine has elicited a strong and polarized response. As of the beginning of 2025, numerous researchers and health professionals have raised concerns due to the high number of adverse events and deaths reported to VAERS—much higher than any vaccine in history. Consequently, many countries have stopped recommending routine COVID-19 booster shots for all citizens, limiting recommendations to those at increased risk. Notwithstanding these concerns, in the United States, the CDC schedule still recommends the vaccine for individuals aged six months and older. Proponents of the COVID-19 vaccine emphasize that VAERS is a self-reporting system and that, under the vaccine's EUA, reporting any perceived adverse event was mandatory, which does not conclusively link reported events directly to vaccine side effects.

There does appear to be some disconnect between the CDC recommendation and public perception of the vaccine. According to the CDC, during the 2023–2024 respiratory virus season, coverage with COVID-19 vaccination was *only 15.3% among acute care hospital personnel and 10.5% among nursing home personnel.* As of January 31, 2025, the percentage of the population reporting receipt of the updated 2024–2025 COVID-19 vaccine was just 11.4% for children and 22.6% for adults over the age of eighteen. When it comes to the COVID-19 vaccine, the information seems to vary and depends largely on who disseminates it. The general population and, apparently, even most health-care workers do not seem to agree with the CDC recommendations for annual COVID-19 vaccines.

Several years after its introduction, the mRNA technology remains polarizing: Some extol the technology as a marvel of medical science, while others view it as detrimental—going so far as to call for its withdrawal from the market. A fact upon which most would likely agree, the COVID-19 vaccine has single-handedly brought the vaccine debate to the forefront of public discourse. Indeed, but for the COVID-19 vaccine, this book might not even exist . . .

7

WHAT IS THE BOTTOM TURTLE STANDING ON?

THE WAY VACCINE MANUFACTURERS HAVE SET UP VACCINE TRIALS FOR SUCCESS

Blind belief in authority is the greatest enemy of truth.

—ALBERT EINSTEIN

Clearly, there are a *lot* of vaccines on the market. They are intended to and do protect against debilitating and oftentimes fatal diseases. But how are these vaccines tested? And how do we know that they are, as we are repeatedly assured, safe?

A vaccine is promoted as safe only after it has undergone extensive prelicense testing, which is carefully designed to identify the vaccine's efficacy and any potential adverse effects. The gold standard for evaluating any medical intervention, including vaccines, is the double-blind, placebo-controlled trial. It results in a more objective comparison of outcomes by minimizing bias and ensures neither participants nor researchers know who is receiving the active treatment versus a placebo.

Most of us are familiar with the meaning of the word *placebo*. Because the definition is indispensable to our understanding of vaccine safety testing, I will remind you that a placebo is a substance or treatment that is specifically designed to have *no therapeutic value*. In clinical trials, placebos such as sugar pills, saline (salt water), or just plain old water are used to compare the effects of a new treatment to the fake placebo treatment. By administering the therapeutic to the treatment group and the placebo to the control group, researchers determine the effectiveness of a drug or vaccine and ascertain any side effects. This is fairly straightforward stuff.

In the context of vaccine safety, the *choice* of placebo is critical. When there is no existing treatment or vaccine for the disease being studied, an *inert placebo*, like saline, is optimal. An inert placebo sets a clear baseline, allowing researchers to comparatively evaluate the true safety and efficacy profile of a new vaccine without interference from other variables. This method provides the most reliable data for assessing the risk of side effects. Any observed differences between the treatment and placebo groups may be confidently attributed to the vaccine.

Here's where it gets a bit more complicated. In cases where an established vaccine or therapeutic exists, regulatory and ethical considerations may lead researchers to use the current standard of care as the placebo control. Instead of testing the new vaccine against saline, it is tested against an *older version of that same vaccine*. The rationale behind this is rooted in the ethics of research. Originally developed by the World Medical Association in 1964, the Declaration of Helsinki is a set of ethical principles that guides human experimentation. Widely regarded as the benchmark in human research, the Declaration of Helsinki essentially provides that injecting a trial participant with saline would leave him or her unprotected against a disease for which a vaccine exists and would, thus, be deemed withholding the standard of care. Consequently, many vaccines are tested against existing therapeutics (i.e., other vaccines and not inert placebos).

While this approach helps determine whether the new vaccine offers *improved or similar* safety or efficacy relative to the existing vaccine, it also carries with it obvious limitations. If both the new and existing vaccines share similar ingredients or mechanisms of action, they could share similar safety concerns. Adverse reactions that are common to both vaccines may go unidentified, obscuring potential risks. Without an inert placebo, it is challenging, if not altogether impossible, to distinguish between reactions caused by the vaccine, those occurring naturally, and those due to the vaccine being tested.

This distinction is particularly important when vaccines contain components, such as adjuvants, preservatives, or other additives designed to enhance their effectiveness or stability. These components themselves may cause side effects independent of the vaccine's primary active ingredients. Comparing one vaccine to another that also contains adjuvants or similar ingredients does not provide clarity on whether the new vaccine is safe or simply no worse than the existing one.

Safety claims arising out of studies that use active comparators (i.e., another vaccine or other active compounds) must be interpreted with caution. Such studies demonstrate *relative safety*—that is, whether the new vaccine appears safer or equally safe compared to the standard of care. These studies do *not* establish *absolute safety*, which requires a true or inert placebo to set a baseline for comparison.

For vaccines administered to healthy individuals and young children, ensuring the highest safety standard is especially critical because the recipients are healthy. When millions of doses are administered, side effects, even if rare, can have significant implications. Accordingly, comprehensive trials using *inert* placebos are necessary to identify and understand the *true* potential risks, if any.

This principle is masterfully explained in the book *Turtles All the Way Down.* The book is written by an anonymous author who, sadly, deemed the topic of vaccines too controversial to reveal his or her identity. The expression "turtles all the way down" originates from a story that has been attributed to different sources over time, including early Hindu and Chinese mythologies. Most often, it is linked to the philosopher and mathematician Bertrand Russell. The story goes something like this: After a scientist gave a lecture about the Earth's position in the universe, an elderly woman in the audience challenged him, claiming the Earth is actually supported on the back of a giant turtle. When the scientist asked her what the turtle is standing on, she replied, "Another turtle." When pressed further, the elderly woman insisted that it's "turtles all the way down." The scientist gave a self-satisfied smile before asking, "What is the bottom turtle standing on?" The metaphor profoundly illustrates the way in which assumptions that are unsupported or rooted in circular reasoning lack a solid foundation. The allegory is used to critique theories that do not have a clear starting point or grounding principle, as well as to emphasize the importance of questioning our assumptions.

"Turtles all the way down" is a poignant analogy to the way vaccine safety studies are frequently conducted. Studies that rely on assumptions, methodologies, and comparisons that may not fully address foundational issues give rise to concerns over the legitimacy of safety claims and are problematic for several reasons:

1. *Relative comparisons.* Most vaccine trials compare a new vaccine to an existing vaccine or an adjuvant-containing placebo, not an inert

placebo, like saline. This means the observed safety profile is *relative*, not absolute—akin to adding another "turtle" rather than addressing the base question: how does the vaccine perform compared to no intervention at all?

2. *Lack of comprehensive testing.* The full vaccine schedule is often presumed to be safe because individual vaccines are tested. But comprehensive trials evaluating the *cumulative* effects of multiple vaccines on health outcomes are lacking. This is similar to assuming the "stack of turtles" is stable without examining the entire structure.

3. *Post-marketing surveillance.* Though systems like VAERS and the Vaccine Safety Datalink help identify rare or postlicense adverse events, they depend on self-reporting, medical reports, and retrospective analyses. These are valuable but inherently reactive measures, meaning the "base turtle" of robust, long-term, placebo-controlled safety studies is still missing.

Vaccine studies must strive for zealous, independent evaluations with clear baselines (i.e., inert placebo trials, long-term studies of individual vaccines, as well as the entire vaccine schedule). This would provide greater assurance that safety claims rest on a firm, evidence-based foundation, and not an infinite regression of assumptions.

The duration of vaccine studies further illustrates their inherent limitations. Safety claims are frequently based on prelicense trials. Generally, these are not conducted over long periods. Instead, they are designed to evaluate *short*-term safety and efficacy. Most vaccine trials monitor participants for a few days to a few months postvaccination, with follow-up periods typically lasting one to three months. In some cases, these studies may extend to approximately six months to one year. Trials rarely assess safety outcomes beyond this timeframe. Consequently, while short-term side effects like fever, injection-site reactions, or allergic responses are well-documented, potential long-term effects—including autoimmune conditions, chronic illnesses, or delayed-onset reactions—are not systematically studied during the trial phase. Absent long-term safety studies, it is difficult to definitively rule out or fully characterize risks that may emerge years later.

As classically educated scientists and physicians, we are told to trust the science, so we faithfully do. We are trained to review research in top journals and accept the findings of a placebo-controlled study at face value. When the word *safe* appears in the conclusion, we don't think to question. Why would we? However, a closer look at the research on childhood vaccines on the CDC schedule reveals that something is amiss.

When I—a medical doctor, who also holds a master's degree in epidemiology, trained to review research with a critical eye—read through the data, it is woefully apparent to me that most trials are rigged to potentially hide the true rate of adverse events. I know what you're thinking. It's scandalous, right? It can't be true. I thought so too . . . until I *closely* examined the data.

Most clinical trials are blinded—meaning, until the study is complete, neither the participants nor the researchers know whether a participant receives the vaccine or a placebo. Therefore, other than through fraud or deceit, the only way to rig the deck is to study a *new* vaccine against one that is *known to cause similar side effects*. Both groups would likely experience similar side effects, allowing vaccine manufacturers to maximize safety claims and unabashedly represent that there is no increased risk between groups A and B—which, although accurate, is also misleading. Does this automatically render a product unsafe? No. It *does*, however, potentiate a desired outcome, conveniently circumventing proof of true safety.

Demonstrating the flaw in this methodology of testing is the following hypothetical: Researchers hope to develop a new vaccine for Ebola virus. In the trial, they test their Ebola vaccine against the meningococcal conjugate vaccine (MCV), focusing on adverse events that lead to hospitalization. In each respective group, 15% of participants are hospitalized within thirty days for what is considered a serious event—meaning, 15% in the treatment group that receives the Ebola vaccine are hospitalized and 15% in the control group that receives the MCV are hospitalized. At the completion of the trial, researchers conclude that the Ebola vaccine is safe because the rate of hospitalization was equivalent in both groups, and the new Ebola vaccine did not increase the risk of hospitalization. Based on this research, the Ebola vaccine is approved for use. Given there was no other Ebola vaccine on the market to assess true safety, this new Ebola vaccine should have been tested against an inert placebo, such as saline. Alternatively, the new vaccine could have been studied against the MCV *and also* an inert placebo. Had the new Ebola vaccine been tested against *both* the MCV and an inert placebo, it would have been readily apparent that the hospitalization rate in the group receiving the inert placebo was 2.5%, with a 15% hospitalization rate for those receiving the Ebola vaccine and a 15% hospitalization rate for those receiving the MCV. You don't need to be a physician or researcher to recognize the distinction between these two hypothetical studies.

People advocating for stricter vaccine safety testing are referring precisely to scenarios like this one in which the choice of comparator is calculated to yield self-serving outcomes. Those pushing for better vaccine testing are not intrinsically anti-vax; they are merely demanding that new vaccines be tested against true *inert* placebos to prevent the potential dangers inherent in the "turtles all the way down" approach. Vaccine package inserts often refer to the control group as placebo, even though researchers nearly always use another vaccine, multiple vaccines, or a similar bioactive compound (and *not* an inert placebo) in the control group. The word *placebo* is, thus, misleading.

MMR

Earlier, we discussed the GlaxoSmithKline PRIORIX study. As a refresher, PRIORIX was tested against the existing MMR II vaccine, as opposed to an inert placebo. Researchers concluded that PRIORIX elicited robust immunoresponses and raised no safety concerns. It would have been more accurate to say: "We did not find any specific concerns with PRIORIX compared to the MMR II vaccine." While the PRIORIX study was problematic for a number of reasons, the most disconcerting among them remains, perhaps, that the PRIORIX study incorrectly rested on the inaccurate presumption that the prior MMR vaccines underwent robust safety studies.

The package insert for the MMR II vaccine, manufactured by Merck, does *not* specifically provide details regarding safety trials; rather, it displays only the clinical efficacy and immunogenicity clinical studies. The package insert does contain a graph noting some adverse events. It also contains the following paragraph:

> "Proportion of participants reporting solicited adverse reactions following vaccination with M-M-R II, concomitantly administered with VARIVAX, by the Intramuscular vs Subcutaneous Route." It further states: "Unsolicited adverse

events that occurred within 42 days following vaccination were recorded using diary cards supplemented by medical review. Data on unsolicited adverse events were transcribed into the study database during an on-site visit at day 42. The rates and types of reported adverse events (AEs) across groups were similar and included common clinical events that are often reported in the evaluated populations. Serious adverse events occurred at rates of 0.3% and 1% in the intramuscular and subcutaneous groups, respectively."

In *all* MMR II vaccine trials, it seems the control group was *not* an inert placebo, but either the earlier MMR vaccine, the measles rubella vaccine (MR), or a single dose of the rubella vaccine. Although the information is limited, the original MMR vaccine trials ostensibly consisted of just around 1,000 patients, and very few studies were performed. Many of the control subjects were siblings of the vaccinated children—meaning, there was *no randomization*. In some studies, the control group received no injection—meaning, there was *no blinding*. Admittedly, there is not much information regarding the original MMR vaccine trials. I am unclear as to what extent the original MMR vaccine was tested against the single-dose measles and/or the single-dose rubella vaccines—if at all.

The original MMR vaccine contained the *Rubelle* strain of the rubella virus, which was grown in duck embryo cells. In 1979, the original MMR vaccine was replaced by the MMR II. In lieu of the *Rubelle* strain, the MMR II vaccine contained the RA 27/3 rubella strain, grown in human diploid cells.

Based on my research, there is little accessible information on the single-dose rubella or measles vaccine development. I am fairly certain that neither single-dose vaccine was tested in accordance with our current rigorous safety standards.

We *do* know that the measles vaccine was originally developed in 1954. During a measles outbreak at the Fernald School, in Massachusetts, John F. Enders extracted blood from an eleven-year-old student named David Edmonston who had been infected with measles. Using this sample, Enders successfully isolated the virus.

In their quest to create a measles vaccine, Enders, Samuel L. Katz, MD, and several others set out to attenuate the virus, propagating it through various mediums, like human kidney cells, human amnion cells, embryonated hens' eggs, and chick embryo cell cultures. This process led to a virus strain that, when tested in susceptible monkeys, was immunogenic—meaning, it was able to produce an immune response—without causing viremia (a condition where viruses are present in the bloodstream) or overt disease.

Between 1958 and 1960, the Enders group conducted an initial clinical study on a small group of children to assess the vaccine's safety and immunogenicity. Katz tested the lab's measles vaccine on thirteen children with disabilities. Each of the eleven vaccinated children developed measles antibodies; nine also developed a mild rash. Two of the children were given a placebo. The vaccinated children did not contract measles from the vaccine but did experience some symptoms. This study was not blinded, and there was no control group. It consisted of just thirteen participants and was most certainly not randomized. Today, this study would fail to meet robust safety testing standards. Moreover, the fact that it was tested on children with disabilities would unequivocally render it unethical!

After the promising results of these initial studies, several additional small studies were conducted by a variety of research groups. In 1963, the measles vaccine was first licensed, and in March of that year, the first measles vaccines were approved for use in the United States. These included a live attenuated vaccine developed by Merck & Co., marketed as Rubeovax, and a formalin-inactivated vaccine produced by Pfizer, known as Pfizer-Vax Measles–K. The live vaccine was based on the Edmonston-B strain of the measles virus. The live vaccine demonstrated high efficacy; it was also associated with side effects such as fever and rash. In contrast, the inactivated vaccine had fewer immediate side effects but was later found to provide only short-term immunity. In 1967, due to its limited effectiveness, the inactivated vaccine was withdrawn from the market.

In 1966, researchers conducted the cooperative measles field trial. Overall, this seems to have been a fairly good study. It involved 5,210 children. The efficacy of two measles vaccine schedules was tested in a double-blind, placebo-controlled trial. One group of children received three injections of 0.5 mL of inactivated measles virus vaccine. A second group received two injections of inactivated measles virus vaccine followed by a live attenuated virus measles vaccine. Half of the participating children received placebo injections. The contents of the placebo injection are not specified.

In 1968, Maurice Hilleman, at Merck, improved the measles vaccine by developing the Edmonston-Enders strain vaccine, which offered a better safety profile. Since then, this version of the measles vaccine has been the basis for measles vaccination in the United States.

In the 1960s, following a devastating rubella epidemic that swept through the United States and Europe, Stanley Plotkin, MD, along with a group of researchers, developed the rubella vaccine at the Wistar Institute. Plotkin's team successfully weakened a strain of rubella virus known as RA 27/3 by repeatedly culturing it in human WI-38 cells derived from fetal tissue. Their research led to the successful development of a vaccine that provided immunity against rubella while minimizing side effects that had been observed with earlier versions.

Beginning with small-scale studies in children, Plotkin's team conducted a series of clinical trials to assess the effectiveness and safety of the RA 27/3 rubella vaccine. Initially, they vaccinated one child per household in fifteen families, measuring antibody levels before and after vaccination to confirm an immune response. In subsequent trials, they tested a nasal vaccine on thirteen children and one adult, finding it similarly effective at eliciting immunity without spreading the virus. Larger trials followed, involving 123 children and their 170 close contacts. These trials confirmed that vaccinated children developed strong immune responses and unvaccinated contacts showed no signs of infection.

Thereafter, Plotkin's team worked with medical researchers and health officials across the United States, United Kingdom, Switzerland, France, Israel, Iran, Japan, and the (now former) Soviet Union. In total, researchers vaccinated 500 people subcutaneously, of which 392 were children, and 275 people nasally, of which 236 were children. The vaccine's effectiveness was over 99% in subcutaneously vaccinated and 84% in nasally vaccinated individuals developing strong immunity.

In 1969, after clinical trials demonstrated its effectiveness, the RA 27/3 rubella vaccine was licensed and, in 1971, was incorporated into the combined measles-mumps-rubella (MMR) vaccine, alongside Maurice Hilleman's measles and mumps vaccines.

If we trace it all the way back, PRIORIX was tested against the MMR II vaccine; the MMR II vaccine was tested against the original MMR or single-dose measles and/or rubella vaccines; the original MMR vaccine was tested against its component vaccines, and most early vaccine trials did not conform to the criteria the scientific community currently deems adequate.

The deliberately careful (and arguably suspect) wording routinely used in vaccine inserts, which often reassures us that the vaccine carries no increased risk relative to the placebo, does little to instill confidence. By this rationale, if, after receiving the original MMR vaccine, a person grew a third leg, then researchers would not deem there to be an *increased risk* when a person also grew a third leg after receiving the MMR II vaccine. I use this hyperbolic and admittedly laughable example to highlight the obvious flaw in the logic: In the case of PRIORIX, we are not even offered such transparency but, instead, told that in trials, PRIORIX raised no safety concerns.

Over the last few decades, the dosing schedule has also changed considerably. Originally, only a single dose of the MMR vaccine was recommended at fifteen months. In 1989, a second dose was recommended for ages four to six. In 1998, the age at which the first dose was recommended was switched to twelve to fifteen months. These modifications all occurred *post*license. Additionally, the combined measles, mumps, rubella, varicella (MMRV) vaccine was licensed in 2005. At the time, it was the preferred vaccination. However, in 2008, due to the increased risk of febrile seizures, the recommendations regarding this vaccine were retracted. The MMRV is not generally given as the first dose of MMR and varicella. Instead, it is administered at the time of the booster dose, between four and six years of age.

One thing remains clear: The safety profile of the MMR II vaccine that children receive today is predicated upon the presumption that the MMR and other vaccines against which it was tested were also tested in accordance with today's rigorous standards. PRIORIX was merely one "turtle" resting on the back of many others. That is not to say PRIORIX or the MMR II vaccines are unsafe, though the way they were tested does raise questions.

HEPATITIS B

Let's reexamine another vaccine on the schedule—hepatitis B. In my practice, there is no singular vaccine on which I receive more pushback from parents—perhaps because the hepatitis B vaccine is given to babies at birth and protects against a disease that is largely transmitted sexually or through intravenous drug use. (You haven't heard? Newborn babies are a promiscuous bunch.) All joking aside, one would assume (or at least hope) that we would not give a vaccine to a newborn baby unless we had compelling research proving its unequivocal safety—particularly when newborn babies are not typically sexually active or intravenous drug users and expectant mothers are routinely screened for hepatitis B.

According to the handout, ENGERIX B—the hepatitis B vaccine—was studied in thirty-six clinical studies. A total of 13,495 doses of ENGERIX B were administered to 5,071 individuals, including adults and children. *All subjects were monitored for four days post-administration.* Yes. You read that correctly. *Four days.*

ENGERIX B is manufactured by GlaxoSmithKline. The insert offers a very brief section on safety testing, which states: "The incidence of local and systemic reactions was comparable to those of plasma-derived hepatitis B Vaccines." Again, this language reveals that ENGERIX B was tested against a plasma-derived hepatitis B vaccine and *not* an inert placebo, thereby allowing GlaxoSmithKline to conclude that ENGERIX B does not pose more safety concerns than other plasma-derived hepatitis B vaccines. This, of course, does not shed any light on the side effects and safety concerns potentially associated with those other plasma derived hepatitis B vaccines.

Moreover, the subjects were apparently actively monitored for a mere four days post-administration. This begs the inescapable question: Based on the documented studies in the vaccine handout, do we really know anything about the *long-term* side effects of ENGERIX B?

Another hepatitis B vaccine, RECOMBIVAX HB, is manufactured by Merck. In three clinical studies, 434 doses of RECOMBIVAX HB, at 5 mcg, were administered to 147 healthy infants and children up to ten years of age, who were *monitored for five days after each dose.* In a group of studies, 3,258 doses of RECOMBIVAX HB, at 10 mcg, were administered to 1,252 healthy adults, who were actively monitored for just five days after each dose. This information is taken directly from the RECOMBIVAX HB insert. This is, quite literally, all it says. Perhaps I'm missing something. One would presume that, prior to deeming a vaccine sufficiently safe to administer to fragile newborn babies, it would have undergone robust, prelicense and postlicense studies. At a minimum, I would expect extraordinarily robust safety trials, specific to newborn babies—even amid such skewed noninert placebo trials.

Vaccine advocates are quick to point out that numerous postlicense studies conducted on the hepatitis B vaccine demonstrate its safety. This is accurate, albeit, again, *not* the same as prelicense testing and far from double-blind control trials. There are epidemiological *post*license trials, like the Kaiser Permanente Study, conducted between 1991 and 1994, which involved *only* healthy, full-term newborns. In this study, 3,302 infants were vaccinated with the hepatitis B vaccine within twenty-one days of birth and 2,353 were not. The study assessed whether the hepatitis B vaccine increased the incidence of fever or suspected sepsis. The findings indicated no significant increase in these conditions, allergic reactions, seizures, or other neurologic events among vaccinated infants, supporting the vaccine's safety profile in newborns. Nevertheless, this study does *not* examine any long-term concerns, and the research is of moderate scientific quality—far from the gold standard. Furthermore, this study was conducted in 1991, *after* the CDC recommended the hepatitis B vaccine for all newborns. Surely, for any product recommended for healthy newborns, safety should be established *before*, as opposed to after, the fact.

If the duration of hepatitis B safety testing was not already of sufficient concern, then the origin of the hepatitis vaccines may just be the icing on a very revolting cake. Between 1955 and 1970, Saul Krugman, MD, and Joan Giles, MD, led experiments at the Willowbrook State School, a New York state–supported institution for children with intellectual disabilities. As part of these experiments, more than fifty children with mental disabilities, between the ages of five and ten, were deliberately infected with hepatitis to study immunity and vaccine development. Some were injected with the virus; others were made to consume chocolate milk mixed with feces from infected children. Such reprehensible testing was justified on the basis that, due to overcrowding and poor sanitation, hepatitis was already rampant at Willowbrook. Krugman believed his work could lead to a vaccine for a disease that plagued US troops during World War II and claimed millions of lives globally.

Krugman, a respected pediatrician, secured approval for his studies from the Armed Forces Epidemiological Board, defending that such experimentation would result in better medical care for these children than they would have otherwise received. In a 1958 paper published in the

New England Journal of Medicine, Krugman wrote, "The decision to feed hepatitis virus to patients at Willowbrook was not undertaken lightly." Thankfully, as time passed, the ethical implications of the experiment came under scrutiny. In 1966, a leading medical ethicist, Henry K. Beecher, MD, condemned the study in his landmark paper, "Ethics and Clinical Research." Beecher asserted, "There is no right to risk an injury to one person for the benefit of others."

Around the same time, the Tuskegee Experiment—in which black men were exposed to syphilis and deliberately left untreated even after a cure was known—was exposed. These revelations sparked a national reckoning over the treatment of vulnerable populations in medical research.

Despite the controversy, Krugman's career flourished. He later became the head of pediatrics at New York University School of Medicine, was elected to the National Academy of Sciences, coauthored a leading textbook on pediatric infectious diseases, received the prestigious Lasker Award, and helped develop the first rubella and measles vaccines. To his dying day, he defended the Willowbrook studies, writing in 1986, "I am as convinced today as I was at that time that our studies were ethical and justifiable." The Willowbrook studies serve as a sinister reminder that vaccine development was not always confined by ethical guardrails.

Prior to writing this book, I believed that vaccine approval was subject to the strictest ethical and safety standards. Clearly, that has not always been the case. We have made significant strides in the field of ethics, leaving us with the icing on a far more palatable cake. Still, licensing a vaccine for use after four to five days of testing seemingly leaves room for growth. I was under the (apparently mistaken) impression that we would not recommend any vaccine to newborns unless it had first undergone the most rigorous safety testing in that age group. I am not suggesting the hepatitis B vaccine is unsafe. I am suggesting that, based on the available research, we simply don't know for certain. Though rigorous safety testing may not detect all potential risks immediately, it provides a more comprehensive understanding of a vaccine's safety profile. Don't our babies deserve this level of scrutiny? Going forward, if we are to approve vaccines for newborns, shouldn't we demand scrupulous testing—beyond merely the baseline established for the hepatitis B vaccine? And shouldn't we demand such testing be performed *before* the vaccine is recommended?

DTAP

The story is similar for the DTaP vaccine. As you may recall, GlaxoSmithKline's PEDIARIX is one of those "the more the merrier" combination shots that protects against diphtheria, tetanus, pertussis, hepatitis B, and polio. The package insert mentions fourteen clinical trials involving 8,088 subjects. In the largest study, the trial group received PEDIARIX and the Hib vaccines, and the control group received the DTaP vaccine, INFANRIX, the Hib, and oral polio vaccines. In yet another study, PEDIARIX was tested against INFANRIX, the hepatitis B, and inactivated polio vaccines. According to the PEDIARIX handout, in the twelve other studies, the control group received "comparator vaccines." (I'm pretty sure that's GlaxoSmithKline's way of saying, "Don't worry about it.")

PEDIARIX was not tested against an inert placebo. It was tested against the DTaP vaccine, INFANRIX, among others. "But how was INFANRIX tested?" you so logically ask. In clinical studies, approximately 95,000 doses of INFANRIX were administered. One control group received the older, whole-cell DTP vaccine (you know, the one that was ultimately phased out in the United States in the 1990s due to associated concerns for high risk of febrile seizures and hypotonic-hyporesponsive episodes . . . more on this later). The other control group received the DT vaccine.

So then, how was the whole-cell DTP vaccine tested? The original whole-cell DTP vaccine was introduced in the 1940s and underwent relatively limited clinical trials by current standards. At the time, vaccine development and approval processes were not as rigorously standardized or regulated as they are today. Studies primarily compared disease incidence rates between vaccinated and unvaccinated populations during outbreaks or in specific communities. Early data showed that vaccinated children were significantly less likely to contract pertussis compared to unvaccinated children. Mortality rates from pertussis dramatically decreased after vaccine introduction. While this may prove that the vaccine serves its desired purpose, it does little to address the equally important concern—safety. Researchers did document short-term side effects, such as fever, local injection site reactions, and systemic effects, like irritability. Reports of serious adverse effects, including seizures and hypotonic-hyporesponsive episodes, emerged later, leading to increased scrutiny in the 1970s and 1980s. Randomized controlled trials, as we know them today, were not common practice at the time of the DTP vaccine's development. Early trials often involved smaller groups compared to modern standards. Post-marketing surveillance was minimal, and long-term safety data were not robust. As far as I can best tell, the DTP vaccine was never studied in a modern clinical trial or against an inert placebo.

Similarly, as you may recall, Pentacel, manufactured by Sanofi, is a combination of DTaP, Hib, and inactivated polio vaccine. It was tested in four clinical trials. In three of the trials, the control groups received an array of different vaccines. It remains unclear whether the fourth trial contained a control group.

In trials for yet another DTaP vaccine, DAPTACEL, 18,000 doses were administered to infants and children in nine clinical studies. Between 1992 and 1995, in a randomized, double-blinded pertussis vaccine efficacy trial known as the Sweden I Efficacy Trial, DAPTACEL was tested against the DT and a whole-cell pertussis DTP vaccines. (Again, this was the same DTP vaccine that was discontinued in the United States in the 1990s.) In the study, a standard diary card was kept for fourteen days after each dose, and follow-up telephone calls were made on days one and fourteen after each injection. Thereafter, telephone calls were made monthly, for the two months after the last injection, to monitor the occurrence of severe events and/or hospitalizations.

When we trace the chain of comparators all the way back, we cannot ignore the conspicuous fact that all subsequent trials are based on previous trials that were lacking in a solid foundation.

PREVNAR

Perhaps the most confounding among the "turtles all the way down" vaccine trials is Prevnar. According to the package insert, Prevnar 15 was tested against Prevnar 13. Serious adverse events were observed up to six months after the four-dose series of vaccinations, with 9.6% reported in those who received Prevnar 15 and by 8.9% of recipients of Prevnar 13.

Prevnar 13 was tested against the original Prevnar 7 vaccine. In the trials, serious adverse events were reported in 8.2% of the infants who received Prevnar 13 and 7.2% in those who received Prevnar 7.

The original Prevnar 7 vaccine was studied in a large trial consisting of approximately 17,000 infants in each group. *The trial group received*

Prevnar, while the control group received the meningococcal conjugate vaccine (MCV)—not an inert placebo. Among those participants who received the Prevnar vaccine, one out of thirty-five were hospitalized and one out of sixteen visited the emergency room within thirty days of vaccination. It should be noted that all trial subjects (including those in the control group) concurrently received the DTP or DTaP vaccines.

In 1998, when the original Prevnar vaccine trial took place, Prevanar was the only available potential prophylaxis against pneumococcus. Let's focus ourselves on the timeline. This was 1998, not the 1940s or 1950s, like some of the other original DTP trials. Ethical concerns require researchers to use the current standard vaccine as the placebo in trials where *another vaccine or treatment is available.* In this case, Prevnar was the only existing vaccine or treatment for the disease. Admittedly, this one is a real head-scratcher. To me, this is analogous to giving a cashew to someone with a nut allergy and concluding that the cashew carries with it no increased danger relative to a peanut. At the risk of stating the obvious, if the peanut and cashew both cause anaphylaxis, neither is safe for the person with the nut allergy.

In the Prevnar trial, there should have been no ethical qualms with giving an inert placebo to the control group. So why did researchers choose to give the MCV and not a true inert placebo to the control group? Why would the manufacturer prefer to use an expensive vaccine in the control group instead of salt water, to which there is essentially no cost? Why would the licensing bodies, such as the FDA, accept a trial of this nature?

In the context of Prevnar, I cannot fathom any reason for testing against a noninert placebo other than . . . well . . . one.

VARICELLA

You're starting to get the picture, right?

In trials, VARIVAX, manufactured by Merk, was administered to over 11,000 healthy children, adolescents, and adults. According to the insert, VARIVAX underwent a double-blind, placebo-controlled study consisting of 914 children. Pain and redness at the injection site occurred at a significantly greater rate in vaccine recipients than in placebo recipients. At this point, as you may have (correctly) guessed, the placebo group did not receive an inert placebo, but the test vaccine from which the viral component had been removed.

Another study compared two formulations of the VARIVAX vaccine against each other. The clinical trials involved healthy children who were monitored for up to forty-two days after a single dose. The study did not extend beyond forty-two days and did not test more than this single dose. However, the CDC vaccine schedule recommends that all children receive two doses: the first, between the ages of twelve and fifteen months, and the second, between the ages of four and six years.

In 1995, in the United States, initial studies and the initial licensing were based on a one-dose regimen. The evidence suggested that, over time, a two-dose regimen provided better protection, especially in the context of outbreaks and among certain populations. After further clinical trials and observational studies that indicated improved efficacy and a sustained immune response with a second dose, in 2006, the CDC recommended a routine two-dose regimen for children.

ROTAVIRUS

The next on the list is the rotavirus vaccine. In 1998, the FDA approved the first rotavirus vaccine, RotaShield. In 1999, RotaShield was recalled after it was found to significantly increase the risk of intussusception. (That's a big science word used to describe a life-threatening condition that occurs when a part of the intestine folds into another part, blocking the passage of food and fluids.) Given the unequivocally serious nature of this known side effect, surely, future trials would need to ensure that subsequent incarnations of the rotavirus vaccine did not similarly increase the risk of intussusception.

In the early 2000s, the second generation of rotavirus vaccines underwent preclinical trials. When RotaShield was removed from the market, no other vaccines were available to protect against rotavirus. The rotavirus vaccine is a clear oral liquid. Thus, clear water or a saline solution could and should have been used in the placebo group in all of the safety trials, right? *Wrong.*

In the main ROTARIX trial, which consisted of 63,000 infants, the control group was given the vaccine without the antigen. This means all other vaccine components—Dulbecco's Modified Eagle Medium, di-sodium adipate and sucrose—were still administered to the placebo group, without any inquiry into what effects, if any, these components may have had independent of the antigen.

As for Merck's RotaTeq—the other rotavirus vaccine—infants were evaluated in three placebo-controlled clinical trials, which consisted of 36,165 infants in the group that received RotaTeq and 35,560 infants in the group that received the placebo. It is unclear which placebo was administered in all trials. It seems that in some trials, RotaTeq, minus the antigen, was administered to the placebo group. Subjects in the trial group that received RotaTeq were contacted on days seven, fourteen, and forty-two after each dose to ascertain whether they were experiencing intussusception or any other serious adverse events.

In the phase 3 clinical studies of RotaTeq, in the forty-two-day period after the administration of a single dose of the vaccine, serious adverse events occurred in 2.4% of those who received RotaTeq as compared to 2.6% of those who received the placebo. In the ROTARIX trials, one in thirty experienced a severe medical event, sixteen suffered intussusception, and forty-three died. In the RotaTeq trials, similar rates were recorded: One in forty subjects experienced serious adverse events, fifteen suffered intussusceptions, and twenty infants died. Are these the baseline rates in an unvaccinated population? Maybe.

The ROTARIX package insert states: "No increased risk of intussusception was observed in this clinical trial following administration of ROTARIX when compared to placebo." There are those words again: "no increased risk." So was it that there was no increased risk of intussusception from the new vaccine, or was it just that there was no increased risk of intussusception relative to the *non*inert placebo? Was the placebo purposely similar to ROTARIX to deliberately bolster safety claims?

In another study, the temporal association between vaccination with ROTARIX and intussusception was evaluated in a hospital-based, active surveillance study that identified infants with intussusception at participating hospitals in Mexico. Using a self-controlled case series method, the incidence of intussusception during the first seven days after receipt of ROTARIX, and during the thirty-one-day period after receipt of ROTARIX, was compared with a control period.

This study looked at around 1 million infants under the age of one in various hospitals over the span of two years, predominantly checking for cases of intussusception. Out of those infants, 750 developed intussusception.

The researchers wanted to see if intussusception cases were more likely to occur shortly after infants received the first dose of the ROTARIX vaccine. They found that, within thirty-one days after the first dose, the likelihood of developing intussusception was about 1.75 times higher than during times outside this thirty-one-day window. This means the risk was nearly double in this period. Within the first seven days after the first dose, the likelihood was even higher—6.49 times more than usual, suggesting a stronger association between the vaccine and intussusception within the first week.

Is this getting tedious? Are you screaming, "What in the actual f@$k"? You're not alone.

POLIO

Turning now to the last in our nonexhaustive list of vaccines safety tested utilizing the "turtles all the way down" approach—the polio vaccine. The package insert for the inactive polio vaccine (IPV), manufactured by Sanofi, does not mention *any* prelicense randomized controlled safety trials for the vaccine. Wasn't it tested for safety? According to a 2018 document released by the FDA under the Freedom of Information Act, IPV underwent two clinical trials. These trials did not meet the current requirements for phase 3 randomized controlled trials. The first trial, conducted in 1980, consisted of a combined total of 371 subjects. This includes both the trial and control groups. The control group received OPV by Lederle. In addition, all trial participants received the DPT vaccine.

In a second study conducted in the late 1980s, 114 children were enrolled and underwent a series of three vaccines including either OPV or IPV, or both. Most also received DPT. This trial was not controlled, randomized, or blinded. The OPV vaccine, introduced in the 1960s, has no public documentation of any prelicense clinical trials that meet today's standards.

As you may recall, the original IPV was developed by Salk. For the purpose of this discussion, when I refer to the *original* IPV, I am referring to the Salk version. The version of the IPV currently used in the United States is *different*. The 1954 Salk polio vaccine trial marked a significant milestone in medical history. It involved approximately 1.8 million children to assess the vaccine's efficacy using two distinct methods: The first method was a randomized, placebo-controlled, double-blind design involving about 623,972 children across eleven states. Participants received either the vaccine or a placebo, and neither the children nor the physicians knew who received which. The second method, the observed-control design, involved about 1,080,680 children across thirty-three states. Second graders were vaccinated, and first and third graders served as controls without any blinding or randomization. The trial results, which were announced on April 12, 1955, showed the vaccine to be 80–90% effective in preventing paralytic polio.

Although most would view the Salk IPV trial as robust, the study *still* would not meet today's standards for safety testing. The trial monitored participants for immediate and short-term adverse reactions, such as fever and swelling at the injection site. No serious effects attributable to the vaccine were observed *during* the study. The trial did have its limitations, namely, its focus on short-term safety and insufficient long-term safety evaluation. Half of the trial was unblinded and not randomized. Despite this, the Salk IPV trial was arguably one of the most robust vaccine studies ever conducted. I wish that today, trials were conducted in a manner similar to these polio trials, except that they would additionally be randomized and controlled.

While this original IPV underwent one of the largest studies among all childhood vaccines, it nevertheless falls short. Yes, it was tested on millions of children, providing some solid insights into its safety. Because the current version of the IPV is significantly different from the original formulation, we should not base our claims of safety solely on data from the deficient study of the original (and different) version of the IPV.

In August 2022, the Informed Consent Action Network (ICAN) and Attorney Aaron Siri filed a petition with the FDA to either suspend or withdraw approval of Sanofi Pasteur's inactivated polio vaccine (IPOL) for babies and children. ICAN demanded more rigorous clinical trials, specifically a properly powered, double-blind, placebo-controlled study to adequately demonstrate IPOL's safety.

Six months later, director of the Center for Biologics Evaluation and Research at the FDA, Peter Marks, MD, PhD, responded only to state that the issues needed further review and analysis.

ICAN had initially raised concerns about IPOL in 2017, after discovering that the vaccine's clinical trials for children did not meet what they considered proper safety standards. After a Freedom of Information Act request for the clinical trial data used for FDA approval in 1990, ICAN claimed the data did not substantiate the vaccine's safety, leading to the formal petition.

Perhaps now you understand the reason some people claim "vaccines have never been safety tested." Whereas these people are dismissively labeled "anti-vaccine," in reality, they are just pro-transparent and honest safety testing protocols. Even though all vaccines on the market today have undergone safety testing, they may not have always been tested in the optimal way. *Unfortunately, this leaves room for doubt where none would have otherwise existed had pharmaceutical companies conducted, and had the FDA required, the best possible safety studies.* Until then, we are left wondering, what is the bottom turtle standing on?

8

LET'S TALK ABOUT NEWBORN VACCINES

In 1736 I lost one of my sons, a fine boy of four years old, by the smallpox taken in the common way. I long regretted bitterly and still regret that I had not given it to him by inoculation. This I mention for the sake of the parents who omit that operation, on the supposition that they should never forgive themselves if a child died under it; my example showing that the regret may be the same either way, and that, therefore, the safer should be chosen.

—BENJAMIN FRANKLIN (EXCERPT FROM HIS AUTOBIOGRAPHY)

As a pediatrician, I often get this apprehensive look from new parents. Before their mouths open to speak, their eyes seem to ask, "Is it safe to talk to this guy about vaccines?" While I have not quite mastered the art of telepathic communication, I manage to flash a reassuring glance, signaling that I *am* one of those doctors willing to participate in a respectful discussion. We spend several minutes awkwardly exchanging expressive stares before they finally muster the courage to initiate a conversation.

I keep coming back to that line from *Fight Club*—"The first rule of Fight Club is you don't talk about Fight Club"—except, in my line of work, the first rule of Vaccine Club is you don't talk about vaccines. It's baffling, really. We are told that vaccines are recommended. Nevertheless, first-time parents who attempt to consult with their pediatrician about newborn vaccines are sometimes belittled for inquiring about a medical intervention that is not mandatory—an intervention whereby the very word "recommended" implies choice. In contemplating whether to follow recommendations, these first-time parents rely on the expertise of the very medical professionals who possess the knowledge to help navigate such important decisions. Rather than engage in a dialogue, some medical professionals use their position to berate parents who dare question.

An unfortunate example of this is a recent social media post made by a well-known pediatrician:

> In my practice you will vaccinate and you will vaccinate on time. You will not get your own "spaced-out" schedule that increases your child's risk of illness or adverse events. I will not have measles-shedding children sitting in my waiting room. I will answer all your questions about vaccines and present you with facts, but if you will not vaccinate then you will leave my practice. I will file a CPS report (not that they will do anything) for medical neglect, too.
>
> I have patients who are premature infants with weak lungs and hearts. I have kids with complex congenital heart disease. I have kids who are on chemotherapy for acute lymphoblastic leukemia who cannot get all of their vaccines. In short, I have patients who have true special needs and true health issues who could suffer severe injury or death because of your magical belief that your kid is somehow more special than other children and that what's good for other children is not good for yours.
>
> This pediatrician is not putting up with it. Never have, never will.

Some may laud this doctor. Others will surely recognize that such divisive rhetoric from a health-care provider does not promote vaccination but alienates parents and fosters an adversarial relationship between patients and the professionals entrusted with their care. Of course, physicians have the discretion to exclude patients from their practices. Threatening to report parents who choose not to vaccinate to Child Protective Services raises serious concerns around ethics and compassion and reflects poorly upon the medical profession as a whole. This doctor missed the memo: Vaccines are recommendations, not compulsory directives.

Vaccines are a product manufactured by highly profitable corporations. They are not some omnipotent deity before whom we doctors must loyally genuflect—albeit sometimes, it feels that way. To the dismay of many, the internet has provided a platform for the dissemination of vaccine research and conversation. This marketplace of ideas sometimes leads well-intentioned and intelligent individuals to uncover gaps in our scientific understanding. Despite the frequent repetition of phrases like "safe and effective" or "the science is settled," anyone with a basic understanding of science and the research process knows these statements oversimplify complex realities. There is no shame in admitting that we doctors don't know everything. We don't have to know everything. What better way to honor our human connection to our patients than through honesty and humility?

Most parents who ask questions intend to vaccinate. They just want their concerns addressed first. The simple act of inquiring violates that cardinal rule of Vaccine club—we don't talk about vaccines. In fact, many doctor's offices are unwilling to accept patients who choose not to vaccinate or even those who prefer to follow an alternative schedule.

Vaccine hesitancy is on the rise. We should not overlook the possibility that this growing reluctance is rooted in medicine's unwillingness to participate in these conversations with transparency and candor, if at all. Why are parents so afraid that they are relegated to communicating with their eyes? Becoming a parent for the first time already comes with a concomitance of anxieties. Speaking openly to one's pediatrician should not be one of them.

The medical community, at large, increasingly downplays the risks of vaccines. The CDC website and Vaccine Information Sheets (VIS) do not provide sufficient information. Parents have the right to voice concerns over the known and unknown risks of vaccines—because vaccines *do* come with risks, even when those risks may not be readily apparent. In 1955, Cutter Laboratories produced batches of the OPV vaccine that were not properly inactivated, leading to forty thousand mild polio cases, two hundred cases of paralysis, and ten deaths. Since then, vaccines have been recalled after they were found to cause intestinal blockage; they have been contaminated with the virus SV40 known to cause cancer in lab animals; they have caused myocarditis and menstrual cycle abnormalities. The list goes on . . .

This isn't fearmongering. Both the mild and severe known side effects are printed right there in black-and-white, on the vaccine inserts generated by the vaccine manufacturers. If, by way of example, your newborn baby is one of the small few who experiences an anaphylactic reaction after receiving a particular vaccine, you would want to know that such reaction, though rare, is possible. As a diligent and caring parent, you have every right to thoroughly discuss potential vaccine reactions without fear of criticism, just as, when contemplating cancer treatments, patients are made aware of serious side effects, like hair loss and immune suppression. Oncologists compassionately weigh the risks and benefits of treatment with their cancer patients, ultimately urging their patients to decide which course of treatment to pursue. Even after learning of the potentially severe side effects of treatment, many cancer patients would still choose treatment. However, few would ostracize a cancer patient for opting out of a treatment that could cause serious adverse consequences.

Similarly, notwithstanding the fact that vaccines come with risks, most parents would and do still choose to vaccinate their children. But we should not anathematize parents who are unwilling to assume those risks. Despite medical recommendation, a Jehovah's Witness may refuse a blood transfusion. Informed consent, whether in the context of cancer, heart surgery, blood transfusions, vaccines, or any other medical intervention, is critical because it empowers individuals to make decisions that align with their values and needs. Respect for patient autonomy is fundamental—regardless of whether we may, personally, disagree.

Under very specific circumstances, there is an override switch. The *parens patriae* doctrine allows doctors to supersede informed consent or parental wishes in emergency situations, when a child's life or health is at serious risk. In cases where parents refuse lifesaving treatments, such as blood transfusions, chemotherapy, or insulin, courts have upheld state intervention—often citing the 1944 case *Prince v. Massachusetts*, in which the court ruled that parental rights do not extend to endangering a child's welfare. Public health laws also allow for mandatory vaccinations and quarantines in disease outbreaks. While parental rights are respected, the law prioritizes a child's right to life and health, permitting court-ordered medical interventions when refusal poses imminent harm.

Typically, when we speak of nonemergency vaccine recommendations, we are not referring to the types of scenarios contemplated by the *parens patriae* doctrine. We are talking about everyday medical decisions that do require informed consent. The dictionary defines "recommendation" as a suggestion or proposal for one's consideration, as to the best course of action. Unlike a mandate, a recommendation presumes one has a choice. In a 2024 interview, the former commissioner of the FDA, Scott Gottlieb, voiced concern that routine childhood vaccination may *shift* to "shared clinical decision making"—a category that requires more active involvement and agreement between health-care providers and parents before administration. The implication that the decision to vaccinate is *anything other than a shared clinical decision* is mind-boggling!

Like Gotlieb, the CDC's understanding of the word *recommendation* deviates from the dictionary's. On its website, the CDC differentiates routine childhood vaccinations on the schedule from those that are not recommended on the schedule. Although the CDC deems "shared clinical decision-making" appropriate for vaccines that do *not* fall on the recommended vaccination schedule, it instructs us that, for the routine childhood vaccines on the schedule, the "default decision is to vaccinate."

This distinction is notable. The disconcerting connotation is that, when it comes to the vaccines on the recommended schedule, the decision to vaccinate is *not* made jointly between physician and patient. Given that the decision to vaccinate is a medical decision, I firmly believe that it should be made by the parents, in consultation with their pediatrician.

Coercive methods—whether by intimidation, shaming, or outright silencing—run counter to the idea that parents have a choice in making medical decisions for their children. They vitiate informed consent, without which no medical procedure should ever be performed on any patient. This secret fraternity around vaccines has engendered distrust in the entire institution of medicine. If the concern is truly that the known side effects or the potential for unknown, long term adverse consequences would deter vaccination, then our focus should *not* be on suppressing conversation but on making vaccines safer and studying them more rigorously.

The medical community resolutely condemns vaccine misinformation and disinformation. And yet the medical community stands in the superior position to disseminate *correct* information—provided, of course, it is willing to bend the rules of Vaccine Club and talk about vaccines.

By laying all facts on the table and engaging in thoughtful discussion, we doctors can and must provide parents with the clarity and confidence necessary to make the best choices for their child's health.

HEPATITIS B

Among the various vaccines administered to newborns, the hepatitis B vaccine garners the most questions from parents. Many debate its utility at such a young age and wonder whether the hepatitis B vaccine is truly needed at birth or if it can be postponed until later in life. To address these concerns, we must first understand the bases for the current recommendations and examine the way hepatitis B is transmitted and its risks, along with the history of earlier vaccination efforts.

As a reminder, hepatitis B is a viral infection that affects the liver and can lead to chronic liver disease, liver cancer, and cirrhosis. It is primarily spread through blood and bodily fluids, including through contaminated needles, unprotected sex, and from mother to child during childbirth.

When it was first introduced, the hepatitis B vaccine was recommended *primarily* for high-risk populations, such as health-care workers exposed to blood; intravenous drug users who share needles; people with multiple sexual partners or those in high-risk sexual behaviors; and, due to the high risk of mother-to-child transmission during birth, babies born to mothers who are hepatitis B positive. The focus was on reducing the risk of chronic hepatitis B infection in adults and at-risk infants.

By the late 1980s, despite targeted vaccination of high-risk groups, hepatitis B remained a public health issue in the United States, with tens of thousands of new infections annually. One of the primary challenges remained that many infected individuals did not possess clear risk factors. Some children were being infected without anyone realizing how or where the exposure occurred.

Consequently, in 1991, as a way to prevent the transmission of hepatitis B, the Advisory Committee on Immunization Practices (ACIP) and the CDC decided to recommend universal vaccination of all infants at birth. This marked a major shift from vaccinating only high-risk groups to ensuring that all children were protected from potential infection.

Still, compared to other vaccines, hepatitis B is more controversial. With the 1991 recommendation, the hepatitis B vaccine became one of the first vaccines routinely given at birth. Additional doses are then given at one to two months and, again, at six to eighteen months. In my practice, parents frequently express misgivings about the hepatitis B vaccine, largely because it is administered to newborns within the first day of life. They question the need to vaccinate a newborn whose mother has tested negative for hepatitis B, arguing that the risk of early childhood transmission is minimal, and vaccination could be delayed without significantly increasing the child's risk of infection.

Critics of the vaccine also note the studies that show that antibody levels can decline over time, with approximately 60% of individuals vaccinated at birth retaining detectable antibodies twenty years later, though most experts agree that immune memory remains intact, allowing vaccinated individuals to mount a protective response upon exposure to the virus.

Some have pointed out that a *common* known side effect of the hepatitis B vaccine is fever. In fact, 1–6% of children experience a low-grade fever after receiving the vaccine. While a fever is deemed a mild vaccine side effect, in a newborn, a fever could be an indication of sepsis or meningitis. Accordingly, when a newborn has a fever (regardless of the cause), he or she must typically go to the hospital for a full workup, which frequently includes a lumbar puncture (a procedure whereby a needle is inserted into the lower back to collect cerebrospinal fluid). Often the infant is admitted to the hospital for supervision, where he or she will likely risk exposure to other pathogens and infections. Even if it is ultimately determined that the fever was attributable to the hepatitis B vaccine, the newborn will have been subjected to a battery of invasive tests and hospitalization simply to rule out the possibility of sepsis or meningitis. Because, after the first few months of life, a low-grade fever is no longer considered dangerous in a newborn that otherwise appears healthy, some parents contemplate whether to delay vaccination for several months, particularly when the risk of hepatitis B transmission is low.

Others still argue that the mandatory nature of the hepatitis B vaccine for school attendance is unnecessary for a disease primarily spread through behaviors uncommon in children. Advocates for delayed vaccination suggest waiting until adolescence, when behaviors associated with higher hepatitis B risk (e.g., sexual activity or IV drug use) become more common. This could maximize protection during the years of greatest risk; it may also reduce overall vaccine coverage due to missed opportunities during infancy.

The consensus among public health agencies, including the CDC and WHO, remains that such prophylactic measures are appropriate and even necessary. They continue to strongly advocate for the hepatitis B vaccine's inclusion in routine immunization schedules for several key reasons:

Although hepatitis B is associated with adult risk factors, transmission during infancy and childhood is possible. Many people infected with hepatitis B show no symptoms for years, making it difficult to trace and prevent its spread. Household members can transmit the virus through cuts, scrapes, or open sores. When children contract hepatitis B, they are much more likely to develop chronic infection (up to 90% for infants), leading to long-term complications such as liver cancer.

From a community public health standpoint, universal vaccination against hepatitis B has proven highly successful. Since the vaccine was introduced, the number of new hepatitis B infections in the United States has precipitously dropped by more than 90% among children and adolescents. By vaccinating infants the chances of children developing chronic hepatitis B, and accompanying complications, have reduced significantly. Universal vaccination also guards the broader population, reducing overall transmission rates and protecting individuals who may not be vaccinated or for whom the vaccine is less effective.

The decision to vaccinate newborns against hepatitis B requires parents to weigh the relatively low risk of early childhood transmission against the known and unknown risks from the vaccine. Parents must also take into account the potential benefits of universal coverage and long-term protection. This particular vaccine forces us to balance public health priorities, vaccine risks, and individual rights.

For parents, these decisions generally come down to trust in public health recommendations versus personal risk and vaccine risk assessment. Health-care providers can convey the importance of the hepatitis B vaccine in protecting individual and community health and simultaneously address parental concerns in a respectful and open-minded manner—because a parent's reservations and concerns can be logical, intelligent, and valid *and, at the same time*, the vaccine can be effective. These are not mutually exclusive propositions.

In my clinical practice, parents seem to most frequently decline the hepatitis B vaccine at birth more than any other vaccine on the schedule. Instead, many opt to give the vaccine at a later date. (Don't worry, I haven't reported any of them to Child Protective Services.) While some would debate the correctness of this assessment by the parents, many of these families express to me that, in their view, the known and unknown risks associated with vaccinating a newborn outweigh any personal risk of hepatitis B exposure, which they believe to be near zero, given that neither biological parent is infected with hepatitis B. Typically, they choose to give the vaccine at two months old or closer to school age.

Notably, in a 2025 episode of his podcast, host and CEO of MAHA Action and the Informed Consent Action Network (ICAN), Del Bigtree, interviewed virologist and former Director of the CDC, Robert Redfield. Redfield's discussion of the RECOMBIVAX vaccine insert renders it shockingly apparent that Redfield's view of the hepatitis B vaccine seems to resonate with that of parents opting to delay hepatitis B vaccination:

> BIGTREE: I just really want to get to, no placebo group, 147 children, and a five-day safety review. There's two products like this. The other hepatitis B, I could show you, has a four-day safety review period. This is a product given to 1 day-old babies. Did they establish safety? Is there any way on earth to establish safety of a product in a five-day safety review?

> REDFIELD: I wouldn't come to that conclusion. I suspect what they've done by the committee… is that the FDA [insert]?

> BIGTREE: This is the insert that comes with the vaccine.

> REDFIELD: The FDA probably extrapolated. We can argue whether that is appropriate or not, that data that they had from adults and adolescents. I'm not a big advocate that the hepatitis B vaccine is a vaccine that needs to be prioritized for newborns. I'd rather see that vaccine as a vaccine along with the human papilloma virus vaccine, that we consider for ten, eleven, twelve, fifteen year-olds. But no. I would not say that establishes. It basically just builds on the fact that they had this adult data and I'm actually relatively surprised that then they would change the indication. So I don't know what the indication was before but say the indication was a vaccine was approved for people over the age of two or over the age of five. I'm surprised that based on that limited data they now said it's approved for people. What did you say how many days old?

BIGTREE: One.

Despite the fact that, between 2018 and 2021, Redfield served as the Director of the CDC—the *very* agency responsible for formulating vaccine *recommendations*—Redfield, by his own admission, was unaware of a number of significant details surrounding the hepatitis B vaccine recommendations.

VITAMIN K: IT'S JUST A VITAMIN—OR IS IT?

Like the hepatitis B vaccine, the vitamin K shot is given to newborns; it is administered within a few hours of birth. When first-time parents are introduced to the vitamin K shot, they are often reassured, "It's just a vitamin." Although the shot does contain a vitamin (vitamin K), the sentiment that it is *just* a vitamin is somewhat misleading. It fails to convey the full picture—namely, the way the shot works and the *other* ingredients it contains. Without these significant details, parents are not in the position to make a truly informed decision.

The vitamin K found in the shot is not a natural form of vitamin K1, like that typically found in leafy greens or other dietary sources. It contains phytonadione, a synthetic version of Vitamin K1—used because it is stable, effective, and easily absorbed when injected.

Beyond synthetic vitamin K, the shot also consists of preservatives and stabilizers that help ensure its efficacy and shelf life. These may include polysorbate 80 (an emulsifier that helps mix the components), propylene glycol (a solvent used to stabilize the solution), and benzyl alcohol (a preservative added to some formulations, associated with toxicity concerns in newborns if used in high amounts). For obvious reasons, referring to the shot as "just a vitamin" is not entirely accurate and arguably disingenuous. For many parents, a knowledge of these miscellaneous ingredients could influence their decision to give the shot to their newborn.

Earlier, we discussed the vitamin K shot in the more general sense. However, the shot, its components, and its potential side effects warrant deeper exploration. Specifically, the vitamin K vaccine comes with a black box warning in the prescribing information for AquaMEPHYTON® (Phytonadione). A black box warning is the strictest warning issued by the FDA, signaling potential risks associated with a medication. In the case of the vitamin K shot, though, the black box warning can be misunderstood or misinterpreted. The black box warning on the vitamin K shot states: "Severe reactions, including fatalities, have occurred following intravenous (IV) and intramuscular (IM) administration. These reactions are described as resembling hypersensitivity or anaphylaxis, including shock, cardiac arrest, or respiratory arrest." The warning additionally reveals: "Fatalities have been reported after IV administration, even when precautions were taken to dilute the medication and administer it slowly."

It comes as no surprise that parents may be hesitant to administer a shot to their newborns when the word *fatalities* is prominently listed among the other alarming, possibly severe, reactions. Notably, the black box warning derives primarily from the risks observed from intravenous administration, whereby rapid infusion can lead to severe hypersensitivity reactions, such as anaphylaxis and shock. This is largely irrelevant to newborns, as the vaccine is not given intravenously. Intramuscular administration carries a much lower risk of adverse events compared to intravenous use.

In fact, as far as I am aware, to date, there have been no confirmed cases of death directly attributed to the intramuscular administration of the vitamin K shot to newborns. Moreover, severe allergic reactions, like anaphylaxis, are estimated to occur in about one per one million doses, making them exceptionally rare.

Although not mentioned in the black box warning, of additional concern—and the subject of much controversy—is the possible link between the vitamin K shot and childhood cancers. In the early 1990s, a study published in the United Kingdom by J. Golding noted the potential correlation between intramuscular vitamin K and an elevated risk of leukemia in children. This study was based on a retrospective case-control design, which has limitations, such as bias and confounding factors. In the aftermath of this initial study, several large-scale studies and systematic reviews were conducted in the United Kingdom, Europe, and North America. These studies, which involved thousands of participants and used more rigorous methodologies to address the shortcomings of the earlier research, all consistently found no convincing evidence that the vitamin K shot increases the risk of childhood cancers. For instance, a 2002 study published in the *British Journal of Cancer* analyzed data from multiple trials and found no association between vitamin K administration and childhood leukemia.

The consensus remains that the benefits of the vitamin K shot in preventing life-threatening bleeding far outweigh any hypothetical risk of cancer for which there is currently no solid evidence.

Yet as is true of every medical intervention, we cannot and should not contemplate the risks without simultaneously weighing the benefits. Serving as a horrific reminder of the reason the vitamin K shot is recommended is the story of Judah, who was born on July 15, 2011. The midwife who delivered Judah offered to administer the vitamin K shot to Judah. Judah's parents declined. None of their other five children had received the vitamin K shot, and all five of those children were healthy and thriving.

In fact, prior to Judah's birth, none of his siblings had taken any antibiotics; they had never experienced an ear infection or anything more than the common cold or seasonal flu. Judah's labor and delivery went smoothly and were without any complications. Judah was born at full term. His mother, Krista, characterized her pregnancy as "great" and Judah's birth as "beautiful."

Krista recalled that when Judah's older brother was born, there had been speculation that the vitamin K shot was linked to childhood leukemia, which had since been proven false. She did not fathom that there was the remotest possibility that anything could go wrong because nothing had gone wrong with any of her other five children. The first five weeks of Judah's life were normal.

But on August 20, 2011, when Judah was five weeks old, he started displaying stomach flu–type symptoms. He threw up a few times. By bedtime, Judah seemed very lethargic. His parents attempted to wake him up to eat, to no avail. He was too sleepy. They packed their bags in preparation to leave for the hospital. As Judah's father, Chad, changed Judah's diaper, Judah experienced a seizure and stopped breathing. Chad screamed, "Judah! Judah! Come on, buddy! Krista! Call 911!" A 911 call, transport to the hospital, a whirlwind of tests, another transport to a major hospital, and surgery to place a temporary shunt in Judah's brain led to the nightmarish realization that this was not the stomach flu.

Judah suffered two brain hemorrhages believed to have been caused by vitamin K deficiency bleeding. Judah's parents were told, "Had you given your baby the shot, this probably would have never happened." Krista recounts, "Those words would replay in my mind hundreds and hundreds of times."

Despite stories such as this one, and notwithstanding the recommendations, some parents are quick to note this existential quandary: By deeming newborn babies deficient of a vitamin essential to their survival, does science presume that human design is inherently flawed? Maybe, low vitamin K levels are not a glitch in the machinery but the product of finely tuned evolutionary design. Medicine narrowly focuses on reducing the risk of vitamin K deficiency bleeding. While undeniably important, it fails to consider the biological reason human babies are universally born with lower vitamin K levels and the broader implications of altering natural physiology—to the extent there are any.

While they have not been rigorously studied and proven, several theories offer conceivable explanations for the biological utility of low vitamin K levels at birth. The first of these theories is that low vitamin K reduces the risk of blood clots. Birth is a highly traumatic process that involves significant stress and physical compression for both the baby and the mother. Low vitamin K levels may reduce the risk of clotting complications, like thrombosis, during or shortly after birth. A higher clotting factor at birth could potentially increase the likelihood of dangerous clot formation in the placental vessels or within the newborn's delicate circulatory system.

Another theory suggests that vitamin K may play a role in the development of the gut microbiota. Vitamin K is synthesized naturally by gut bacteria. Since newborns have sterile intestines, it may take time for these microbes to colonize and begin contributing to vitamin K production. This gradual process aligns with the infant's digestive system maturing and adapting to life outside the womb. Artificially boosting vitamin K at birth may bypass this natural progression with unknown consequences to the microbiome.

Still another theory is rooted in evolution. Evolution prioritizes traits that improve overall survival and reproductive success, meaning vitamin K deficiency bleeding could have been too rare to outweigh other advantages of low vitamin K levels at birth.

These theories, while merely speculative, provide several plausible ways that low vitamin K could serve a biological purpose. What if altering the levels of vitamin K at birth has unintended long-term consequences that we are yet to assess? This type of philosophical inquiry is not a rejection of medicine; rather, it is a call for deeper reflection. Open, thoughtful discussion and consideration of legitimate theories not only engenders the trust of skeptical parents; it promulgates greater scientific understanding. It's a win-win, really.

Yes, vitamin K deficiency bleeding is rare. We know the vitamin K shot effectively prevents this life-threatening condition. Choosing to give your child this shot is not synonymous with rejecting nature. It means you are leveraging modern medicine to address an avoidable risk. At the same time, we must respect questions raised by parents regarding natural physiology. Babies are not "born wrong." We can and should acknowledge this while simultaneously understanding that the fact that something is natural does not alone render it preferable. After all, pneumonia is natural, but few would argue against treating it. Medicine can honor the complexity of biology and the valid concerns of parents without undermining confidence in interventions like the vitamin K shot.

TDAP

Unlike the hepatitis B vaccine and vitamin K shot, the Tdap vaccine, which protects against tetanus, diphtheria, and pertussis, is recommended *not* for newborns but for anyone who comes into contact with them. Known as cocooning, this practice is believed to shield the infant from whooping cough.

Calling into question the adequacy of this approach is a 2014 study involving baboons, published by Jason Warfel in the *Proceedings of the National Academy of Sciences*. The purpose of this study was to determine whether vaccinated individuals could carry and transmit *Bordetella* pertussis (the bacterium causing whooping cough) to others, even if these vaccinated individuals were asymptomatic. Using baboons as a model, the study explored the dynamics of *Bordetella* pertussis infection, vaccination, and transmission. Baboons were divided into three groups: those vaccinated with acellular pertussis (aP) vaccine, those with the whole-cell pertussis (wP) vaccine, and unvaccinated controls. All groups were exposed to *Bordetella* pertussis to observe disease severity, bacterial colonization, and transmission potential. Researchers concluded that, though effective in preventing the disease in the vaccinated individual, the Tdap vaccine may not completely prevent a vaccinated individual from carrying the bacteria and inadvertently spreading it, thus challenging the perceived efficacy of the cocooning strategy.

Among other key findings, this study revealed that both vaccinated groups received effective protection against severe symptoms of pertussis. However, the acellular vaccine (aP) group could still be colonized by *Bordetella* pertussis and subsequently transmit the bacteria to unvaccinated baboons. In contrast, the whole-cell vaccine group showed significantly lower bacterial colonization and a reduced likelihood of transmission. Interestingly, baboons that received the aP vaccine carried the bacteria for up to thirty-five days, whereas unvaccinated baboons cleared the bacteria more swiftly—typically within eighteen days after recovering from natural infection.

The implications of these findings for human vaccination are significant. According to this study, while acellular pertussis vaccines effectively prevent severe disease, they do not prevent the colonization or transmission of the bacterium as effectively as the older whole-cell vaccines, which are no longer used. This suggests that vaccinated individuals could act as asymptomatic carriers, potentially contributing to the spread of pertussis among vulnerable populations such as infants who are too young to be vaccinated. This study underscores the need for further discussion on universal recommendations to vaccinate all individuals around a newborn baby. On the one hand, vaccinating close contacts could reduce the risk of pertussis transmission by lowering the severity of symptoms, like the coughing episodes that are a primary driver of transmission. Reduced symptoms might also decrease the risk of aerosolizing bacteria, indirectly protecting the infant. On the other hand, vaccinating close contacts could theoretically increase the risk of transmission to a newborn as asymptomatic carriers might unknowingly transmit pertussis to the baby—particularly if they are less cautious about close contact in the absence of noticeable symptoms. Whereas a person who is actively sick and coughing is (hopefully) likely to stay away from a baby, a seemingly healthy, asymptomatic carrier of whooping cough would have no reason to keep his or her distance.

Subsequent research has explored the implications of these findings in humans. A number of studies, including a literature review in the journal of *Clinical Infectious Diseases* in 2020, have demonstrated that individuals vaccinated with aP vaccines could carry *Bordetella* pertussis asymptomatically. Reinforcing the findings in the baboon studies, these studies similarly indicate a potential for transmission without showing symptoms. Recent research seems to show that cocooning may not be as effective as previously believed.

The evidence does show that maternal Tdap vaccination during pregnancy is highly effective at providing direct protection to the baby through passive antibody transfer and, therefore, may be the optimal method for preventing whooping cough in infants. Despite the questions around its efficacy, cocooning remains widely promoted.

9

TACKLING INDIVIDUAL CHILDHOOD VACCINE CONTROVERSIES

MMR, DTAP, HPV, VARICELLA, AND INFLUENZA

*Global immunization efforts have saved at least
154 million lives over the past 50 years.*

—WORLD HEALTH ORGANIZATION

We turn now from our discussion of newborn vaccines to several other childhood vaccines on the schedule.

MMR VACCINE

Not only the focus of extensive research but the centerpiece of vaccine discourse, MMR is the veritable A-list celebrity of the vaccine world. Everyone seems to have an opinion on it—from "The MMR vaccine is the literal Second Coming of Christ" to "The MMR vaccine killed JFK" and everything in between.

To my knowledge, and despite what some may think, the MMR vaccine is not mixed up in some sordid government conspiracy, nor is it the Messiah. It is, however, the childhood vaccine that garners the most skepticism from parents, which is somewhat puzzling given this specific vaccine's well-established and long-standing history of efficacy. Of course, reluctance stems predominantly from safety and not efficacy concerns. Making informed choices requires us to weigh the potential risks of vaccination against the risks of the underlying disease; our understanding of these respective risks is indispensable to our analysis and consequent decisions.

Regardless of one's stance on vaccines—and the MMR vaccine, in particular—the incontrovertible fact remains: Measles is extremely contagious. The measles virus spreads rapidly through airborne transmission, with an R_0 (basic reproduction number) between 12 and 18—meaning, in unvaccinated populations, one infected person can spread measles to dozens of others. To some, measles conjures horrible imagery of feverish children, covered in head-to-toe painful rashes. Others take a more lackadaisical view of the disease, perceiving it as merely yet another cold or flu. Indeed, the severity and deadliness of this disease remain a point of contention. Both historical and modern data reveal widely varying case-fatality rates across different populations and time periods. Frankly, I'm not quite sure how to make sense of it.

Before widespread vaccination, measles infected an estimated three to four million people in the United States each year. Approximately four hundred to five hundred deaths were attributed to measles annually. In the context of infectious disease, this is a relatively low overall fatality rate. In fact, the word *measly* derives from the word *measles*—connoting that, historically, measles was often perceived as a mild or even insignificant illness. In stark contrast, a 1911 measles epidemic in Rotuma, Fiji, killed 13% of the island's inhabitants. In 1529, measles devastated Cuba's indigenous population, wiping out two-thirds of its population.

These vastly disparate outcomes raise critical questions: Was the *same* disease responsible for the outbreaks in Fiji, Cuba, and the United States? Or were the Fiji and Cuba outbreaks caused by an entirely different infection that presented similar symptoms? Did mutations in the virus cause it to be more or less deadly? If it was, in fact, the same disease, were some populations more genetically or environmentally vulnerable?

The theoretical answer to such questions may perhaps lie in vitamin A. Research shows that children deficient in vitamin A are at a higher risk of severe disease and complications from measles. The WHO recommends high-dose vitamin A supplementation (200,000 IU for children, 100,000 IU for infants) in populations where vitamin A deficiency is common, as vitamin A has been shown to reduce measles-related mortality.

Part of what makes measles so dangerous is that it carries a significant rate of associated complications and hospitalizations. Pneumonia affects one in twenty children who contract measles. Pneumonia is also the leading cause of measles-related deaths. According to CDC data, about one in five unvaccinated people in the United States who contract measles require hospitalization, reminding us that even in modern health-care settings, measles can result in serious illness.

The high rate of transmissibility, together with the potential risk of hospitalization, pneumonia, and long-term health complications, renders measles a disease that requires efficacious prevention strategies. The current version of the MMR vaccine has proven effective prophylaxis against measles. The existing mainstream research, evidence, and data strongly support the MMR vaccine's risk profile to benefit ratio.

Although earlier versions of the MMR vaccine used in other countries did prompt legitimate safety concerns, those versions have been phased out. These previous incarnations contained the Urabe strain of the mumps virus, which was correlated to a higher risk of meningitis. Consequently, in the 1990s, several countries—among them, Japan—stopped using the Urabe strain. Japan replaced the MMR vaccine with a combination measles and rubella vaccine (MR), providing a separate and optional mumps vaccine. The strain of the mumps virus used in the United States is Jeryl Lynn. The evidence shows no significant link between the Jeryl Lynn strain and meningitis.

The Cochrane Review, the veritable gold standard for medical research, found a small but measurable risk of febrile seizures after the MMR vaccine currently used in the United States, with an attributable risk of 1 per 1,150 to 1,700 doses. Seizures are typically mild and transient, mostly affecting children who might otherwise experience febrile seizures due to infections or fevers.

The MMR vaccine has also been associated with a slightly increased risk of idiopathic thrombocytopenic purpura (ITP)—a blood disorder that causes a low platelet count and can lead to bleeding and bruising—at approximately 1 case per 40,000 doses. The risk of vaccine-related ITP is significantly lower than the risk of ITP from natural infections with measles, mumps, or rubella.

Large-scale studies, including the Cochrane Review and numerous independent investigations, have found no evidence linking the MMR vaccine to autism spectrum disorders or developmental delays. We will explore these studies in greater depth in our later discussion of autism.

For now, I will merely note that a review of 1.2 million children showed no increase in autism rates among children vaccinated with MMR. Furthermore, the Cochrane Review found no association between MMR vaccination and conditions like asthma, dermatitis, hay fever, leukemia, or multiple sclerosis.

The MMR vaccine is a live attenuated vaccine—meaning, it contains weakened versions of the measles, mumps, and rubella viruses. Some parents worry that vaccinated individuals may shed the virus and transmit it to others, particularly newborns or immunocompromised individuals. Shedding refers to the release of weakened, vaccine-derived viruses. Research shows that MMR vaccine shedding is extremely rare and has never been shown to cause disease in healthy or immunocompromised contacts. A 2002 study, published in the *Journal of Infectious Diseases,* found that while vaccine-strain measles RNA could be detected in respiratory secretions, no secondary transmission cases have been reported. Similarly, a 2016 study in *Vaccine* found no evidence of person-to-person spread of vaccine-strain mumps.

For rubella, the viral strain from the vaccine can be detected in throat swabs or urine for up to twenty-eight days, albeit, transmission is extremely rare and primarily observed in severely immunocompromised individuals. The CDC, WHO, and ACIP confirm that MMR shedding does not pose a meaningful risk to the general population, and the vaccine is considered safe for household contacts of the vaccinated, including newborns and pregnant women. Given that, at this time, wild-type measles, mumps, and rubella infections pose far greater risks, the benefits of MMR vaccination in preventing outbreaks and protecting vulnerable individuals outweigh any theoretical concerns about shedding.

With an efficacy rate of up to 97%, the MMR vaccine is highly successful at preventing measles. An undeniable testament to this fact, the rates of measles have declined by over 99% from just a few decades earlier. More recently, a decrease in vaccination rates has led to an increase in several minor measles outbreaks. Given measles's long incubation period, if every single person on this planet was vaccinated against it, the disease would, in all likelihood, be eradicated.

There can be no doubt that widespread vaccination against measles has played an instrumental role in mitigating the rates and transmission of a highly contagious and terrible disease. The question many vaccine-hesitant and anti-vax parents are left asking is, "At what cost?" There is a palpable growing pushback against the MMR vaccine, which, in some areas, is causing a resurgence of measles. The solution to this problem is not to point fingers at vaccine-hesitant and anti-vax parents but to utilize their concerns as an opportunity for reflection and improvement. Vilifying parents who feel the risks of vaccination outweigh the benefits isn't convincing anyone to vaccinate. It's actually deterring them, leaving pockets of children increasingly susceptible to measles infection.

Despite the tremendous efficacy of the MMR vaccine, critics often advocate for a stand-alone measles shot. They argue that, among the three diseases it targets, measles poses the greatest threat because outbreaks are more common. While a solo measles vaccine could provide an option for vaccine-hesitant individuals concerned with combining three vaccines, it does not exist for several key reasons—namely, combining vaccines into a single shot improves compliance and ensures broader protection. Moreover, creating and maintaining separate vaccines for each disease increases costs and presents logistical challenges for health-care systems. Still, to the extent it could mitigate outbreaks, I believe a solo measles vaccine warrants exploration.

DTAP

In my experience, parents are typically less reluctant about the DTaP vaccine than the MMR. Due to observations of waning immunity over time, their concerns usually center on the efficacy of the pertussis component and particularly, the acellular pertussis vaccine. Initially, the DTaP vaccine is effective in preventing pertussis. Yet studies indicate that, after the final dose of the childhood series, the DTaP vaccine's protection diminishes by approximately 10% each year. This decrease in efficacy has led to instances of pertussis outbreaks, *even among populations with high vaccination rates.* You may recall the 2014 Warfel study involving baboons, which suggested we might wish to rethink our position on cocooning newborns against pertussis.

An argument I frequently hear in opposition to the DTaP vaccine is, "It isn't working." Adherents to this theory claim that mainly vaccinated children are contracting pertussis. In 2019, at the prestigious Los Angeles private school Harvard-Westlake, thirty students came down with pertussis. Of the 1,600 students attending the school, only eighteen were unvaccinated.

Surprisingly, these eighteen unvaccinated students were *not* to blame for the outbreak. All thirty students who contracted pertussis had been vaccinated—a fact you wouldn't necessarily glean from reading the CBS news article "LA Countywide Outbreak of Whooping Cough Hits Exclusive Harvard-Westlake Hard." The author wrote: "*None of the 30 students who contracted whooping cough were not vaccinated.*" I'm going to go out on a limb here and assume that the convoluted verbiage and use of double negatives was intentional. The mental gymnastics I had to perform to decipher this sentence could have easily earned me an Olympic gold medal. None were not vaccinated? Huh? Any seasoned (or even unseasoned) journalist would know that the correct way to have written this sentence is: "All thirty students who contracted whooping cough were vaccinated." Then again, between January and April of 2023, CBS received $363 million from medical and pharmaceutical advertisements. This may just explain the confusing double negatives.

Yes, due to the waning efficacy of the DTaP vaccine, children vaccinated against pertussis can still contract pertussis. Before we disparage a vaccine's efficacy, we need to go one step further. We must acknowledge the vaccine's broader impact on reducing the rates of the target disease. Most vaccines are not 100% effective—meaning, even if a majority of the population is vaccinated, a number of breakthrough cases may still occur in vaccinated individuals. With pertussis, it is clear that unvaccinated individuals can contract and spread pertussis to vaccinated individuals and vaccinated individuals can spread it to one another. This does not automatically mean the vaccine is ineffective. For instance, if, in a given population of 102 people, a vaccine that is 95% effective is administered to 100 people, then approximately five vaccinated individuals may still become infected. Let's assume the two unvaccinated individuals in this scenario contract the disease. More vaccinated individuals (five) will have gotten the disease than unvaccinated individuals (two). However, the critical factor is not whether vaccinated individuals contract the disease but the overall reduction in cases. If none of the 100 individuals had been vaccinated, then potentially eighty or more of them would have become ill. This hypothetical illustrates the way that even in spite of breakthrough infections, vaccines significantly lower the risk of disease.

Though the now phased-out DTP vaccine was highly effective, it is no longer used in the United States. Instead, we are left with an imperfect product. Should we make efforts to find a more efficacious version of a pertussis vaccine for those who want it? It seems odd to administer the same vaccine five times in early childhood and then, subsequently, every five to ten years thereafter. This isn't simply a mildly flawed vaccine; it is an extremely imperfect one, particularly when we consider that the other components—tetanus and diphtheria—do not necessarily require so many boosters.

Perhaps we can develop a vaccine that provides more lasting efficacy without the adverse side effects. Maybe we could offer a pertussis antibody shot, similar to the RSV shot, during the first year of life when pertussis poses the greatest risk.

HPV

The human papillomavirus (HPV) vaccine is another one high on the list of distrusted vaccines. Like placing objects on opposite sides of a balance scale, our discussion of HPV will weigh common parental concerns against the vaccine's known benefits and existing research so that you can ultimately decide whether the scale tips in favor of the recommendations.

For starters, the HPV vaccine is widely recognized for its effectiveness in preventing cervical cancer and other HPV-related diseases. Tipping the scale very much in favor of vaccination is the research which shows that, when administered early, the HPV vaccine is estimated to prevent up to 90% of cancers caused by HPV.

Tipping the scale somewhat in the other direction, critics of the HPV vaccine note that the clinical trials primarily focused on the vaccine's role in the prevention of precancerous cervical changes, known as cervical intraepithelial neoplasia (CIN), rather than on preventing cervical cancer itself. These changes are recognized as precursors to cervical cancer. Yet the distinction between these precursors and cancer is important.

The pivotal studies that led to the approval of HPV vaccines, such as Gardasil and Cervarix, assessed the efficacy of these vaccines in preventing high-grade cervical lesions (CIN2 and CIN3). These high-grade cervical lesions *are* significant risk factors for developing cervical cancer. By preventing these high-grade lesions, the vaccine *indirectly* aims to prevent cervical cancer. However, the principal endpoints in these studies were the *prevention of these lesions* and other HPV-related diseases, like vulvar and vaginal cancers, anal cancers, and genital warts—depending on the HPV vaccine type. Notably, the *direct* study of cancer development would require longer-term studies due to the slow progression from HPV infection to cancer, which can take decades. Therefore, the trials used these precancerous changes as a surrogate marker to evaluate the efficacy of the vaccine in a shorter time frame.

Using precancerous changes as endpoints in HPV vaccine trials as opposed to actual cervical cancer outcomes is controversial for several reasons, the first and most significant of which is that precancerous changes do *not* usually progress to cancer. Most regress without treatment. Therefore, while preventing these conditions is beneficial, it does not necessarily equate to preventing cancer. Some argue that the efficacy of the vaccine in truly preventing cancer might be an overstatement if, in fact, those efficacy claims are based solely on the intermediate markers.

Over 91% of CIN 1, or low-grade lesions, are considered mild dysplasia and regress spontaneously without intervention. Whereas most CIN spontaneously regress, progression to invasive cancer occurs in approximately 1% of CIN1, 5% in CIN2, and around 12% in CIN3.

Using precancerous changes as surrogate endpoints is based on the assumption that reducing these will reduce cancer incidence. Surrogates sometimes fail to capture the complexity of disease progression or the significance of other health interventions. For example, improvements in screening and treatment might also contribute to reductions in cancer rates, convoluting the assessment of the vaccine's direct impact.

Tipping the scale back in favor of vaccination is compelling data showing the dramatic impact of public health initiatives around the HPV vaccine. For instance, in England, younger children vaccinated at school showed an 87% lower rate of cervical cancer compared to older, unvaccinated groups. These data strongly support the vaccine as a cornerstone of cancer prevention efforts.

The scale dizzyingly tips back yet again: In 2013, Japan temporarily suspended proactive recommendations for the HPV vaccine after reports of adverse events, including chronic pain and neurological symptoms. Subsequent studies failed to establish a causal link, and the recommendations were reinstated with additional informed consent measures.

Globally, the HPV vaccine has encountered varying levels of acceptance. In some countries, including the United States and much of Europe, the vaccine is widely recommended. Within the United States, Rhode Island, Virginia, Puerto Rico, and Washington, DC, currently mandate the HPV vaccine for school entry. Legislative efforts to expand mandates, such as New York's 2019 proposal to require HPV vaccination for school-age children, have faced significant resistance and ultimately failed to advance.

Indeed, the teetering scale is indicative of the polemical nature of the HPV vaccine, which has been and remains the subject of ongoing debate and controversy. Reports of adverse reactions, like chronic fatigue, neurological symptoms, and other health issues, have led some families to question the vaccine's safety, especially for individuals with a history or predisposition to chronic or autoimmune conditions. Although large-scale studies have not conclusively established a causal link between the vaccine and these side effects, the concerns have persisted. These disputes, by and large, center on balancing the undeniable benefits of cancer prevention with potential risks of adverse effects.

When the HPV vaccine was introduced in 2006, the volume of reports submitted to VAERS was relatively higher than for other vaccines administered to adolescents. By 2008, VAERS had received over twelve thousand reports of adverse events after HPV vaccination, raising public concerns. Fainting, dizziness, nausea, and headaches were most commonly reported. But more severe events, like blood clots, autoimmune conditions, and even deaths were also reported.

Several follow-up studies have been conducted to address concerns raised by the data from VAERS. Among them, a 2009 study by Barbara Slade et al. reviewed VAERS data spanning from 2006 to 2008. It revealed that 94% of the reported events were nonserious. This analysis found no new or unexpected safety concerns, affirming that the HPV vaccine's safety profile was consistent with what was observed during prelicense clinical trials. (As a quick aside, "et al." is an abbreviation for the Latin phrase "et alia," which means "and others." It is used to refer to a group of people when there are too many to name individually. "Et al." is commonly used when citing research because most research studies are conducted by too many authors to list in the body of the text. Instead, only the primary author is listed, followed by "et al." This is the part where that "the more you know" rainbow and star flash across the screen).

Additionally, a 2011 study by Nizar Souayah et al. examined neurological adverse events, including Guillain-Barré Syndrome (GBS), reported to VAERS. The study found no evidence of an increased risk associated with the HPV vaccine when compared to the background rates observed in the general population. A 2018 systematic review, published in the *British Medical Journal*, examined the efficacy and safety of the HPV vaccine, ultimately concluding that the HPV vaccine significantly reduces the risk of cervical cancer precursors without increasing the risk of serious adverse events. A noteworthy 2013 study by Arnheim-Dahlström et al. found no significant increase in autoimmune disorders after HPV vaccination, albeit, the study did find that the vaccine could theoretically trigger autoimmune responses in individuals who are genetically predisposed.

A 2020 Cochrane Review conducted a comprehensive review of HPV vaccine safety, analyzing 138 studies with over 23 million participants. The review found no evidence of an increased risk of serious adverse events, autoimmune conditions, or neurological disorders.

On the flip side of the balance scale, research, including a 2016 study in *Clinical Rheumatology*, conducted by Louise Brinth, explored the link between the HPV vaccine and postural orthostatic tachycardia syndrome (POTS), a condition characterized by an excessive increase in heart rate (tachycardia) when standing up from a lying or sitting position. While causality was not established, the study found a temporal association in some cases between the HPV vaccine and POTS.

Syncope (fainting) appears to be another relatively common side effect of the HPV vaccine, especially among adolescents. VAERS data suggest that fainting, often related to anxiety over the injection, typically occurs shortly after vaccine administration or the injection process and further indicates rare instances of fainting, accompanied by seizures or injuries, postinjection. Moreover, some vaccine recipients report persistent symptoms of chronic pain, brain fog, and fatigue, which are particularly challenging to study due to their subjective nature and the absence of standardized diagnostic criteria.

Epitomizing the nuance and complexity of the vaccine debate, the HPV vaccine is one that tips the scale both in favor of and, possibly, against vaccination. This vaccine seems to be a battle between the existing research and individual reporting. The HPV vaccine does appear to have benefits, but at what cost? The science and data suggest the risks associated with the HPV vaccine are rare. Nonetheless, critics of the vaccine are noisy—and getting increasingly more raucous. You'll have to determine for yourself which way the scale tips.

On her show, *Shot in the Dark*, Candace Owens shared a personal anecdote, recounting her experience with the HPV vaccine. Owens candidly detailed the significant health challenges she experienced after receiving the shots. She reported fainting after her first dose, attributing it to the fact that she had not eaten breakfast that morning. Her second dose was followed by a more severe reaction: fainting accompanied by possible seizure activity and vomiting. These reactions led her doctor to advise against completing the third dose in the series. Owens also described lingering symptoms such as fatigue and brain fog, which she associated with her vaccine experience.

Personal stories like this one resonate with many families and contribute to the hesitancy surrounding the HPV vaccine. Such anecdotes should not be dismissed outright merely because they don't align with the current scientific consensus. They remain an unequivocal reminder of the importance of informed consent and transparent communication about *not only* the benefits but also the potential risks of vaccination.

VARICELLA

Somewhat less controversial than the HPV vaccine, the varicella vaccine is the newer kid on the vaccine block. As recently as when I was a kid, parents hosted something called chicken pox parties. Not your typical party with cakes and piñatas, a chicken pox party was the less fun kind, where parents brought their children to catch chicken pox from that one kid lucky enough to come down with it. Before the varicella vaccine existed, we wanted kids to get the chicken pox, and we wanted them to contract it at a young age because the virus carries more serious complications for adults.

I remember having chicken pox. I didn't feel all that bad. My body was covered in itchy pockmarks that I was repeatedly reminded not to scratch. I took soothing oatmeal baths for about a week. I recovered. Yes, back in my day, parents strangely rejoiced when their kids contracted chicken pox—as though it was some sort of rite of passage. It seemed like no big deal to me, but chicken pox, also known as varicella, can pose serious health risks.

Many parents today hail from the "chicken pox party" generation, when catching and then getting over chicken pox was a so-called badge of honor. It's really no wonder then that some of these same parents question the need for the varicella vaccine, particularly when the benefits are considered along with the potential long-term side effects.

The varicella vaccine was introduced in 1995, and just like that, along with Blockbuster Video, VHS, and casette tapes (RIP), those delightful chicken pox parties went by the wayside, a long forgotten relic of the past. A testament to its efficacy, the varicella vaccine significantly reduced the incidence of chicken pox, preventing a once-common childhood illness. Oatmeal manufacturers were forced to reevaluate their marketing strategies, shifting from baths to the ever-popular oat milk. (Okay, I'm kidding about that last part.)

Despite the undeniable success of the varicella vaccine, critics often wonder whether it increases the risk of herpes zoster (shingles) in older adults—the reason being, after a person recovers from chicken pox, the virus remains dormant in nerve tissues and can reactivate later in life, causing shingles. Some studies suggest that widespread varicella vaccination in children might reduce the natural boosting of immunity in adults due to reduced exposure to circulating chicken pox. This potentially increases the risk of developing shingles.

However, data on shingles incidence trends provide a mixed picture. The CDC has observed that, in the United States, the rates of shingles among adults have gradually increased over time, though the reasons are not entirely clear. The temporal correlation between initial varicella vaccinations and the rise in shingles does not automatically implicate the vaccine. The surge in shingles could very well be attributed to a slew of other factors. We simply don't have enough evidence to say one way or another. Perhaps leaving us with more questions than answers, recent data also indicate that, in some cases, the rates of shingles have plateaued or even declined across various age groups.

No, this chapter is not about the potential long-term adverse effects of certain vaccines. (That chapter is coming.) But the long-term consequences are indispensable to the conversation as they *are* the very reason so many parents have misgivings about the varicella vaccine. Parents want to know whether preventing chicken pox today comes at the price of shingles or some other long-term complication later in life. They want to know this because shingles tends to be more severe than chicken pox, especially in older and immunocompromised individuals. Complications from shingles, such as postherpetic neuralgia (PHN), can cause significant and persistent pain. The personal suffering caused by shingles—severe pain, lasting discomfort, and disability due to PHN—can profoundly impact the quality of life for affected individuals. Furthermore, the economic burden of shingles and its complications is tremendous, with annual direct medical costs and productivity losses in the United States estimated to exceed $2.4 billion.

Whereas the varicella vaccine helps prevent chicken pox, its potential link to shingles incidence in older adults presents a difficult conundrum. For many parents grappling with the decision to give the varicella vaccine, ongoing research would provide better guidance. Studying the link between varicella vaccination and shingles is imperative to both our understanding of the correlation between them and developing comprehensive vaccination strategies that effectively balance the prevention of chicken pox and shingles.

Of course, as always, we must weigh the potential adverse side effects from the vaccine against the real-world risks posed by the disease, even if uncommon. While chicken pox is often considered a mild childhood illness that many parents brush off as "just a minor rash I had when I was a child," the varicella-zoster virus can cause severe skin infections, such as cellulitis, abscesses, and necrotizing fasciitis (flesh-eating bacteria), requiring hospitalization and intravenous antibiotics. Additionally, varicella pneumonia and bacterial superinfections can occur and lead to life-threatening complications. Neurologically, varicella can cause encephalitis (brain inflammation), meningitis, and cerebellar ataxia, which may result in long-term neurological damage. According to the CDC, before the introduction of the varicella vaccine, about 10,500 hospitalizations and between 100 and 150 deaths were attributed annually in the United States to complications from chicken pox, even in previously healthy individuals.

INFLUENZA

The influenza vaccine or, as it's more commonly referred to, the "flu vaccine" was developed in 1938 and first licensed for public use in 1945. The flu vaccine has long been a cornerstone of public health efforts to reduce the burden of seasonal flu. It is widely recommended for individuals six months and older to prevent severe illness, hospitalization, and death, most notably in high-risk populations (i.e., the elderly, pregnant women, immunocompromised individuals, and young children). Despite its widespread use, the flu vaccine remains the subject of much contention.

One of the primary controversies surrounding the influenza vaccine is its variable and often modest efficacy. The efficacy of the vaccine varies from year to year, depending on how well the strains included in the vaccine match the circulating viruses. Studies have shown that vaccine effectiveness can range from as low as 10% to as high as 60%, depending on the flu season and the individual's age and health status. A 2019 meta-analysis, published in *Vaccine*, found that the vaccine's effectiveness is typically lower in older adults and children. Ironically, these are the demographics most at risk for severe complications from the flu. This variability has led to some skepticism regarding the vaccine's utility.

In 2018, the Cochrane Review evaluated the efficacy of live attenuated and inactivated influenza vaccines in children up to sixteen years of age, focusing on their ability to reduce confirmed influenza cases, influenza-like illnesses (ILI), and associated harms. Live attenuated vaccines likely reduce lab-confirmed influenza from 18% to 4% and may reduce ILI from 17% to 12%, requiring vaccination of seven children to prevent one case of influenza and the vaccination of twenty children to prevent one case of ILI.

This is an epidemiological concept known as the number needed to treat (NNT), which is the number of patients who need to receive a treatment or intervention for one additional person to benefit compared to a control group.

Inactivated vaccines reduce confirmed influenza cases from 30% to 11% and reduce ILI from 28% to 20%, with five children requiring vaccination to prevent one case of influenza and the vaccination of twelve children for ILI. Nevertheless, according to the review, the absolute benefits varied across populations and seasons, and limited data were available for children under two years old.

The review also noted a 2009 H1N1 pandemic vaccine that was linked to rare cases of narcolepsy (a chronic neurological disorder that affects the brain's ability to regulate sleep-wake cycles) and cataplexy (sudden and transient episode of muscle weakness, typically triggered by strong emotions including laughter, excitement, surprise, or anger) in children. The review underscores the need for standardized reporting of adverse events and more comprehensive studies to assess vaccine safety and efficacy.

Another area of concern stems from research that suggests that the flu vaccine could actually increase susceptibility to other respiratory infections. A 2012 study by Benjamin Cowling et al. found an increased risk of non-influenza respiratory virus infections, such as rhinoviruses and coxsackieviruses, in vaccinated individuals compared to those who received a placebo. This phenomenon, referred to as viral interference, suggests that the immune system's response to the vaccine may temporarily render individuals more vulnerable to other respiratory pathogens. Other studies have challenged this finding, though, emphasizing the need for more robust research to clarify the extent and mechanisms of viral interference.

While the influenza vaccine is recommended for children as young as six months old, there is limited data on its efficacy and safety in this age group. The Cochrane Review articles on influenza noted this gap, pointing out that evidence supporting the vaccine's efficacy in children under two years of age is scarce and of low quality. This absence of robust evidence for infants has raised concerns among some parents and health-care professionals, particularly given that this age group is already at higher risk for complications from respiratory infections.

The influenza vaccine remains a tool in reducing the global burden of seasonal flu. But its variable effectiveness, potential for viral interference, and limited research in infants under two years of age warrant further investigation. Addressing these concerns through transparent communication and high-quality research is essential to maintaining public trust and improving vaccine uptake.

THE REMAINING DROPS IN THE SYRINGE: FINAL THOUGHTS ON INDIVIDUAL VACCINES

In his book *Vaccines and Your Family*, pediatrician and internationally recognized expert in the fields of virology and immunology, Paul Offit, MD, writes:

> Parents who choose not to vaccinate their children or choose to
> delay or withhold vaccines are taking a risk. It's not a big risk; in

fact, the odds are in their favor. In all likelihood, their children will not suffer permanent harm or die from an infectious disease. Polio has been eliminated from the United States; so has rubella. Diphtheria occurs in only a few people a year. And although measles cases occur every year in the United States, and we witnessed significant measles epidemics in 2015 and 2019, no one died.

At this time, I agree with Offit's assessment. I would add that circumstances can change quickly, which, as you will recall, they did in 2019 Samoa. Herd immunity, while effective, is not guaranteed indefinitely, especially if vaccination rates decline.

Offit is quick to point out: "So what's the harm of not vaccinating? The fact is that every year vaccine-preventable diseases still kill children in the United States." Again, I agree. There is an unequivocal risk inherent to not vaccinating. Vaccine-preventable diseases, while rare in the United States, can and do cause harm.

Offit goes on to suggest:

> Choosing not to vaccinate is like playing Russian roulette, except instead of having a gun with five empty chambers and one bullet, it's a gun with hundreds of thousands of empty chambers and one bullet. But why take the chance? Why play?

This is the part where my perspective slightly diverges from Offit's. The struggle to balance disease prevention and safety is a dance. Both vaccinating and not vaccinating carry consequences; *each* represents a game of Russian roulette that requires us to weigh the statistical odds.

Although I appreciate the metaphor, I would submit that parents concerned about vaccine safety view this same Russian roulette analogy from the opposite vantage point. For these parents, the *vaccine* represents the gun, and the potential for severe side effects, the bullet. Indeed, "why take the chance" that your child will have a vaccine-induced side-effect? If, as Offit suggests, the risk of contracting a vaccine-preventable disease is like playing Russian roulette with one bullet in a gun containing hundreds of thousands of empty chambers, then concerned parents wonder if the risk of vaccine-related side effects is like playing Russian roulette with one bullet in a gun containing a thousand empty chambers. They are left weighing which game of Russian roulette poses less risk to their child. Some parents are simply unwilling to pull the proverbial vaccine trigger.

10

HEAVY QUESTIONS
THE ROLE OF METALS IN VACCINES

*These walls don't just look good. They're yummy too! New
flavored lead-based paint and varnish. Great Flavors! Pistachio
(shown), cotton candy, lemon, marshmallow.*
—DUTCH BOY LEAD PAINT ADVERTISEMENT

For many parents, the fear of vaccine side effects stems from the other
ingredients inside the syringe—specifically metals. Cynics question whether
metals contribute to or even cause acute reactions, chronic conditions, and
autism. Aluminum—which, as a reminder, is a common adjuvant used to
enhance the body's immune response to vaccine antigens—has garnered
substantial recent attention. Just as parents and health advocates previously
questioned the impact of mercury and lead exposure, today, they question
the long-term health implications of injecting aluminum into our children.

As research illuminated the neurotoxic effects of lead, the levels of
exposure deemed acceptable decades ago are now deemed hazardous. Thus,
our understanding of what constitutes "safe" exposure is continuously
evolving. Similarly, since 2001, the mercury-based preservative thimerosal
has been largely phased out of pediatric vaccines in the United States due
to apprehension over its cumulative neurotoxicity. Making informed health
decisions is, in part, predicated on our recognition of the role metals play
in vaccine technology. We should simultaneously acknowledge that, as new
data emerges, public health recommendations are constantly refined, often
resulting in the reassessment of acceptable risk levels.

Recently, I came across several photographs from the 1950s, depicting two smiling nurses standing by a patient's bedside. These nurses are offering the patient an impressive variety of cigarettes to choose from. In another photograph, a friendly nurse lights a cigarette for her patient as he lies in a hospital bed. Modern medicine routinely brushes aside concerns about aluminum. In light of our growing understanding of the dangers of lead and other metals, we must consider the possibility that aluminum *may* pose a risk of which we are currently unaware.

Although parents who question the safety of aluminum are frequently dismissed as "anti-vax" or "conspiracy theorists," the sordid history of metals lends credence to their skepticism. We cannot overlook the potential long-term effects of any substance administered early in life into the delicate, rapidly developing systems of young children. Aluminum adjuvants have a long track record of use and are generally regarded as safe. But our expanding awareness of metals and health raises valid questions over cumulative exposure to and long-term impacts of metals.

LEAD

Lead is a prime example of the benefit of hindsight. Lead was never used in vaccines (at least I hope it wasn't). Yet the shift in our understanding of lead poignantly illustrates the way our perception of risk changes. A product we were once assured was perfectly safe may later be proven unsafe or even hazardous.

In the early twentieth century, lead was widely used in products like paint, gasoline, and plumbing. Now, this sounds laughable. Back then, it didn't. At the time, there were no federal regulations in place governing lead levels in the environment or consumer products.

In 1971, after growing evidence linking lead exposure to severe health effects, including cognitive impairments, developmental delays, and behavioral issues in children, the United States passed the Lead-Based Paint Poisoning Prevention Act, restricting the use of lead-based paint in federal housing.

In 1970, when lead in gasoline had been identified as a major contributor to environmental contamination, the United States passed the Clean Air

Act, resulting in the phased reduction of lead in gasoline starting in 1973, with a full ban on leaded gasoline for on-road vehicles by 1996.

In 1986, the Safe Drinking Water Act established standards for lead in public drinking water systems, limiting the allowable concentration of lead to fifty parts per billion in tap water. In 1991, under the Lead and Copper Rule, the US Environmental Protection Agency (EPA) lowered the maximum allowable level of lead in drinking water to fifteen parts per billion.

Current regulations aim to eliminate or drastically reduce lead exposure in consumer products, air, water, soil, and paint, with particular attention to protecting vulnerable populations. In stark contrast to the early 1900s, today the dangers of lead are common knowledge. This demonstrates the way scientific advancements shift our understanding of safety.

MERCURY/THIMEROSAL

The same is true of our perception of mercury, particularly in the form of thimerosal in vaccines. Over the past few decades, thimerosal has been the focus of vaccine safety discussions. An organic mercury compound, thimerosal was (and occasionally still is) used as a preservative to prevent bacterial and fungal contamination in multidose vials. This is particularly true of vaccines distributed to areas with limited refrigeration. Developed in the 1920s by the Eli Lilly company, thimerosal was introduced in vaccines in the 1930s. Thimerosal contains ethylmercury, which the body processes differently than methylmercury, the toxic form of mercury associated with environmental exposure, such as in fish.

In the late 1990s, growing awareness of the neurotoxic effects of methylmercury in food led to increased concern over mercury exposure from thimerosal—namely, in infants and children. At the time, thimerosal was present in several vaccines commonly given to infants, including the hepatitis B, DTP, and Hib vaccines.

The EPA's reference dose for methylmercury was set at 0.1 mcg/kg of body weight per day. This guideline was based on studies of methylmercury exposure, predominantly from dietary sources, and intended to prevent adverse neurological effects in developing infants and children. While ethylmercury (from thimerosal) and methylmercury are chemically distinct, the EPA's reference dose was used as a comparative standard, as no specific guidelines existed for ethylmercury. Under the standard vaccine schedule at that time, cumulative mercury exposure from vaccines could exceed this guideline.

Thimerosal breaks down into 50% ethylmercury and thiosalicylate. In the 1990s, limited pharmacokinetic data existed on ethylmercury and its toxicity and excretion. Though it is known to potentially cause neurologic and renal toxicity, including death from overdose, and while ethylmercury is largely recognized to cross the blood-brain barrier, there is sparse data on its effects.

Estimates suggested that by six months of age, cumulative exposure to mercury from vaccines could reach approximately 187.5 mcg for children who received all recommended vaccines containing thimerosal. For reference, the EPA's reference dose for methylmercury is 0.1 mcg per kg of body weight per day. For a six-month-old infant, who typically weighs around 7.5 kg (16.5 lb), this equates to an estimated safe daily intake of approximately 0.75 mcg of methylmercury per day.

You don't need to worry about the minutia. The takeaway and salient point is, there was no direct evidence that thimerosal caused any harm, yet simultaneously, children who received all recommended vaccines were exposed to *more* mercury (through the thimerosal in vaccines) than regulatory agencies considered safe for oral ingestion from food.

These concerns led to the formation of multiple panels in the 1990s, designed to look into the safety profile of thimerosal. Established in 1991, with three sites and a fourth added in 1992, the Vaccine Safety Datalink (VSD) is a collaboration between the CDC and four large health maintenance organizations (HMOs). The VSD's purpose is to address rare, potential vaccine safety issues across more than six million enrolled patients.

The VSD was used to research mercury from thimerosal-containing vaccines and potential neurodevelopmental or renal (kidney) disorders focusing on children born between 1992 and 1999. The initial results indicated a statistically noteworthy correlation between exposure and outcomes, such as developmental delays and attention deficit disorder, supporting a possible link between increased exposure and certain risks. There was some concern that this analysis was biased by the fact that children who visited health-care providers more often were more likely to receive vaccines and, consequently, more likely to be diagnosed with medical conditions.

The consensus was that there was insufficient evidence to show a causal relationship between thimerosal exposure and observed outcomes; further studies were recommended. The potential for litigation and public concern emphasized the need for thorough research. Multiple panel discussions and reports on thimerosal, including an Institute of Medicine (IOM) report, ensued. Generated by the IOM's Vaccine Safety Forum, such reports are designed to evaluate critical issues relevant to the safety of vaccines used in the United States and address methods for improving the safety of vaccines and vaccination programs.

In response to the ongoing debate around the safety and efficacy of thimerosal and the cumulative impact of mercury exposure, between June 7 and June 8, in 2000, representatives from the WHO, CDC, NIH, FDA and pharmaceutical companies, vaccine developers, and researchers met at the Simpsonwood Retreat Center, in Norcross, Georgia. At this Simpsonwood meeting, vaccine researchers presented their findings in a report entitled "Scientific Review of Vaccine Safety Datalink Information."

In a 2024 appearance on the Joe Rogan podcast, episode number 1999, guest Robert F. Kennedy Jr. shared:

> And then somebody handed me a transcript of a secret meeting that took place in 1999. And it was 1999. It might have been 2000. But it's called the Simpsonwood meeting.

> So they found this retreat center, a Methodist retreat center in Norcross, Georgia, called Simpsonwood. And they assembled, I think there was seventy-two people there. And they were from the WHO, CDC, NIH, FDA, and all the vaccine companies and all the big academics, the people who basically develop vaccines in the academic institutions. And they were all there. And they spend the first day, they give them all a copy of the first-hand study, but they have to give it all back because they don't want it out there. And then they have a day of talking about it where they're all saying, "holy cow, this is real and, you know, the lawyers are going to come after us. We're all in trouble."

> And then they spend the second day talking about how to hide it.

When Rogan interjected and asked Kennedy, "How do you know this?" Kennedy responded:

> Because somebody made a recording of it and I got a hold of the transcripts. And I published excerpts from those transcripts in *Rolling Stone* and anybody can go and read these now on our website. It's called Simpsonwood and you can read through the whole thing or you can read my *Rolling Stone* article, which is also on the website, which summarizes it.

The transcript is, in fact, available, and I have personally read it from cover to cover. I did not note any information to suggest this meeting was secret. Nor did I find anything that indicated the report was given covertly. (Perhaps the transcript does not cover everything discussed at Simpsonwood. I simply don't know.) What is apparent from the transcript is that the Scientific Review of Vaccine Safety Datalink Information was circulated at the meeting. The report primarily examined the effects of thimerosal in vaccines, especially those administered early in life, such as the hepatitis B, DTP, and the Hib vaccines.

The Simpsonwood meeting also briefly addressed aluminum in vaccines. The Scientific Review of Vaccine Safety Datalink Information report highlights a need for ongoing examination and better data on mercury and aluminum adjuvants in vaccines and their cumulative impact on developing brains.

Despite the fact that thimerosal had not been proven to cause harm at the levels used in vaccines, in July 1999, the US Public Health Service and the AAP recommended the removal or reduction of thimerosal from vaccines as soon as possible as a precautionary measure. This decision was made to reduce exposure to mercury in infants and children. By 2001, the vaccine manufacturers began transitioning to thimerosal-free formulations for all routine childhood vaccines, with exceptions of some multidose flu vaccines, which continued to use thimerosal due to the difficulty in preventing contamination in these vials. However, thimerosal-free flu vaccines were also made available.

Outside the United States, thimerosal continues to be used in vaccines, especially in multidose vials in developing countries, due to its effectiveness as a preservative and the logistical difficulties of using single-dose vials. The

WHO has maintained that the small amounts of thimerosal in vaccines are safe and that removing it from vaccines in low-resource settings could disrupt immunization programs, leading to more deaths from preventable diseases.

ALUMINUM

Congratulations! You've made it through the semi—okay, maybe *very*—boring science lecture and arrived at the highly anticipated, juicy topic you really came for: aluminum.

The safety of aluminum is complex. We are exposed to aluminum from a myriad of sources, including food, water, medications, cosmetic products, and vaccines. The average daily dietary intake of aluminum for adults, whether from foods, water, or food additives, is estimated to be between 1 and 10 mg.

Interestingly, not only have a number of regulatory agencies set limits on the amount of aluminum exposure deemed acceptable in everything from the air we breathe to the food and water we consume, but the FDA has acknowledged that bottled water should contain no more than 0.2 mg/L. To avoid health concerns, the WHO recommends keeping aluminum levels in drinking water within 0.1 to 0.2 mg/L. In fact, according to the WHO, the provisional tolerable *weekly* intake for aluminum *from all sources* (i.e., water, food, etc.) is 2 mg/kg of body weight. For a 70 kg (154 lb) adult, this translates to 140 mg per week, or 20 mg *per day* across all sources.

Additionally, due to concerns over neurotoxicity in infants, particularly preterm infants, the FDA recommendation is that aluminum exposure does not exceed 5 mcg/kg of body weight per day. The Agency for Toxic Substances and Disease Registry of the US Department of Health and Human Services has set the minimum risk level for oral aluminum intake to 1 mg/kg per day. Occupational Safety and Health Administration (OSHA) set a legal limit of 15 mg/m3 (total dust) and 5 mg/m3 (respirable fraction) of aluminum in dusts averaged over an eight-hour workday. If these numbers sound confusing to you, you're not wrong. They are. The takeaway here is, the FDA, EPA, and WHO recommendations signify that aluminum is not entirely without risk and that aluminum exposure in excess of certain amounts may prove hazardous to human health.

Of course, vaccines contain aluminum—albeit, at much lower doses than most of the above regulations. When comparing exposure to aluminum in the hepatitis B vaccine versus other sources of aluminum (presented in consistent units for clarity), it becomes readily apparent that we cannot entirely ignore the toxicity concerns. Each pediatric dose (0.5 mL) of the hepatitis B vaccine contains 0.25 mg of aluminum, as aluminum hydroxide. For the purpose of comparison, 0.25 mg/0.5 mL is equivalent to 500 mg/L of aluminum. Vaccines are not 1 L though. So we want to be sure we are, as they say, "comparing apples to apples." If you diluted the aluminum from the vaccine into a 1L solution, you would have 0.25mg/1 L, which is *slightly over* the FDA-recommended limit for aluminum in drinking water (0.2 mg/L). Wait, what? How do we reconcile these contradictory recommendations?

Yes, the amount of aluminum in vaccines is *higher* per dose than the aluminum concentration limits set for drinking water. These limits are based on different contexts and forms of exposure. This paradox has been explained away as follows: (1) Vaccines are single exposures that are not comparable to chronic and consistent daily exposures from water (i.e., one receives just one vaccine but drinks water multiple times per day, every day); and (2) when ingested orally, through drinking water or food, 0.1–1% of the aluminum is absorbed into the bloodstream—the rest is excreted in stool. When injected directly into the muscle tissue, aluminum is gradually absorbed into the bloodstream, processed by the body over time and mostly excreted in the kidneys. Healthy kidneys efficiently eliminate aluminum, reducing the risk of accumulation. This may not be true for individuals with impaired kidney function.

Aluminum is also commonly found in over-the-counter antacids, which can contain 500 mg or more per dose. Although it is ingested rather than injected, this far exceeds the amount of aluminum in a hepatitis B vaccine.

Aluminum adjuvants have been used in vaccines for decades, and based on extensive research, the amount used is deemed safe by health authorities like the CDC, FDA, and WHO. These organizations argue that the aluminum in vaccines is a tiny fraction of the amount infants ingest daily through formula or breast milk, and it is rapidly excreted from the body.

Notwithstanding the scientific consensus on the safety of aluminum in vaccines, critics argue that more research is needed to establish the cumulative effects of aluminum from all sources, especially on infants who receive multiple vaccinations.

The conversation around aluminum is further convoluted by research that shows that an adjuvant—in this case, aluminum—is more critical in primary immunization than in boosters. Multiple studies have found that, in a primary immunization, aluminum enhances immune response by promoting antigen-presenting cells. Once immune memory forms, adjuvants may not be required to elicit an immune response. Adjuvant-free boosters were actually shown to be *effective* in animal models. If removing aluminum from boosters may still elicit an immune response and simultaneously reduce concerns over cumulative aluminum exposure, why not offer adjuvant-free boosters? Seems like an obvious and resounding *yes*!

Unfortunately, due to the regulatory complexities, human studies don't often compare adjuvanted to non-adjuvanted boosters. We simply don't have sufficient information to conclude that adjuvant-free boosters are as effective or effective at all. We *do* know that while aluminum enhances the immune response in the primary dose of the vaccine, its necessity in boosters appears less pronounced. I believe the reason adjuvant-free boosters have not been heavily researched is that their development would require vaccine manufacturers to expend tremendous additional resources without a justifiable guarantee of increased return. Quite possibly, it could result in a loss in revenue. When the primary dose formulation can be given, there is little incentive to develop adjuvant-free boosters.

Moreover, some question the accuracy of the stated aluminum content in vaccines. In 2021, a team of aluminum experts at Keele University conducted a study guided by Christopher Exley—a professor of bioinorganic chemistry of twenty-nine years and author of over two hundred peer-reviewed articles on aluminum. This study, published in the *Journal of Trace Elemental Biology*, analyzed thirteen infant vaccines. The findings showed discrepancies between the actual aluminum content in each vaccine and the amounts specified by the manufacturers. Only three vaccines matched the manufacturer-stated levels. Six vaccines contained *significantly more* aluminum than disclosed, and four contained *significantly less*. The aluminum content varied widely within the same vaccine, exemplified by variations from 0.172 to 0.602 mg per vaccine in HAVRIX (hepatitis A). This inconsistency in aluminum levels is not just a regulatory concern. Given aluminum's known potential for toxicity, it raises serious questions about the implications for vaccine efficacy and safety. The variability in aluminum content could lead to unexpected biological responses.

So where does this leave us with aluminum? Although there is no consensus over what constitutes a universally safe limit for aluminum exposure, the amounts used in vaccines are based on extensive research and data and considered safe by global health standards. Ongoing research continues to address public concerns and explore any potential long-term effects. The conspicuous parallels between the current conversation around aluminum and the previous discourse around lead and thimerosal are inescapable. That is not to say the aluminum found in vaccines is harmful. But when viewed alongside other metals once believed to be safe, aluminum, and the cumulative impact it may have on long-term health, should not be so casually dismissed.

11

MISINFORMATION, DISINFORMATION, AND MALINFORMATION, OH MY!

RETHINKING THE VACCINE CONVERSATION IN AN ERA OF DOUBT

I'm generally pretty pro-rolling out vaccines. I think on balance the vaccines are more positive than negative. But I think that while they were trying to push that program [COVID-19 vaccine rollout], they also tried to censor anyone who is basically arguing against it. And they pushed us super hard to take down the things that were honestly, were true. Right, I mean they basically pushed us and said anything that says that vaccines might have side effects, you basically need to take down.

—MARK ZUCKERBURG

The counter to misinformation is better information.

—ELON MUSK

I don't believe it serves my patients or any child to follow silently in lockstep with the scientific gospel. The brilliant Henry David Thoreau wrote: "How vain it is to sit down to write when you have not stood up to live." As a scientist and physician devoted to the well-being of his patients, I deem it my moral responsibility to stand up and ask questions—because my pursuit of knowledge did not end with my medical training.

In the midst of what feels like a concerted and well-organized effort to silence dissenting viewpoints, speaking up may prove difficult. Trendy buzzwords are liberally used to disparage any conversation around vaccines that deviates from the sanctioned narrative. Sometimes, it seems the people who indiscriminately use these buzzwords don't truly know what they mean. So let's get clear on their definitions:

Vaccine hesitancy. Often stemming from concerns about vaccine safety, efficacy, or necessity, vaccine hesitancy refers to the reluctance or refusal to vaccinate despite the availability of vaccines.

Misinformation. False or misleading information that spreads without malicious intent, typically due to a misunderstanding or lack of comprehensive knowledge.

Disinformation. Deliberately spreading false information with the intent to deceive or manipulate public opinion, frequently exacerbating the public's concerns and fueling hesitancy.

Malinformation. The spread of truthful information that is shared with the intent to harm, manipulate, or mislead people. In contrast to misinformation or disinformation, which involves false or deceptive content, malinformation presents facts in a context designed to cause unnecessary fear, outrage, or distrust. For example, sensitive data, such as details about medical risks of a vaccine or medical product, may be viewed by some as malinformation and consequently censored. On social media, malinformation is frequently demoted or suppressed not because it is untrue but because it challenges popular narratives or sparks controversy. This suppression can create a chilling effect, discouraging open dialogue and preventing people from accessing critical information that might influence their decisions. In a landscape where algorithms prioritize popularity, important and possibly uncomfortable truths are periodically sidelined, leading to an incomplete public understanding of significant issues.

The problem with maligning and censoring people who question scientific gospel is twofold: First, it does not stop them from questioning; and second, it *validates* their skepticism. Why would anyone actively silence reasonable questions unless they seek to hide the answers?

A 2023 film, *Shot in the Arm*, by Scott Hamilton Kennedy, and executive produced by Neil deGrasse Tyson, explores vaccine hesitancy both historically and in the context of the COVID-19 pandemic. The riveting (and frankly condescending) slogan used to advertise the film was "Disinformation is its own disease." When did vaccine *hesitancy* become synonymous with *disinformation*? Is the implication here that the vaccine-hesitant are a disease? Who is the omniscient arbiter of what is or isn't disinformation?

We cannot continue to categorize information as "misinformation," "disinformation," or "malinformation" simply because it does not conform to settled dogma. Clearly, the current strategy isn't working. People are now more vaccine-hesitant than ever. This isn't the result of misinformation or disinformation. Rather, I believe it to be the unfortunate consequence of a growing distrust of a pharmaceutical industry that has engaged in deceptive practices and massively profited from them at the expense of public health.

For instance, in 2007, Purdue Pharma paid out $634 million—one of the largest fines ever levied against a pharmaceutical firm at that time— for misleading the public about how addictive the drug OxyContin was compared to other pain medications. In 2012, GlaxoSmithKline pleaded guilty for unlawfully promoting prescription drugs and failing to report safety information. This settlement was $3 billion. In 2009, Pfizer entered into a $2.3 billion settlement as a result of the alleged false promotion of Bextra (valdecoxib) tablets, Geodon capsules, Lyrica (pregabalin), and Zyvox. Pfizer faced allegations of paying kickbacks and submitting false claims to the government.

The COVID-19 pandemic further eroded trust in public health messaging. The phrase "safe and effective" was frequently regurgitated during vaccine campaigns. This unintentionally cultivated skepticism, which was further exacerbated by the fact that the adverse effects of the COVID-19 vaccines weren't fully presented in balance with the purported benefits. As the unwitting guinea pigs of a massive public health experiment, recipients of the vaccine experienced firsthand the dubious long-term efficacy of the COVID-19 vaccine together with the side effects that, for many, followed.

Through social media, recipients of the vaccine were able to draw conclusions by communicating with others who shared similar experiences. In general, vaccines have a well-established track record of saving lives and preventing diseases. However, public discourse should focus on transparently discussing known risks alongside those benefits, as opposed to relying on one-sided messaging that arrogantly thumbs its nose at the public's intelligence.

To say that the increase in vaccine hesitancy is attributable solely to misinformation or disinformation is itself misinformation (if not outright disinformation)—a convenient deflection from the bevy of other identifiable, potential causes. *It's gaslighting.* The pharmaceutical industry would be better served regaining the public's trust than vilifying skeptics.

If the medical community hopes to convert the vaccine-hesitant, I believe it will achieve far greater success by acknowledging the difficult questions and responding to them in a compelling and respectful way.

This book aims *not* to promote vaccine hesitancy but rather to offer a *solution* to it. And although it is considered complete heresy to utter the word *choice* in the same sentence as the word *vaccines*, I believe in bodily autonomy and in providing clear information that empowers individuals to make informed decisions. More likely than not, people will make the decision to vaccinate if the information presented is *truthful*, complete, and transparent. Just as disparaging hesitant parents has brought us to this unfortunate juncture, encouraging communication around vaccines may very well have the opposite effect.

From a public health standpoint, I understand the impetus to silence and denigrate anyone who questions vaccine efficacy. The medical community will argue that the mere act of promoting inquiry breeds hesitancy. I am not here to promulgate doubt. I strive to foster understanding. If, after reviewing the data, readers become hesitant, this is a reflection of the data and its undeniable complexities. The medical community will likely wage a bitter crusade against me for writing this book.

In doing so, it will succeed *only* in inciting further distrust and emboldening the vaccine hesitant. In my opinion, the optimal pathway forward is to reestablish trust through open dialogue—where we, the medical community, hear and seek to understand the concerns voiced by so many parents with an open mind and willingness to discuss.

The data speaks for itself. According to the CDC, in 2024, routine childhood vaccinations among kindergartners in public and private schools in the United States were down from the previous school year. During the 2023–2024 school year, overall coverage declined while the exemption rate increased.

The CDC noted:

> The number of jurisdictions with exemption rates greater than
> five percent increased from two in 2020 to fourteen in 2024.

The agency added that roughly 280,000 kindergartners "did not have documentation of 2 MMR doses." In its report, the CDC acknowledged:

These results could indicate changes in attitudes toward routine vaccination transferring from hesitancy about COVID-19 vaccination, or toward any vaccine requirements arising from objections to COVID-19 vaccine mandates, as well as a potential for larger decreases in coverage or increases in exemptions.

A 2024 Gallup survey found that in the United States, far fewer people than in recent history believe childhood vaccines are important. About 40% agreed that it is extremely important for kids to receive childhood vaccines. This is down from the 58% in 2019 and the 64% in 2001. Only 51% of those Americans surveyed emphatically felt the government should mandate that children receive vaccines, which is down eleven percentage points from 2019.

In Toronto, Canada, where I grew up, the story is similar. According to Toronto Public Health data, during the 2023–2024 school year, coverage for the DPTaP vaccine (diphtheria, pertussis, tetanus, and polio) for twelfth-grade students was 46.5%. This was down from 81% during the 2017–2018 school year. More recently, the rate of coverage for vaccines provided through the School Immunization Program is among the lowest, with 42% of students receiving hepatitis B, 35% receiving human papilloma virus (HPV), and 59% receiving meningococcal vaccines. Public Health Ontario data reveals that, as of 2024, just 70% of seven-year-olds were fully vaccinated against measles—this compared to the 86% who were fully vaccinated against the measles during the 2018–2019 school year. Vaccination rates for pertussis have also dropped significantly in this age range, from 85% between 2018 and 2019 to 69.8% between 2023 and 2024.

In Romania, 4,594 cases of measles were reported between March 2023 and February 2024, making up close to 80% of the total cases of measles collectively reported in the European Union during that time. The latest figures show that just 71% of the population had received a second measles vaccine. In Estonia, reported vaccination rates for a second dose of the measles vaccine fell 20% from 2018 to 2022. In Iceland, they fell 15%.

You may or may not be surprised by some of these statistics. However, you will likely be shocked to learn that, according to a 2022 study published by Timothy Callaghan in the prestigious journal *Vaccine*, 10.1% of primary care physicians did not believe that vaccines are generally safe, 9.3% doubt their effectiveness, and 8.3% question their importance. Of the US adults surveyed for this study, 47.7% strongly agreed that vaccines are safe.

Don't shoot the messenger! I didn't conduct these studies. I am merely relaying the findings. If you disagree with anything I say in this book, the solution is not to censor; it is to participate in healthy debate. Provide better information. Prove me wrong. If you can't because the data doesn't exist, demand more and better research to support your position. Don't gaslight parents. Use real data to convince them—convince me.

I might be mistaken. I will humbly admit if or when I am. I have made every effort to be thorough. There may be a study of which I am unaware or a data point I may have overlooked. I have attempted to present information as accurately and precisely as possible, but I stand willing to accept and invite respectful debate.

Rather than directly address the concerns that precipitated the decline in vaccination rates, some governments have come up with creative solutions. In Canada, pursuant to the Infants Act, a child under the age of nineteen may consent to a medical treatment—this, of course, includes vaccination. If the health-care provider is certain that the treatment is in the child's best interest and the child understands the details of the treatment, a child is designated a mature minor, deemed capable of giving consent. While in most circumstances, parents or guardians must give consent for children twelve years of age and younger, there is no set age for when a child can give mature minor consent for immunizations. Under extenuating circumstances, even a child who is twelve or younger may still consent to a medical treatment.

In parts of Canada, school-based immunization programs have become a mechanism for the routine administration of vaccines in schools. In 1992, British Columbia initiated a school-based program to administer the hepatitis B vaccine. And in 1994, Quebec, Yukon, and Ontario did the same. In 2007, school-based programs were instituted to administer the HPV vaccine for girls in all provinces except Quebec. In 2017, these school-based programs were extended to boys. It should come as no surprise that the Infants Act was enacted in 1996, just four years after the commencement of the first school-based immunization program. Of course, under the authority of the Infants Act, schools may administer vaccines to children without first obtaining parental consent.

In 1992 (the same year British Columbia began its school-based immunization programs), the California Legislature enacted *Family Code* Section 6926. On January 1, 1994, the statute went into effect. Section 6926 allows a minor who is twelve years of age or older to consent to medical care related to the prevention of a sexually transmitted disease. This law allows children twelve and over to obtain the hepatitis B or HPV vaccines without their parents' consent.

Before I am lambasted by the vaccine police, I will note that school-based immunization programs and the enactment of California *Family Code* Section 6926 *predated* the steep decline in vaccination rates. However, school-based immunization programs still exist in Canada, and Section 6926 (and legislation similar to it) remains in effect. Today, these loopholes can—and are being used to—circumvent parental consent to vaccination.

Proponents of school-based immunization programs and legislation similar to Section 6926 argue that some sexually active children may feel uncomfortable or be unable to discuss sensitive topics with their parents. Allowing children to obtain vaccines without first requiring them to seek consent from their parents provides important prophylaxis against vaccine-preventable, sexually transmissible diseases.

In contrast, opponents of such programs and legislation point out that bright-line rules exist for a reason. Each jurisdiction has defined the age of majority, which, in many places, is eighteen. Lawmakers do not deem minors capable of making adult decisions. In the United States, minors cannot vote, purchase cigarettes, get married, get a tattoo, purchase firearms, or make other major health-care decisions for themselves. In some places, even a seventeen-year-old cannot participate in a school field trip without a permission slip signed by a parent or guardian. Despite the fact that society perceives these minors as lacking the maturity to make decisions typically reserved for adults, the Infants Act and California *Family Code* Section 6926 make an interesting exception.

When a growing number of parents are opting their children out of vaccination, legislation that allows children to receive vaccines without parental consent can prove effective in combating declining immunization rates. To me, this is not the solution. The medical community is undoubtedly discouraged by the climbing rates of vaccine hesitancy while parents are frustrated that they and their concerns are marginalized. The medical establishment has its marching orders: promote vaccines and foster trust to increase vaccination rates among children. The way we are going about implementing these edicts is backfiring. It's time to reevaluate the strategy.

12

THE DOUBLE STANDARD

There is no greater warrior than a mother protecting her child.

—N. K. JEMISIN

By championing vaccines as "safe and effective," we perpetuate a flawed perception of them. This incantation is repeated over and over as though to hypnotize the masses into believing vaccines are 100% efficacious and completely without risk. Many of us know this isn't entirely true. Even a substance as innocuous as water can be dangerous if consumed in excessive quantities. There is some risk to virtually everything we do. The level of risk depends on a number of variables. Perhaps the growing distrust of vaccines is, at least in part, attributable to the double standard in the discourse around them. When aluminum salts, formaldehyde, and polysorbate 80, among many other unpronounceable compounds, are given to a newborn in a tiny syringe and called a vaccine, they are touted as safe. If a parent encountered the same compounds in a list of baby food ingredients, he or she would likely shudder at the idea of feeding them to his or her infant. A few vaccines, including influenza, contain ovalbumin, a protein derived from eggs, but we advise against feeding babies solids before six months, following guidelines that suggest their digestive systems aren't ready for *any* food. I am deeply fascinated by the way we reconcile such paradoxes.

Let's consider a thought-provoking anecdote: A person (let's call her Jane) contacted Poison Control claiming a child she knew (let's call him Henry) may have ingested some aluminum and mercury. Because Jane was unable to articulate the amount of aluminum and mercury Henry might have consumed, the alarmed Poison Control agent advised Jane to immediately rush Henry to the emergency room. After a several-minute conversation, the agent established that Henry had not ingested these ingredients orally but through a vaccine. The agent was no longer concerned; the agent no longer suggested that Jane rush Henry to the emergency room or that Jane seek any medical intervention for Henry. Why is it that we are so troubled by the prospect of a baby having ingested aluminum and mercury orally yet are unfazed when these ingredients are injected directly into a baby's bloodstream?

Surely, the medical community will be quick to point out that most vaccines contain only trace amounts of aluminum and mercury, which in such small doses have been found to have no adverse consequences. While the level of concern *is* indeed proportional to the amount of aluminum or mercury ingested, in this scenario, the Poison Control agent was alarmed by the mere notion that Henry *may* have *orally* ingested aluminum or mercury in *any* amount.

The way we respond to adverse reactions from medications, versus the way we respond to similar adverse reactions from vaccines, underscores a disconcerting double standard. For instance, if a few days after starting a medication, like amoxicillin, a person develops hives, these symptoms are commonly ascribed to an allergic reaction to the medication. Due to concerns over the potential for future allergic reactions, the person is typically advised to avoid amoxicillin. Conversely, if a person experiences a seizure, severe rash, or other moderate to severe symptoms shortly after receiving a vaccine, often, the reaction is not as readily attributed (if at all) to the vaccine. In many cases, health professionals will not advise the patient to avoid future doses of that or a similar vaccine.

This glaring disparity in our response to possible reactions from medications versus possible reactions to vaccines is poignantly addressed by Suzanne Humphries, MD in her book, *Dissolving Illusions*. Humphries—a prominent nephrologist—was dismissed by her colleagues for pointing out the potential correlation between vaccines and kidney damage. Calling into question whether our responses to adverse health events is inconsistent when vaccines are involved, Humphries writes:

> This was the first time in my career that my opinion regarding kidney failure was not respected. Any other time I suggested that a drug was responsible for kidney damage, that drug was immediately discontinued—no questions asked. This happens

routinely with certain blood pressure drugs, antibiotics, pain killers, etc. Sometimes kidneys can react to drugs in an allergic fashion—to any drug at any time—and that drug would have been stopped. Some drugs cause direct toxicity to the kidneys, and in the past if I suggested to stop or avoid them, they were always avoided. But now I was unable to protect my own kidney-failure patients from vaccinations given in the hospital. Questioning the vaccines seemed to open an entire Pandora's box that apparently had yellow forensic tape over the lock.

I get it. The public health implications are monumental. People cannot be led to believe vaccines are anything but safe and effective; otherwise, vaccination rates will decline, and diseases that were, at one time, mostly eradicated will reemerge. Despite the optics around them, vaccines are outing themselves. They *are* fallible. This isn't disinformation or faux scientific alarmism or . . . [insert your favorite trendy buzzword here]. The answer lies in plain sight. A number of vaccines previously deemed safe were subsequently pulled from the market as a result of safety concerns. For instance, the DTP vaccine (diphtheria, tetanus, and whole-cell pertussis) was widely used in the mid-twentieth century and was the standard prophylaxis against these diseases.

By the late 1970s, reports—fueled by anecdotal cases of serious conditions like encephalopathy (brain inflammation), linking the DTP vaccine to neurological issues—began gaining public attention. These concerns were amplified by the 1982 documentary *DPT: Vaccine Roulette*, which noted cases of developmental delay, seizures, and neurological damage after DTP vaccination. This led to a surge in lawsuits against vaccine manufacturers, causing some companies to exit the vaccine market. (Of course, this was just before the National Childhood Vaccine Injury Act bestowed virtual immunity against liability upon vaccine manufacturers.)

In the 1980s, studies examining the DTP vaccine's safety yielded mixed results. Some studies suggested a potential risk of rare neurological side effects; others found no causative link. The high rate of minor adverse reactions led researchers to seek alternatives.

By the late 1990s, due to concerns over adverse effects, the original DTP vaccine was gradually phased out in most countries and replaced with the DTaP vaccine, which is regarded as the safer standard. *The shift was promulgated by the confluence of public outcry and scientific findings, emphasizing not only that we should listen to parents, but more significantly demonstrating that, when we do so, we have the ability to strike a happier balance between safety and disease prevention.*

Similarly, when RotaShield was introduced in the United States in 1998, it was the first vaccine to prevent rotavirus. Within a year, postmarket surveillance identified a potential link to intussusception—a serious condition in which part of the intestine telescopes into itself, leading to obstruction. Early studies suggested that after RotaShield vaccination, the risk of intussusception in infants was approximately 1 in 10,000 doses, with cases most frequently occurring within one week after the first dose. By 1999, as reports mounted (over 100 cases were reported within the first year), the CDC and FDA suspended the vaccine's use. After further studies confirmed the increased risk associated with the RotaShield vaccine, it was voluntarily withdrawn from the market.

After RotaShield's withdrawal, researchers developed two new vaccines, RotaTeq (licensed in 2006) and ROTARIX (licensed in 2008). Both were designed to retain the benefits of rotavirus prevention while minimizing adverse effects. Large-scale studies and trials for these vaccines demonstrated a significantly lower risk of intussusception.

The case of RotaShield highlights yet another disconcerting inconsistency in vaccine safety protocols. In 1999, RotaShield was pulled from the market due to an associated risk of intussusception, with studies showing an incidence of approximately 1 in 10,000 doses. Despite the vaccine's benefits in preventing severe rotavirus infections in infants and young children, this was deemed an unacceptably high risk. The fact that RotaShield was promptly withdrawn after its relatively low risks were identified raises an existential quandary: *Are we consistent in addressing vaccine safety when it comes to other potentially serious or long-term adverse effects?*

After the mRNA COVID-19 vaccinations, there has been increasing concern over a number of possible side effects, most notably myocarditis. Studies indicate that the risk of myocarditis, especially in younger males under thirty, may be around 1 in 5,000 to 1 in 10,000 doses, depending on age and dose schedule. In some studies, the rate has been as high as 1 in 2,500 in specific high-risk groups (i.e., adolescent males after the second dose). Myocarditis, an inflammation of the heart muscle, can range from mild to severe and has prompted ongoing discussions about the long-term health implications for affected individuals.

This discrepancy—where a vaccine like RotaShield was withdrawn, while the COVID-19 vaccine remains in use in spite of potentially similar or even higher risks in some populations—indicates that our current approach may lack consistency.

If some risks for severe, long-term outcomes from vaccines are indeed more frequent than 1 in 10,000—possibly even approaching 1 in 1,000—then these should be considered with the same level of scrutiny historically applied to other vaccines. The precedent exists. Vaccines that pose identifiable risks have been pulled or altered to mitigate those risks. We seem to be more and more hesitant to concede that identifiable risks exist and, accordingly, take the appropriate precautionary measures. This has contributed to a deep distrust of the medical community and pharmaceutical industry. To regain trust and, more importantly, to ensure the public remains safe, we must stop hiding behind the words "safe and effective" and balance the benefits of widespread immunity with the need for robust safety standards.

13

EXEMPTIONS

There is no such thing as freedom of choice unless there is freedom to refuse.

—DAVID HUME

Vaccination requirements vary by location. Common vaccines mandated for grade-school entry include MMR, DTaP/Tdap, polio, varicella, and hepatitis B. College entry often requires meningococcal vaccines, especially for students living in dormitories, along with Tdap and MMR boosters if not previously received. Health-care practitioners typically require influenza, hepatitis B, MMR, Tdap and varicella vaccines, as well as, in some settings, tuberculosis screenings, to minimize the risk of transmitting infections to vulnerable patients.

The growing concern over childhood vaccines has led many parents to seek exemptions. Across various regions in the United States, there are three primary types of vaccine exemptions. Each allows individuals to forgo otherwise required vaccination for a specified reason:

Medical exemptions. These are granted when a person has a health condition that contraindicates vaccination, such as severe allergies to vaccine ingredients, immunodeficiencies, or a history of adverse reactions to vaccines. Medical exemptions require documentation from a licensed health-care provider and are typically the most accepted exemption across states and countries.

Religious exemptions. This type of exemption allows individuals to opt out of vaccinations based on sincerely held religious beliefs that oppose immunization. Documentation requirements vary by region. Some areas may request proof of authenticity or verification from a religious leader, while others accept self-attestation.

Philosophical or personal belief exemptions. These exemptions are based on personal or philosophical objections to vaccination, which are not rooted in religion or medical reasons. They are the broadest and most variable category available in some US states but restricted in others.

These exemptions differ widely by jurisdiction. Some allow all three; others restrict or eliminate specific categories.

MEDICAL EXEMPTIONS

In recent years, obtaining a medical exemption has become increasingly difficult. In some states, like California, strict laws have drastically altered the landscape. The pendulum has swung so far in one direction that even doctors who genuinely believe a child qualifies for a medical exemption are, at times, reluctant to write one due to the potential professional ramifications.

In 2019, California passed SB 276 and SB 714, requiring doctors to submit all medical exemptions to a state database. The legitimacy of the exemptions notwithstanding, if a physician writes more than five in any given year, he or she must automatically face a mandatory review by the state health department. This has (perhaps intentionally) had a chilling effect. Physicians now fear potential investigations or losing their medical license if their exemptions are deemed inappropriate by state regulators. Consequently, many doctors, even those acutely familiar with their patients' medical histories, are hesitant to write *any* exemptions, leaving parents feeling helpless.

Parents—who have contacted multiple doctors, only to learn that none are willing to so much as discuss exemptions—frequently share their frustration with me. These parents feel that their child's complicated medical history warrants an exemption.

I often speak to parents who believe their child has suffered from a severe reaction to a vaccine and, thus, should qualify for an exemption. Given the lack of definitive evidence that the reaction resulted from the vaccine (something rarely provable), the child is required to obtain further vaccines to attend school.

Despondent parents of children with complex neurological conditions, like seizure disorders, have tearily told me they are unable to procure an exemption. Fully informed and well aware of the possible risks associated with diphtheria, tetanus, and pertussis, these parents nonetheless feel the risks to their child posed by the DTaP vaccine (including the risk of seizure, which is enumerated among the list of rare but possible side effects on the DtaP vaccine insert) outweigh the benefits the vaccine offers. The physician caring for a child who suffers from seizures may agree that the child should be exempt from receiving the DTaP vaccine. Yet the physician may be constrained by the legal consequences or threat to his or her livelihood and, therefore, decline to write an exemption. Seemingly, parents are reasonably justified in declining to give a child afflicted with seizures a vaccine that has been known to cause seizures.

With zero appreciation for this child's unique medical history, a group of strangers on the medical board may conclude that this child's condition does not meet the criteria for an exemption. These parents have intelligently weighed and assessed the known risks for their child but are unlikely to receive an exemption in California or any other jurisdiction that imposes Draconian penalties on physicians who write them. Is this right or wrong? While there may be arguments in favor of and in opposition to, I believe these parents should have the right to make this difficult medical decision on behalf of their child. As the DTaP vaccine *may* cause seizures, a child afflicted by a seizure disorder has a small, *increased* risk of experiencing seizures. Should this not qualify for an exemption if, after full and difficult consideration, the parents seek it? I wonder whether lawmakers would feel differently if they helplessly watched their own child convulsing uncontrollably.

One mother shared with me that her youngest child experienced a severe cardiac reaction after receiving a routine vaccination. The child's heart rate was so fast, she was rushed to the emergency room where she was diagnosed with supraventricular tachycardia, with a heart rate over 200. (Just so we're clear, this is *really* high.) A few hours later, the symptoms subsided. Despite the conspicuous timing, the supraventricular tachycardia was *not* deemed a vaccine reaction. Two months later, this child's parents, who had always followed the regular vaccination schedule without questioning vaccine safety, found themselves in a difficult position. Their pediatric office had a policy of dismissing patients who did not adhere to the CDC's vaccine schedule. Reluctantly, and after a reassuring consultation with their pediatrician, who affirmed the safety of continuing vaccinations, these parents proceeded to vaccinate their child. Again the child experienced the *same* symptoms. *Still* the child was not given the diagnosis of a vaccine reaction by the emergency room or her primary doctor. Now deeply distressed by their child's serious reactions that resulted in two emergency room visits, these parents sought to pause further vaccinations until their child was older. They requested a vaccination exemption from their doctor but were denied. Although these parents were not opposed to vaccines and had an older child that was fully vaccinated, they were informed that if they decided against continuing with recommended vaccinations, they would need to find a new medical practice. After hearing this story (and so many like it), I was heartbroken. Sadly, this family was unable to secure an exemption for further vaccines. Opting not to further vaccinate their child, these parents were left with little choice other than to homeschool her.

Another parent, whose child was diagnosed with a complicated combination of autoimmune disorders, recounted to me that her child was denied an exemption—this, not only after multiple specialists *agreed* vaccinations could exacerbate the child's condition, but that the mother herself had a history of severe vaccine reactions as a child.

I share these few, among countless, stories to illustrate the growing conflict between parents who seek medical exemptions for what they believe are legitimate reasons and the current legal framework that restricts physicians from issuing them. The inability to secure medical exemptions— even when they are ostensibly warranted—leaves many families in an unenviable position, grappling with the possibility of risking an adverse vaccine reaction or otherwise facing barriers to school enrollment due to noncompliance with vaccine mandates. For most households that rely on two incomes to support it, homeschooling is not a viable option. Relocating to a state that allows exemptions could mean moving away from friends, family, and other support systems.

Conventional doctors and medical boards maintain that medical exemptions are still permitted for valid reasons. However, the criteria they deem valid are quite narrow. Providers and parents may significantly disagree over the definition of the word. Parents might perceive risk differently. Some may be unwilling to accept the increased likelihood of their child experiencing seizures or cardiac events. The decision should not be made for them by a group of strangers who, though medical experts, do not personally know the family seeking the exemption or its unique reasons for doing so. These members of the medical board have little to no familiarity with the patient's particular history. They do not have the opportunity to meet the patient and parents or to participate in a meaningful discussion regarding the true necessity of the exemption. By placing doctors in proverbial handcuffs, state regulatory agencies interject themselves into the sacred provider-patient relationship, effectively forcing a desired outcome. Parents are told they have the discretion to make medical decisions for their children. In this case, the decision is not so simple as to vaccinate or not vaccinate. Rather, it is whether to vaccinate or forego attending school. For many families, this isn't financially feasible or practical. The choice is, therefore, essentially made for them.

As policies around exemptions continue to evolve, lawmakers, physicians, and public health experts must find a way to safeguard public health while simultaneously addressing the individual needs of children with legitimate medical risks. If you are a parent whose child is at greater risk of being rushed to the emergency room with a cardiac event or experiencing a seizure after receiving a vaccine, you should not feel that your sole option is to deliberately subject your child to these probable risks.

So too, doctors should not be afraid to write valid exemptions or face existential repercussions. These laws have successfully served their deterrent function. I personally know doctors who have been reviewed for writing exemptions. I am aware of doctors who have altogether lost their ability to write exemptions. I know doctors who have been placed on probation or even lost their licenses for writing exemptions they viewed as medically warranted. These didactic tales intimidate physicians from writing *any* exemptions; the prospects of facing the medical board, jeopardizing our livelihoods, and losing our licenses are consequences that most doctors consider far too onerous. Altogether abstaining from writing exemptions is just easier and safer.

RELIGIOUS FREEDOM AND VACCINES: SHOULD SCHOOLS ALLOW RELIGIOUS EXEMPTIONS?

One of the most contested issues in the vaccine debate is whether schools should allow religious exemptions. Although I am married to an attorney, I myself am not one. I am not qualified to delve into the legal complexities of religious freedom, nor is this the appropriate place to do so. I will, however, note that the First Amendment to the US Constitution explicitly states, in relevant part: "Congress shall make no law respecting an establishment of religion, or prohibiting the free exercise thereof."

On January 11, 2018, one of the world's leading virologists and vaccinologists, who is widely recognized for his pivotal role in the development of the rubella vaccine and his significant contributions to vaccine science, Stanley A. Plotkin, MD, was deposed by Attorney Aaron Siri. Plotkin was asked, "Do you believe that someone can have a valid religious objection to refusing a vaccine?"

He responded, "No."

Siri next posed the question, "Do you take issue with religious beliefs?"

Plotkin replied, "Yes."

Plotkin was asked, "You have said that, quote: 'Vaccination is always under attack by religious zealots who believe that the will of God includes death and disease?'"

Plotkin answered, "Yes."

Siri then inquired, "You stand by that statement?"

Plotkin said, "I absolutely do."

Siri asked, "Are you an atheist?"

He answered, "Yes."

Siri pried further: "Do you accept that some people hold religious beliefs that are inherently unprovable?"

Plotkin responded, "Yes, I'm sure they do."

Plotkin's unapologetic testimony poignantly highlights the philosophical dissonance between the scientific and religious communities, which lies at the crux of the religious exemption debate.

In the vaccine-manufacturing process, viruses need a host to replicate. Human fetal cell lines provide the reliable, human-compatible medium to grow viruses necessary for vaccine production. The viruses are propagated in these cells, harvested, purified, and then inactivated or weakened (depending on the vaccine) prior to being added to the vaccine formula. In the context of vaccines, the concern over religious freedom arises in part from the use of aborted fetal cell lines in the development of certain vaccines, including those for rubella (found in the MMR vaccine), chicken pox, and hepatitis A. These vaccines contain traces of human diploid cells derived from abortions. Some individuals with strong religious or moral beliefs oppose these vaccines due to their origins. The use of human fetal cells in vaccine development is rooted in the creation of cell lines from elective abortions in the 1960s, specifically the WI-38 and MRC-5 cell lines. WI-38 comes from lung tissue of a twelve-week-old female fetus, and MRC-5 from the lung tissue of a fourteen-week-old male fetus.

Notably, fetal cell lines are not continuously sourced from new abortions. WI-38 and MRC-5 cell lines have been propagated in laboratories for decades—meaning, they have been replicated many times without the need for new fetal tissue. The common misconception is that ongoing use of fetal cells requires continuous abortions. Due to their unique biological properties, these cell lines offer a consistent environment for viral cultivation, which is the reason they have remained in use for over half a century.

The Vatican and several other religious authorities have addressed this issue, noting the distinction between remote cooperation with evil (i.e., using vaccines with no direct involvement in the abortion) and the obligation to protect public health. Still for some, this has not settled the debate.

The refusal of religious exemptions raises ethical and legal concerns about discrimination and the right to religious freedom. Some institutions argue that no major religion explicitly prohibits vaccination, but this perspective can be viewed as an imposition of one's interpretation over the individual's beliefs. By denying religious exemptions, these policies effectively prioritize a generalized interpretation of religious doctrine over the personal convictions of the individual. Furthermore, such denials can alienate families with sincere religious beliefs, creating a divide where those who hold alternative views on health practices may feel marginalized or coerced. In a society valuing religious freedom, the debate over religious exemptions underscores the need for a respectful balance between public health priorities and individual religious rights.

Although we typically think of religious exemptions in the context of school vaccine requirements, they also play a role in other medical decision-making. In 2024, a twelve-year-old girl, Adaline, was denied placement on the heart-transplant list at a major children's hospital in Ohio because she was unvaccinated. Adaline's parents, who adhere to a nondenominational religious belief that opposes vaccination, sought a religious exemption. Nevertheless, the hospital maintained its stance that vaccinations—specifically flu and COVID-19—are essential for post-transplant survival due to the lifelong immunosuppressive therapy required after transplantation. Reading this may upset you—though you may be upset that Adaline was not vaccinated, or you may be upset that Adaline was denied a potentially lifesaving treatment due to her religious beliefs.

From a medical perspective, hospitals prioritize organ recipient success rates and long-term survival. Since transplant recipients are highly immunocompromised, vaccines are seen as critical to preventing life-threatening infections. Allowing an unvaccinated individual to receive a transplant could be viewed as a high-risk allocation of a scarce resource. Donor organs are limited, and the hospital must ensure donor organs are utilized in ways that maximize survival chances. (Given that the COVID-19 vaccine is a sensitive subject for many, some reading this may strenuously argue—okay, might be foaming at the mouth—that the opposite is true.)

This policy raises ethical and even philosophical questions about religious freedom, medical autonomy, and access to care. Whereas hospitals argue that their duty is to protect patient safety, families like Adeline's contend that their personal beliefs should not bar their child from receiving a lifesaving procedure. Should hospitals have the right to deny transplants based on vaccine refusal, or should alternative options exist for families with religious or philosophical objections?

Recently, several legal challenges have tested the boundaries of religious freedoms and medical mandates. In a 2024 landmark legal decision led by Informed Consent Action Network (ICAN) attorneys, the University of California (UC) system was forced to allow religious exemptions for all 295,000-plus students. The ruling marked a significant victory for those advocating for the protection of religious rights. The court held that UC's policy of allowing secular exemptions but denying religious ones violated the First Amendment. This precedent could pave the way for future legal battles concerning elementary through high school students, whose parents may fight to reinstate similar religious exemptions.

The question remains, should states and schools have the right to deny religious exemptions, especially given the precedent set in these university cases? Denying these exemptions can lead to further erosion of religious liberty, which has historically been protected under the US Constitution. Of course, the reinstatement of personal belief and religious exemptions would come with a corresponding trade-off. We must contemplate whether we are prepared to handle potential increases in outbreaks of vaccine-preventable illnesses among a growing population of unvaccinated children in schools.

The ongoing tension between individual choice, religious beliefs, and public health policy continues to raise difficult ethical and legal questions. As legal precedent evolves, religious exemptions may find stronger footholds even in the face of mounting pressure for universal vaccine mandates.

Stanley Plotkin is widely regarded as one of the key figures in modern vaccine advancement. He played a crucial part in shaping immunization programs worldwide. Given Plotkin's preeminence in the field, his thoughts on ethics and religion perhaps lend insight into a more pervasive ethos shared by his peers—the very people responsible for shaping vaccine policy. Plotkin's secular views are an affront to people of faith who believe their religious freedoms extend to medical decisions.

One of the most contentious debates in vaccine discourse involves the use of human-derived materials, such as fetal cell lines and human serum, in vaccine production. While many dismiss these concerns as irrelevant to public health, others see them as deeply significant ethical and moral issues. Do religious belief exemptions invite exploitation by those surreptitiously obtaining them for personal belief reasons? Does it qualify as overreach when the government intervenes in the sanctity of the doctor-patient relationship, or is it necessary to prevent systemic abuses that may imperil public health? What value do we place on bodily autonomy and the right to choose?

Offering greater insight into these questions is a thought-provoking excerpt from Plotkin's January 2018 deposition:

SIRI: Do any vaccines on the childhood vaccine schedule contain MRC-5 human diploid cells?

PLOTKIN: Yes.

SIRI: What are these?

PLOTKIN: Rubella, varicella, hepatitis A.

SIRI: What are MRC-5 cells?

PLOTKIN: They are human fibroblast cell strain.

SIRI: So cell strains from an aborted fetus?

PLOTKIN: Yes. Yeah. They're not immortal.

SIRI: And then how is more MRC-5 created?

PLOTKIN: Well, a seed stock is made of early passage cells so that one can go back to the seed stock, which is, let's say, at the, more or less the eighth passage and make new cells at the twentieth passage and use those to make the vaccine.

SIRI: Okay. So these are, these cell strains are human cells?

PLOTKIN: Yes.

SIRI: Do any vaccines on the childhood vaccine schedule contain WI-38 human diploid lung fibroblast?

PLOTKIN: Well, they used to, but I don't think anything is made in those cells anymore. They have been replaced by MRC-5. [Note: This answer is incorrect. These cells are still used in the manufacturing process of several vaccines, including those for rubella, hepatitis A, varicella (chicken pox), and zoster (shingles).]

SIRI: They took the lung tissue from the aborted fetus?

PLOTKIN: Yes.

SIRI: Do any vaccines in the childhood vaccine schedule contain human albumin?

PLOTKIN: Oh, yes.

SIRI: What is human albumin?

PLOTKIN: Human albumin is part of human serum.

SIRI: And what is human serum?

PLOTKIN: What is human serum? Human serum is part of the blood that is liquid.

SIRI: Right. It's the non-red blood cell part of the blood, right?

PLOTKIN: Yes.

SIRI: From where was it obtained?

PLOTKIN: The human serum.

SIRI: Do any vaccines in the childhood vaccine schedule contain recombinant human albumin?

PLOTKIN: Yes.

SIRI: What is recombinant human albumin, A-L-B-U-M-I-N?

PLOTKIN: So it's a component of human serum which is useful to stabilize cells and keep them healthy, and it's made by genetic engineering.

SIRI: Okay. So it's genetically engineered human serum basically?

PLOTKIN: Part of human serum, yes.

PERSONAL BELIEF EXEMPTIONS: A QUESTION OF FAIR CONSIDERATION

Much like religious belief exemptions, personal belief exemptions are a contentious area in the vaccine debate. Personal belief exemptions raise important ethical and philosophical questions about individual rights and respect for deeply held values. For instance, vegans and those with certain religious or ethical beliefs may point out that some vaccines contain ingredients derived from animals (i.e., gelatin, which is sourced from the skin and hooves of pigs.) For those who strictly avoid animal products or pig-derived products, using these vaccines may pose a moral dilemma.

In most other areas of life, society tends to accommodate such beliefs. Yet when it comes to vaccines, these personal beliefs are dismissed in favor of public health priorities. While the collective good of vaccination cannot be understated, this dismissal can feel like an infringement on personal freedoms.

The debate over vaccine exemptions and their impact on disease outbreaks is, of course, such as all other conversations around vaccines, nuanced, with research offering insights on both sides. A *JAMA* study published in 2016 showed that states allowing personal belief exemptions had higher rates of measles and pertussis outbreaks compared to states with more stringent vaccine policies. The study found that areas containing high exemption rates often had clusters of unvaccinated individuals, creating pockets where herd immunity was insufficient. For example, in California, before the state removed personal belief exemptions in 2016, clusters of unvaccinated children contributed to the 2014 measles outbreak that originated at Disneyland. These findings, which are supported by common sense, suggest that in areas with many unvaccinated children, disease transmission is more likely.

Those in favor of personal belief exemptions have routinely argued: "If vaccines work and your child is vaccinated, then you shouldn't worry if mine isn't. Your child is safe." In reality, though vaccines are effective, they are not infallible. Public health advocates express concern that pockets of unvaccinated individuals can undermine vaccine efficacy, particularly affecting those with waning immunity or underlying health conditions. This risk extends to individuals for whom vaccines are less effective or who cannot be vaccinated due to health limitations. The argument that vaccinated individuals should not worry about the unvaccinated is fundamentally flawed because it erroneously presumes that vaccines are 100% effective.

However, providing mechanisms for circumventing vaccine mandates may prove too slippery a slope, as was the case in Texarkana. Between 1970 and 1971, Texarkana, a city divided by the Texas-Arkansas state line, experienced a measles outbreak. During this outbreak, Texarcana reported 633 measles cases, noting a significant disparity between the number of cases in the Texas versus the Arkansas sides of the city. In 1968 and 1969, Arkansas had implemented mass vaccination campaigns and school vaccination policies, which resulted in over 99% immunization coverage among children aged one to nine. In contrast, Texas had not conducted similar community or school vaccination initiatives, resulting in approximately 57% coverage. Consequently, 606 (95.7%) of the measles cases occurred in Texas, demonstrating the effectiveness of widespread vaccination efforts in preventing outbreaks in the Arkansas side of the city. Opponents of personal belief exemptions deem examples such as this one compelling didactic evidence in support of universal vaccine mandates.

Other studies present a more complex picture, suggesting that exemption policies do not universally lead to outbreaks. Some states that permit religious or personal belief exemptions have not seen a significant increase in vaccine-preventable disease rates. For instance, despite allowing exemptions, states like Maine and Maryland have maintained high vaccination coverage and have not experienced large-scale outbreaks in recent decades. This indicates that, while exemption policies can contribute to outbreaks in areas with concentrated clusters of unvaccinated individuals, they do not necessarily lead to widespread public health crises across entire states.

Another notable consideration inextricable from the exemption debate is the "social contract"—the unspoken understanding that we must all get vaccinated to protect society as a whole from infectious diseases. The counterpoint to personal belief exemptions, the social contract is perceived, by some, as a moral obligation; others grapple with its implications for personal freedoms. The social contract poses a difficult philosophical conundrum, forcing us to reflect on our personal values.

Proponents of the social contract firmly adhere to the view that vaccines safeguard the weak and vulnerable. If a child or elderly person is immunocompromised and cannot receive a vaccine, we protect them by vaccinating ourselves. Though this viewpoint is undeniably salient, it fails to acknowledge the slew of other easily transmissible communicable diseases, for which no vaccines exist. For instance, we are not vaccinated against the common cold. A person with cancer who contracts the common cold could ultimately die from complications, such as pneumonia. That is not to say we shouldn't protect immunocompromised people from as many vaccine-preventable diseases as possible. However, to suggest that ubiquitous vaccination provides blanket protection to the immunocompromised is not entirely correct.

Moreover, in a broader sense, the social contract asks us to contemplate the existential question: Just how far should we go to help others? Is your child responsible for protecting other children at school or in the community? Because everyone's moral barometer is different, this question is, of course, rhetorical. Years ago, we were asked to take a handful of vaccines. That number continues to increase seemingly *ad infinitum*. The potential for known and unknown adverse short- and long-term side effects are real. At some point, the imposition on our personal freedom and bodily autonomy becomes excessive. We may be asked to take a medical intervention that contravenes with our personal beliefs—a product we deem too dangerous to swallow, inject, or connect to our brains.

In early 2025, Louisiana decided to stop actively promoting mass vaccination. The state's surgeon general, Ralph Abraham, MD, justified the move, stating:

> There is a need to rebuild trust from COVID-19 "missteps" and that people have less trust in institutions like the Centers for Disease Control and Prevention over COVID vaccination requirements.

He further emphasized that *"conversations about specific vaccines are best held between an individual and their health-care provider."*

Criticizing this decision, Paul Offit passionately argued that prioritizing individual choice and medical freedom over collective responsibility and public health is dangerous. Offit stated:

> On its surface, it makes no sense. If there was an outbreak of measles, for example, and it started to sweep through the state . . .Would you then say, "No, you can do what you want. If you want to get a vaccine, fine. If you don't, that's fine," knowing that there are people in the state of Louisiana who can't be vaccinated, knowing that they depend on those around them to protect them?

He continued:

> This sort of medical freedom notion that you do what you want, the rest of society doesn't count, your neighbor doesn't count, is at best shortsighted, and at worst sort of absents you from any sort of societal responsibility.

Offit added:

> Do you have any responsibility for the person you sit next to on the bus or you stand next to on the elevator? You do and you benefit, and they benefit.

Offit certainly makes valid points. But his position reflects his personal moral beliefs. Beliefs, by their very nature, are subjective—meaning, others may and likely will feel differently. A belief is not inherently wrong simply because it doesn't align with another's.

If, suddenly, the government issued a mandate requiring everyone with two working kidneys to donate one to a person in need of a transplant, many of us would be unwilling to undergo a surgical procedure that leaves us with one working kidney to save the life of a person we don't know. Would this qualify as a "responsibility for the person you sit next to on the bus or stand next to on the elevator"?

What if, in order to attend school, your child was required to give up a kidney? If you sought an exemption for your child, would that be immoral?

Admittedly, a nephrectomy is more invasive than a shot, but is it more invasive than 200 shots? What if your child is the 1 in 100,000 who gets encephalitis or seizures from a vaccine? What if your child is medically complex and fragile? Should you be forced to take a vaccine that has a real risk of side effects to your child to potentially and theoretically protect another through herd immunity? As a parent, should you have the right to make decisions for your child, even if that means prioritizing your child over others? In the greater sense, is any mandate that *forces* a medical procedure justified to protect others?

These are difficult questions. Candidly, I grapple with the answers. Reasonable, loving, and moral parents may hold vastly different opinions.

Studies show that, in states that offer exemptions, most families adhere to vaccination schedules. According to the CDC, in 2024, the exemption rate for kindergartners was only around 3%. The vast majority of children are vaccinated, even in areas where exemptions are permissible.

Although higher exemption rates may result in increased vulnerability and localized outbreaks in a given area, they do not typically translate to statewide epidemics. Many outbreaks—most notably, pertussis—affect both vaccinated and unvaccinated individuals. Lying at the crux of our debate over exemptions is a broader philosophical question: Do we place greater value on personal freedoms or public health? Just as those who answer "personal freedoms" deem *themselves* correct, those who answer "public health" deem *themselves* correct. What if I told you that each is wrong and both are right? Because there is validity to each of their positions.

We must acknowledge the perspectives of those who raise ethical concerns about vaccines much in the same way we acknowledge the perspectives of those who raise public health concerns. Earlier, I shared excerpts from Stanley Plotkin's January 11, 2018, deposition, taken by Aaron Siri. Plotkin's testimony reveals the ways that, for some, vaccination could conflict with deeply held beliefs and should, therefore, warrant exemption consideration. The following further excerpt from Plotkin's deposition reminds us of the importance of respecting personal and religious beliefs, even when they don't necessarily align with our own.

Fair warning: some may find this testimony deeply disturbing.

SIRI: I'm going to hand you, I'm going to hand you what's been marked Plaintiff's Exhibit 41. Okay? Are you familiar with this article?

PLOTKIN: Yes.

SIRI: Are you listed as an author on this article?

PLOTKIN: Yes.

SIRI: This study took place at the Wistar Institute, correct?

PLOTKIN: Yes.

SIRI: You were at the Wistar Institute, correct?

PLOTKIN: Yes.

SIRI: How many fetuses were used in the study described in this article?

PLOTKIN: Quite a few.

SIRI: In your work related to vaccines, how many fetuses were involved in that work?

PLOTKIN: There were only two fetuses involved in making vaccines. When fetal strains of fibroblast strains were first developed, I was involved in that work trying to characterize those cells; but they were not used to make vaccines.

SIRI: So this study involved seventy-four fetuses.

PLOTKIN: Yes.

SIRI: Okay. These included fetuses that were aborted for social and psychiatric reasons, correct?

PLOTKIN: Correct.

SIRI: What organs did you harvest from these fetuses?

PLOTKIN: Well, I didn't personally harvest any, but a whole range of tissues were harvested by co-workers.

SIRI: And these pieces were then cut up into little pieces, right?

PLOTKIN: Yes.

SIRI: Included the lung of the fetuses?

PLOTKIN: Yes.

SIRI: Included the skin?

PLOTKIN: Yes.

SIRI: Kidney?

PLOTKIN: Yes.

SIRI: Spleen?

PLOTKIN: Yes.

SIRI: Heart?

PLOTKIN: Yes.

SIRI: Tongue?

PLOTKIN: I don't recall, but probably yes.

SIRI: So I just want to make sure I understand. In your entire career—this was just one study. So I'm going to ask you again, in your entire career, how many fetuses have you worked with approximately?

PLOTKIN: Well, I don't remember the exact number, but quite a few when we were studying them originally before we decided to use them to make vaccines.

SIRI: You're aware, are you aware that the, one of the objections to vaccination by the plaintiff in this case is the inclusion of aborted fetal tissue in the development of vaccines and the fact that it's actually part of the ingredients of vaccines?

PLOTKIN: Yeah, I'm aware of those objections. The Catholic church has actually issued a document on that which says that individuals who need the vaccine should receive the vaccines, regardless of the fact, and that I think it implies that I am the individual who will go to hell because of the use of aborted tissues, which I am glad to do.

SIRI: Do you know if the mother's Catholic?

PLOTKIN: I have no idea.

SIRI: Okay.

PLOTKIN: But she should consult her priest.

SIRI: I'm just asking you, some of the fetuses that you did use did come from abortions from people who were in psychiatric institutions, correct?

PLOTKIN: I don't know that. What I'm telling you is that I got them from a co-worker; and if it's stated in the paper, it's true. But, otherwise, I do not know.

SIRI: Okay. Have you ever used orphans to study an experimental vaccine?

PLOTKIN: Yes.

SIRI: Have you ever used the mentally handicapped to study an experimental vaccine?

PLOTKIN: I don't recollect ever doing studies in mentally handicapped individuals. At the time in the 1960s, it was not an uncommon practice.

SIRI: So you're saying—I'm not clear on your answer. I'm sorry. Have you ever used mentally handicapped to study an experimental vaccine?

PLOTKIN: What I'm saying is I don't recall specifically having done that, but that in the 1960s, it was not unusual to do that. And I wouldn't deny that I may have done so.

SIRI: Well, there's an article entitled "Attenuation of RA 27/3 Rubella Virus in WI-38 Human Diploid Cells." Are you familiar with that article?

PLOTKIN: Yes.

SIRI: In that article, one of the things it says is thirteen seronegative mentally retarded children were given RA 27/3 vaccine?

PLOTKIN: Okay. Well, then that's, in that case that's what I did.

SIRI: Have you ever expressed that it's better to perform experiments on those less likely to be able to contribute to society, such as children with handicap, than with children without or adults without handicaps?

PLOTKIN: I don't remember specifically, but it's . . .

SIRI: I'm going to hand you what's been marked as Exhibit 43. Do you recognize this letter you wrote to the editor?

PLOTKIN: Yes.

SIRI: Did you write this letter?

PLOTKIN: Yes.

SIRI: Is one of the things you wrote: The question is whether we are to have experiments performed on fully functioning adults and on children who are potentially contributors to society or to perform initial studies in children and adults who are human in form but not in social potential?

PLOTKIN: Yes.

SIRI: It may be objected that this question implies a Nazi philosophy, but I do not think that it is difficult to distinguish nonfunctioning persons from members of ethnic, racial, economic, or other groups.

PLOTKIN: Mm-hmm.

SIRI: Have you ever used babies of mothers in prison to study an experimental vaccine?

PLOTKIN: Yes.

SIRI: Have you ever used individuals under colonial rule to study an experimental vaccine?

PLOTKIN: Yes.

SIRI: Did you do so in the Belgian Congo?

PLOTKIN: Yes.

SIRI: Did that experiment involve almost a million people?

PLOTKIN: Well—well, all right, yes.

Plotkin's admissions to testing on vulnerable populations and using fetal tissue and human serum in vaccine research are astonishing, particularly given that he is one of the most influential and prominent figures in modern vaccine development. Plotkin's testimony details the utilization of aborted fetal tissue in vaccine production, cutting fetal tissue into small pieces for vaccine testing, research on orphans and people with disabilities, and even experimentation conducted on babies born to incarcerated mothers and individuals in colonial territories. While Plotkin's testimony may not change opinions on the importance of vaccination, it does shed some light on the reason certain individuals feel so strongly about exemptions. His testimony challenges the prevailing assumption that all vaccine opposition stems from "misinformation," instead shining a disturbing spotlight on the ethical, moral, and philosophical considerations inextricable to the vaccine debate.

14

VACCINATED VS. UNVACCINATED TRIALS

Nothing has such power to broaden the mind as the ability to investigate systematically and truly all that comes under thy observation in life.

—MARCUS AURELIUS

Given the undeniable health implications, vaccines must undergo rigorous safety and efficacy testing. The medical community and vaccine manufacturers maintain that existing testing protocols adequately and rigorously assess the safety of vaccines. However, critics contend that the use of noninert placebos—in combination with the administration of other vaccines—leads to self-serving findings that fail to *thoroughly* identify risks. To briefly refresh your recollection (because, yes, that was many, many chapters ago and *so* much has happened since then), when another therapeutic or vaccine exists, a new vaccine will be tested against the existing therapeutic or vaccine, as opposed to an *inert* placebo (like saline or water).

Are we doing it right? Is the current approach really the *best* approach?

The methodologies used to test many vaccines are inherently flawed. A number of vaccines on the current CDC schedule were initially tested at a time when we did not demand the same rigorous safety testing standards we do today. Earlier, we rather extensively addressed the drawbacks of testing vaccines against *noninert* placebos.

Although I will not rehash the studies detailed in previous chapters, I will, just by way of example, remind you that the MMR II vaccine was tested against the original MMR vaccine, which was tested against the original individual measles and/or rubella vaccines. This, of course, presumed that the original vaccines did not carry their own safety risks or that the studies met today's standards. Most of the children in these studies also received the other vaccines recommended at that time, including DTP and polio, further convoluting the results. This does not automatically render the MMR II vaccine unsafe. Yet the fact that the comparator vaccine was not tested against unvaccinated children casts doubts on an assertion that researchers were in a position to ascertain the actual risks associated with the MMR II vaccine. When Prevnar was first tested, no other pneumococcal vaccine existed. Ordinarily, this would mean that the control group should receive an inert placebo. In the Prevnar study, that was not the case. The placebo group received the meningococcal conjugate vaccine.

Ethical considerations have since been imposed on medical research that now require participants in the control group to receive not only the current recommended standard of care vaccine but also *all* vaccines on the schedule. The Belmont Report provides the framework for ethical research in human subjects, emphasizing three fundamental principles: respect for persons (autonomy), beneficence, and justice. Conducting a study that involves withholding vaccines is believed to violate the principles of beneficence (doing good) and justice, particularly if the population left unvaccinated disproportionately contains vulnerable groups. Modern ethical standards in research focus on minimizing harm and ensuring scientific validity.

You see the conundrum here, right? Most of the vaccines that we use today were not tested against inert placebos. At the same time, ethical considerations now preclude us from testing vaccinated individuals against unvaccinated individuals to ascertain whether vaccines are *truly* safe in their own rights. For most vaccines, all we know is that studies showed no increased risk relative to the noninert placebo. We are stuck. And we are being told that the obvious solution is not a viable one.

Many parents, researchers, and health-care professionals have voiced concerns over the lack of robust, comparative data between fully vaccinated, partially vaccinated, and unvaccinated children. At the heart of this discussion is the dilemma: How do we study vaccine safety and effectiveness in a way that maintains scientific rigor, without compromising the rights and well-being of participants?

What is the optimal way to test vaccines? No doubt, many of you are screaming, "Vaccinated versus unvaccinated!" You're not wrong. But the logistics are not as simple as they may appear, no matter how emphatically you shout. Because the control group receives the comparator vaccine *and* all vaccines on the schedule, it may be difficult to ascertain whether side effects are attributable to the new vaccine or the battery of other vaccines, each of which may be accompanied by its own respective laundry lists of possible minor to severe side effects. Seemingly, the only way to definitively determine whether any observed side effects are traceable to the new vaccine is to do precisely what we are being told we cannot: Use unvaccinated children in the control group and administer an inert placebo, like saline.

The dilemma doesn't end there though. Let's put aside the ethical considerations for just a moment. Randomized, controlled, clinical trials are the gold standard for evaluating safety and efficacy. One could theoretically set up a trial with a comparison of those who choose to vaccinate versus those who do not. Yet conducting a controlled trial that compares vaccinated and unvaccinated children, while meeting today's scientific standards, is virtually impossible. By placing unvaccinated children in the control group, the study inherently ceases to be blinded or randomized.

Selecting a control group that consists of similar participants removes the randomized component of the randomized, controlled trial. Randomization ensures that any observed differences between the trial group and the placebo group are truly due to the new vaccine itself and not due to preexisting differences between the participants in each group. Randomization further helps distribute any possible confounding variables equally across both groups. Hypothetically speaking, parents who choose not to vaccinate their child may, on the whole, feed their child healthier foods, which, in turn, positively impacts the child's overall health. Perhaps some of these unvaccinated children are homeschooled. As they are not exposed to the onslaught of viruses school-age children encounter on a daily basis, these unvaccinated children could have more delicate, underdeveloped immune systems. Or maybe homeschooled, unvaccinated children have stronger immune systems because they are not incessantly bombarded by viruses. Whatever they may be, the similarities among a self-selecting and definitely *not* randomized group could skew data by diminishing variability. Voluntary participation studies may also attract participants with strong opinions or unique circumstances, which has the further potential to affect the results.

Blinding is equally important to help eliminate researcher and participant bias. If participants know they are receiving a placebo, their expectations and psychological response can influence the results of the study, possibly obscuring the data and making it difficult to accurately assess the efficacy of the actual treatment being tested.

We momentarily digressed from the ethical considerations to address the significance of randomization and blinding in controlled studies. Let's now return to ethics. Vaccines are widely accepted as the standard of care for preventing serious illnesses. On the one hand, randomly assigning children to an unvaccinated group could leave them vulnerable to potentially life-threatening diseases. This is most notably true for diseases like measles or pertussis, which can spread rapidly and lead to significant morbidity and mortality. On the other hand, randomly assigning children to a vaccinated group could require giving vaccines to individuals or families who do not want them, violating the principles of informed consent and bodily autonomy. Forcing vaccination would undermine trust in the health-care system. The ethical principle of beneficence requires researchers to maximize benefits and minimize harm to participants. Both withholding vaccines and administering them without consent violate ethical principles. Thus, traditional, randomized, controlled trials to compare vaccinated and unvaccinated groups are widely believed to be unethical and impractical.

However, there *are* ethical and scientifically sound ways to gather meaningful data on vaccination outcomes. Despite the obvious scientific shortcomings of a nonrandomized and nonblinded study comparing vaccinated versus unvaccinated participants, I do believe such a study still holds scientific value. After all, many vaccines, including the original MMR and measles vaccines, were tested in nonrandomized, nonblinded trials. The MMR vaccine currently in use was tested against the original MMR vaccine. We know the original MMR vaccine was tested in a way that did not comport with today's rigorous safety testing standards. This suggests that, in certain circumstances, we *do*, in fact, accept research and studies that fall short of the gold standard. It is somewhat hypocritical to accept a nonblind, nonrandomized study in one context (such as in the case of the original MMR vaccine) but refuse to conduct studies comparing vaccinated and unvaccinated individuals.

A voluntary participation study would allow parents who choose not to vaccinate their children to *elect* to enroll their families. These children could be compared to fully vaccinated peers in a nonrandomized, open-label design. While these studies have their inherent limitations, they provide a way to ethically gather comparative data without forcing or denying vaccines. Moreover, increasing the number of participants in such a study could contribute to more reliable findings. If we observe adverse events in a trial group of one hundred participants, the data is less compelling than if we observe the very same adverse events in a trial group of one hundred thousand participants.

Another way to address these ethical concerns while also satisfying the demand for better evidence are observational studies that use existing datasets. These types of studies use preexisting data to examine the relationship between an exposure and an outcome. In the case of vaccine research, large health-care databases and vaccine registries already collect extensive information on vaccination status, health outcomes, and demographics. Researchers can analyze this data to compare health outcomes in vaccinated, partially vaccinated, and unvaccinated children. For instance, comparing the rates of asthma, allergies, or autoimmune conditions among different groups could provide some understanding of the potential long-term effects of vaccines or vaccine schedules.

Variations in vaccine uptake, due to geographic, cultural, or socioeconomic factors, also provide researchers with additional opportunities for natural experiments. Researchers can study health outcomes in communities with high vaccination rates versus those with low vaccination rates without directly intervening.

Alternatively, rather than studying vaccinated versus unvaccinated, researchers may focus on comparing different vaccine schedules. Studies could assess whether spacing out vaccines or delaying certain shots impacts the overall risk of adverse events or the effectiveness of immunization. Many countries collect vaccination and health outcome data through national health systems. Researchers can analyze this data to identify trends, correlations, and potential safety signals without the cost and effort of conducting new trials.

Can you imagine if vaccines were studied in one or several of these ways? Could you fathom a world in which a vaccine insert plainly stated that based on preclinical trials, a vaccine is safe as opposed to vaguely reassuring us that it poses no increased risk relative to the noninert placebo? Wouldn't stricter scrutiny impose greater accountability on vaccine manufacturers? Shouldn't it?

As with any medical intervention, the possibility of side effects is inevitable. This is true of even the most relatively innocuous medications, like over-the-counter pain relievers and antacids. For the most part, we are willing to assume some risk when it is outweighed by the benefit. Obscuring potential risks by testing vaccines in a self-serving way does little to instill consumer confidence. It raises suspicion and promulgates vaccine hesitancy, leading some to question whether the benefits of vaccination indeed outweigh the risks. The solution is simple. Reassure concerned parents and the medical community alike. Test vaccines in a way that engenders trust in the findings. Rather than gaslighting parents, prove to them that vaccines are, in fact, safe. So why not do it?

Conducting meaningful research on vaccines and vaccine schedules in vaccinated versus unvaccinated trials, while simultaneously upholding ethical standards, is not only possible; it is necessary. Observational studies, voluntary participation, and the use of large datasets allow us to gather valuable evidence without compromising the principles of informed consent and standard of care. The goal is not to promote division between those who vaccinate and those who do not but to foster a shared commitment to scientific inquiry and ethical responsibility. By addressing these questions thoughtfully and respectfully, we can advance vaccine science while honoring the values of autonomy, safety, and evidence-based medicine.

15

THE COMPLEX LANDSCAPE OF VACCINE RESEARCH AND ITS LONG-TERM IMPLICATIONS

NAVIGATING THE NUANCES OF VACCINE SAFETY: BEYOND IMMEDIATE DISEASE PREVENTION

Medical science has made such tremendous progress that there is hardly a healthy human left.

—ALDOUS HUXLEY

The paucity of vaccinated versus unvaccinated studies is not the only conspicuous gap in the current vaccine research. For many vaccines, long-term safety studies do not exist. Surprising, right? Vaccine safety is initially assessed through prelicense clinical trials. Preapproval vaccine trials often span months to a year. The lengthiest prelicense trials typically monitor participants for approximately six months postdosing for safety and efficacy outcomes. Thereafter, long-term safety follow-up usually takes place postlicense, *not* through prospective clinical trials (the gold standard for safety research) but through *passive* surveillance systems.

Why is this significant? As the name implies, passive surveillance is precisely that—passive. It relies on voluntary disclosure from sources, such as the Vaccine Adverse Event Reporting System (VAERS), and health datasets, such as the Vaccine Safety Datalink (VSD). This form of surveillance depends on individuals and institutions to report adverse events. It lacks the standardization found in clinical trials, which could result in incomplete, delayed, or a dearth of reporting. Furthermore, systems like the VSD cover a mere fraction of the population, failing to capture all demographic groups equally.

That is not to say they are entirely ineffective though. By scanning for safety signals, these systems are competent at identifying short-term concerns or adverse events reported en masse. Recent examples of their success are the detection of the risks of myocarditis arising from the COVID-19 vaccines and intussusception from the rotavirus vaccines. This leaves many wondering (myself included): From an ethical perspective, should we wait until after so many people have experienced adverse consequences before making vaccines safer? How do we balance the exigent demand to make a vaccine widely available with the need to sufficiently study its safety profile prior to marketing it?

Whereas postmarket surveillance is deemed adequate for detecting most short-term consequences that go unnoticed in prelicense studies, it has its undeniable shortcomings. Prospective clinical trials are more effective at revealing long-term and nonspecific consequences that may otherwise slip through the cracks.

Most individuals are unlikely to make the connection between a vaccine received months or years ago and nonspecific or attenuated adverse consequences. Frankly, unless actively studied, most scientists wouldn't either. For instance, nearly *all* vaccine inserts state: "Carcinogenesis, mutagenesis, impairment of fertility has not been evaluated." Carcinogenesis is the process by which healthy cells transform into cancerous ones. What if ten years after it is administered, Vaccine X causes a specific type of cancer? A whole decade later, few, if any, would identify any correlation between Vaccine X and the cancer. The cancer would not be reported through surveillance systems and the link would, thus, go undetected. In contrast, a prospective clinical trial may reveal that, over time, an increasing percentage of vaccinated participants developed the same type of cancer as compared to controls, signaling researchers to investigate its potential link between Vaccine X and cancer.

Some will undoubtedly argue that the current infrastructure for monitoring vaccine safety postlicense is comprehensive and sufficient. They would be quick to point out that, where surveillance systems fall short, longitudinal and cohort studies, as well as meta-analyses, fill the gaps. However, these mechanisms, too, have their limitations. The lack of funding and resources dedicated to long-term studies restricts the ability to conduct extensive research over time.

Moreover, conducting postlicense studies presumes that interest exists in researching a specific issue. Returning to our earlier example of Vaccine X and cancer, a researcher would first need to formulate the hypothesis that, over the span of a decade, Vaccine X might contribute to a certain type of cancer. Next, he or she must perform a retrospective study using an existing dataset, if one exists, or devote upward of ten years to conducting research and risk the possibility that his or her hypothesis was incorrect and research for naught. The researcher must secure considerable resources to conduct such an ambitious study, which may prove impossible. And all this rests on the assumption that the researcher has made the correlation between Vaccine X and the cancer; otherwise, he or she would have no impetus to study it in the first place. I suspect that most scientists conduct studies not in consultation with their crystal ball but rather based on observable potential correlations between A and B. If the link is not apparent, why would a researcher think to study it?

And, given that many studies showing a connection between vaccines and adverse consequences have been discredited, researchers may be altogether deterred from conducting studies on the subject.

According to this researcher-dependent model, if nobody chooses to study a specific problem or side effect, it might remain unidentified until it becomes significant enough to draw attention—*if* it is ever identified. By the time adverse events are recognized and acknowledged, the delayed response may prove too little too late.

Yes, practical considerations might render prospective postlicense clinical trials difficult, if not entirely infeasible. The potential long-term or tangential consequences do not cease to exist merely because we fail to study them. We cannot turn a blind eye to the very distinct probability that adverse events could manifest well beyond the initial trial period or that adverse consequences could go undetected by our surveillance systems. The current infrastructure for postmarket surveillance is simply insufficient to competently identify long-term or nonspecific adverse events. Long-term consequences are another piece of the vast and complex vaccine puzzle . . . or maybe they're that pesky missing puzzle piece without which we cannot sufficiently weigh the benefits and risks of a given vaccine.

I will likely (okay, definitely) receive criticism for suggesting that our methods for studying long-term vaccine consequences are deficient. But long-term safety studies aren't some radical notion I've concocted. I am far from the only one to draw attention to them.

Since 1982, the National Vaccine Information Center (NVIC) has advocated that well-designed, independent, ongoing scientific studies are needed to:

1. define the various biological mechanisms involved in vaccine injury and death;
2. identify genetic and other biological high-risk factors for suffering chronic brain and immune system dysfunction after vaccination; and
3. evaluate short- and long-term health outcomes of individuals who use many vaccines and those who use fewer or no vaccines to determine the health effects of vaccination on individuals and the public health.

I trust few among us would disagree with these recommendations. Practically speaking, once a vaccine receives FDA approval and hits the market, it is seemingly presumed to warrant little further exploration—this, despite the fact that approval of that vaccine was predicated on trials that were relatively limited in duration and usually performed by the vaccine manufacturer itself. This leaves us reliant on surveillance systems as virtually the exclusive means of identifying vaccine complications and long-term side effects.

We *know* that some vaccines cause certain safety risks because long-term adverse events are well-documented. As the NVIC has urged for over forty years, we must improve our monitoring and increase our study of the long-term health implications of vaccines. One solution is to implement a more robust safety monitoring system that adapts to the growing number of vaccines being introduced, quickly investigates adverse events, provides clearer conclusions, and strengthens public confidence in vaccines. While there is little harm in improved monitoring and studying long-term vaccine consequences, there is great harm in *not* doing so.

The debate over long-term vaccine risks earns its rightful place among the wide range of other hot-button topics in the divisive realm of vaccine discourse. It marks yet another instance in which we feel like spectators at a nail-biting tennis match, watching the ball rally back and forth between "vaccines are totally safe and effective" and "vaccines are the Antichrist." In this match, serving the proverbial ball is team "no long-term risks associated with vaccines." Although few studies have specifically examined long-term vaccine safety, one such study, published in *Pediatrics* in 2010 by Michael J. Smith et al., looked at whether children who received recommended vaccines on time during the first year of life experienced different neuropsychological outcomes at seven to ten years of age as compared to children with delayed receipt or nonreceipt of these vaccines. Ultimately, it concluded that timely vaccination during infancy has no adverse effect on neuropsychological outcomes seven to ten years later.

Returning the tennis ball back over the net and offering a slightly different perspective is a 2024 opinion piece published in the *New England Journal of Medicine*, one of the most highly respected medical journals, which raised important questions over the lack of long-term vaccine safety data. The article noted that long-term vaccine side effects may only become apparent (if at all) *after* a vaccine is widely used.

The authors of this opinion piece—among them, Stanley Plotkin, whose deposition testimony you may recall from our earlier discussion of religious exemptions—argue that additional long-term safety data are crucial to maintaining public trust. They emphasize the need for increased funding for ongoing post-authorization safety research, contending:

> Despite widespread vaccine use, there has been insufficient investment in long-term safety research to match the pace at which new vaccines are developed and distributed. Increasing funding and improving active surveillance systems are critical to ensure that long-term safety data is available to the public and to better understand the biological mechanisms behind rare adverse events.

Not only corroborating that vaccines may cause unintended, unknown, long-term consequences, but also highlighting the imperative for prospective clinical trials, is the COVID-19 vaccine, which, postmarket, was discovered to adversely impact menstruation. In a *New York Post* article, NICHD director Diana Bianchi stated: "Nobody expected [the COVID-19 vaccine] to affect the menstrual system, because the information wasn't being collected in the early vaccine studies." Bianchi further defended: "They weren't doing this type of research," because "changes to the menstrual cycle are really not a life-and-death issue." (Respectfully, I must disagree with Bianchi. *The menstrual cycle is quite literally a life issue.*) As a reminder, vaccines are not studied for impairment of fertility. We know this because the manufacturers routinely tell us in the vaccine inserts. In this same article, Bianchi claimed, "We were worried this was contributing to vaccine hesitancy in reproductive-age women." This raises the question of whether, sometimes, there may be incentives to avoid long-term safety research.

Still, the scientific community widely rejects the notion that vaccines cause or contribute to chronic disease or other maladies. Urging us to perhaps consider otherwise are the Institute of Medicine's (IOM) reports spanning over two decades. In the 1990s, Congress asked the IOM to assemble independent physician committees to review the medical literature for scientific evidence of a causal relationship between childhood vaccines and immune and neurological dysfunction. Between 1991 and 2013, the IOM published a series of reports on evidence for adverse effects of vaccines, confirming: "*Vaccines can and do carry risks for complications that can be greater for some individuals than others and may lead to chronic brain and immune system damage or death.*"

In 1991, 1994, and 2012, IOM committees published reports finding that the following health problems are causally related to vaccination:
- Acute encephalopathy (brain inflammation)
- Chronic nervous system dysfunction (brain damage)
- Anaphylaxis (whole-body allergic reaction)
- Febrile seizures (convulsions with fever)
- Guillain-Barre syndrome (peripheral nerve inflammation)
- Brachial neuritis (arm nerve inflammation)
- Deltoid bursitis (shoulder inflammation)
- Acute and chronic arthritis (joint inflammation)
- Syncope (sudden loss of consciousness/fainting)
- Hypotonic/hyporesponsive episodes (shock and unusual shocklike state)
- Protracted, inconsolable crying and screaming
- Vaccine strain infection (smallpox, live polio, measles, varicella zoster vaccines)
- Death (smallpox, live polio, measles vaccines)

In 2012, the IOM published a report that revealed continuing and significant gaps in scientific knowledge regarding the biological mechanisms of vaccine injury and death—notably, a point that was previously made two decades earlier in the 1991 and 1994 IOM reports. *The IOM committee could not arrive at any definitive conclusions regarding causation for many of the reported vaccine reactions involving chronic brain and immune system dysfunction and even death.* Twenty years later, our scientific understanding of the biological mechanisms of vaccine injury and death remained no less enigmatic.

In fact, for eight routinely used vaccines—among them, the MMR, DTaP, hepatitis B, hepatitis A, varicella-zoster, and meningococcal—the IOM *did* determine there were too few scientifically sound studies published in the medical literature to conclude whether more than a hundred serious brain and immune system problems are or are not caused by vaccines, including diseases such as multiple sclerosis, arthritis, atopy, allergy, autoimmunity, learning disorders, communication disorders, developmental disorders, intellectual disability, attention deficit disorder, disruptive behavior disorder, tics and Tourette's syndrome, seizures and febrile seizures, epilepsy, lupus, stroke, SIDS, autism, and asthma.

Of course, the IOM's inability to conclude whether vaccines caused these diseases does not mean that vaccines do cause these diseases. It does, however, mean that there could be a causal link between vaccines and long-term, nonspecific consequences that may not have been identified in the postdosing and postmarket surveillance periods. Given the serious nature of many of these diseases, the possibility that they could in some way be correlated to vaccines stresses the importance of more attenuated, long-term research, preferably through prospective clinical trials.

Despite the IOM's findings, a common argument against long-term or attenuated vaccine-related side effects is the lack of biological plausibility. Vaccine proponents often assert there is little to no evidence suggesting *any* mechanisms through which vaccines could contribute to long-term health complications. Yet some researchers and studies have challenged this position. While such ideas remain speculative and are not broadly supported by the scientific community, I mention them to illustrate that the discourse is (not surprisingly) more nuanced than it may be presented.

I will briefly touch upon several theories that have emerged in the research not to advocate for their validity but to emphasize that this topic merits ongoing exploration. The first of such theories is based on various studies observing the effect of vaccines on animal brains. A 2010 study by

Laura Hewitson et al. found that infant rhesus macaques monkeys that received the complete pediatric vaccine schedule demonstrated significantly altered amygdala growth and increased brain volume. The amygdala is the region of the brain associated with social and emotional behavior.

In a separate study, the same team observed that newborn rhesus macaque monkeys given the hepatitis B vaccine within twenty-four hours of birth experienced delays in acquiring neonatal reflexes such as rooting, sucking, and snout reflexes compared to unvaccinated controls. If, as the study posits, the region of the brain associated with social and emotional behavior is altered by the complete pediatric vaccine schedule, then chronic diseases associated with the brain—namely, the laundry list of behavioral issues cited in the 1991, 1994, and 2012 IOM reports—*could* manifest years after a child is vaccinated. Before I am pilloried by the vaccine police, I must again make clear that this is mere conjecture on my part, an extrapolation from the nonhuman findings of the Hewitson studies.

Another theory postulates that vaccines may cause inflammatory responses, which, over time, could lead to the development of autoimmune diseases. One such study by Lluís Luján et al. found that sheep repeatedly vaccinated against various diseases developed autoimmune and inflammatory symptoms, like acute meningoencephalitis, poor response to stimuli, and neurological issues.

Ken Tsumiyama et al. proposed the theory of "self-organized criticality," whereby repeated vaccination in mice overstimulated the immune system, leading to autoimmune injury resembling systemic lupus erythematosus. The mice also produced autoantibodies associated with autoimmunity. The greatest takeaway from his research was that "systemic autoimmunity appears to be the inevitable consequence of overstimulating the host's immune system by repeated immunization with antigen, to the levels that surpass system's self-organized criticality."

In the Luján and Tsumiyama studies, autoimmune conditions were observed in lab animals after vaccination. If autoimmune diseases are the possible side effects of vaccine-induced inflammation in lab animals, there may be some biological plausibility to the theory that humans could develop autoimmune conditions in the months or even years after receiving vaccines. Notably, lab animals are vastly different from human children in the real world, and therefore, these studies, while interesting, are not sufficiently definitive evidence of the correlation between vaccines and autoimmune conditions.

Yet another, and quite possibly the most interesting, theory suggests that vaccines may alter the balance between Th1 (cell-mediated immunity) and Th2 (antibody-driven immunity) responses. Though vaccines are designed to mimic natural immune responses, some hypothesize that vaccines might tilt the immune system toward a Th2-dominant state, increasing susceptibility to autoimmune conditions or allergies. This hypothesis stems from the observation that vaccines often induce strong antibody, or Th2 responses, which potentially suppress Th1 pathways critical for fighting intracellular infections. The concerns over excessive stimulation of Th2 responses is based on the way the immune system develops and functions. The balance between Th1 and Th2 responses is critical for maintaining an appropriate immune reaction to pathogens while avoiding overreactions that could lead to allergies, asthma, or autoimmune conditions.

This theory is explained as follows: At birth, the immune system is naturally skewed toward a Th2-dominant state (antibodies). This is thought to protect the fetus during pregnancy by reducing the likelihood of inflammatory Th1 responses. After birth, exposure to environmental microbes, infections, and other immune challenges helps the immune system shift toward a balanced Th1/Th2 state.

Vaccines that predominantly stimulate Th2 pathways, such as some inactivated or subunit vaccines that focus on antibody production, could reinforce the Th2 dominance rather than promoting a balance, thus interfering with the natural development of the immune system.

Th2 dominance is closely linked to the production of cytokines (small proteins secreted by various cells in the body, primarily immune cells, that play crucial roles in regulating immune responses, inflammation, and other physiological processes). These cytokines promote the production of IgE antibodies and recruitment of eosinophils—key players in allergic reactions. If the immune system remains skewed toward a Th2 response, the body may be more likely to overreact to harmless environmental antigens, such as pollen, dust mites, or food proteins, resulting in allergies or asthma.

Many vaccines also contain adjuvants to enhance the immune response. These adjuvants may preferentially amplify Th2 responses. If this occurs repeatedly through multiple vaccinations, it could theoretically contribute to immune imbalances in susceptible individuals.

Pervasive among these theories is the belief that long-term and even nonspecific vaccine consequences are biologically plausible. For the time being, such theories have been rejected by the scientific community, which continues to maintain that the diseases prevented by vaccines generally pose a much greater risk of immune-related complications than the risks associated with vaccines. To me, these are not mutually exclusive premises. How can we rule out unexpected and tangential long-term side effects when the vaccine inserts themselves admit to and enumerate the recognized mild and severe side effects? Side effects are not only possible but *known*. So how is it that unknown side effects are biologically implausible? For the love of science, somebody please make this make sense!

Certain FDA-approved medications have the potential to cause long-term effects. The symptoms manifest later in life, even once treatment has ceased. For instance, chemotherapy agents, such as doxorubicin, cyclophosphamide, and cisplatin, can lead to late-onset cardiotoxicity, possibly increasing the risk of heart failure years after cancer treatment. Corticosteroids, like prednisone, may cause conditions such as osteoporosis, adrenal insufficiency, and cataracts long after discontinuation. Isotretinoin, used for severe acne, can result in joint pain and digestive issues persisting post-treatment. Similarly, bisphosphonates, used for osteoporosis, can lead to complications, which include osteonecrosis of the jaw and atypical femoral fractures years after initiation. Medications, including certain antibiotics, such as fluoroquinolones, are linked to long-term tendon problems that can occur well after treatment. Drugs, such as hydralazine and procainamide, are known to induce systemic lupus erythematosus; allopurinol, certain anticonvulsants, and some antibiotics can cause Stevens-Johnson syndrome, a serious disorder of the skin and mucous membranes. When such reactions are possible with medications, why not with vaccines? Why is it inconceivable that a vaccine, or multiple vaccines given regularly over several years, could potentially trigger chronic conditions or serious reactions outside the short list defined by the IOM?

We know that vaccines can cause seizures. They can cause encephalitis. This isn't conspiracy theory. The inserts say so. If, in rare cases, certain vaccines may cause seizures or encephalitis, isn't it also possible that vaccines are capable of causing other severe damage to the brain? How can it be argued there is no biological plausibility?

Some believe that vaccines may weaken the overall immune system or interfere with natural immune development. Such theories are rooted in the belief that vaccines disrupt the immune system's maturation and potentially increase susceptibility to unrelated conditions. Does this theory also have zero biological plausibility? By repeatedly stimulating the immune system with an adjuvant like aluminum, is it plausible that, at least in a small subset of individuals, this could have broader consequences on the maturation of the immune system than are currently understood?

In the late 1960s, children in Washington, DC, received an RSV vaccine in which the virus was inactivated with formalin. After immunization, 80% of the children were hospitalized with a variety of severe respiratory diseases, and two children died. Researchers at Johns Hopkins explained that the vaccine did not elicit a strong enough initial immune response, instead leading to a prolonged immune response that caused enhanced respiratory disease (ERD). The investigation revealed that the antibodies produced were not sufficiently potent to protect against RSV. Rather, this vaccine actually pulled the inactive virus into the body and provoked a severe immune reaction in the children who received it.

In 2024, Moderna halted its pediatric RSV vaccine trial after increased hospitalizations occurred during the study. According to an FDA briefing, two experimental Moderna RSV vaccines were given to infants aged five to eight months. The phase 1 trial was paused after five cases of severe to very severe lower RSV respiratory tract infections were reported among the forty babies who received the vaccine dose—this, compared with the one case in the placebo group of twenty babies. Five infants in the treatment group required hospitalization, and one needed mechanical ventilation.

The Moderna RSV study successfully identified severe side effects. The same may not be true of other studies. The undeniable correlation between the Moderna RSV vaccine and a severe reaction serves as a reminder that unexpected vaccine complications are, in fact, biologically plausible. If the RSV vaccines can cause severe immune complications, then other vaccines may (and *do*, as we know) also trigger similar immune responses in a small subset of children. When example upon example provides us with theoretical mechanisms by which vaccines could cause long-term complications, we simply cannot deny the biological plausibility.

The current scientific consensus remains that vaccines play a role in strengthening the immune system. Lobbing the tennis ball over the net yet again, the research shows that vaccines teach the immune system to recognize and combat specific pathogens. With the exception of a few isolated studies, vaccinated populations are not thought to be at higher risk for unrelated diseases, and vaccines have been shown to reduce long-term health complications by preventing severe infections that can damage the body.

Is it conceivable that vaccines could succeed in warding off the diseases they are designed to prevent, while also weakening the immune system, affecting the body in an unintended way, or leaving the body more susceptible to autoimmune conditions and other infectious diseases in a select population? Is this merely another highly contested topic in the vaccine battle royale that is neither as black nor as white as the proponents on either side emphatically deem it to be?

Sometimes, it may not be readily apparent that a particular adverse consequence is the result of a vaccine. Unless we perform clinical trials to actively identify these nonspecific events, we are left to rely solely on passive postlicense surveillance. Though effective at times, surveillance systems can easily overlook long-term and nonspecific vaccine consequences. Illuminating this point is an excerpt from a 2024 news segment in which Secretary of Health and Human Services, Robert F. Kennedy Jr., stated:

> Let me just give you one quick other example. The most popular vaccine in the world is the DTP vaccine, diphtheria, tetanus and pertussis. We banned, we got rid of it in this country because it was causing injuries, brain injuries, severe brain injuries or death to one in every 300 children.

> We used it in the 80s, and that's why there was all this litigation against vaccine companies that precipitated the passage of the Vaccine Act, that then gave them immunity from liability, but in Europe, they don't use it. In America, they don't use it. But we give it to 161 million African children a year.

> So Bill Gates asked the Danish government to support that program and said it saved 30 million lives. The Danish government said, show us the data. He wasn't able to. So they went to Africa and did their own studies. And they looked at

thirty years of DTP data. And what they found shocked them all.

They found that girls who got the DTP were dying at ten times the rate of unvaccinated girls. But they were dying of things that nobody had ever associated with the vaccine. They were dying of anemia, malaria, bilharzia, pulmonary disease, respiratory disease and pneumonia. And nobody noticed for thirty years that it was the vaccinated girls and not the unvaccinated girls who were dying.

And what had happened is these girls were not dying of diphtheria, tetanus, and pertussis. The vaccine had protected them against those. But it had also ruined their immune systems. And they were unable to defend themselves against other just minor diseases that other kids who had hearty immune systems were able to fend off.

So that's why you need these long-term studies, and that's why I'm worried that we don't do that here in the United States.

Before I heard this interview, I was unaware of this study. So of course, ever-insatiably curious, I looked it up. Insofar as the whole-cell DTP vaccine continues to be administered in Africa, Kennedy is correct. As a reminder, the whole-cell DTP vaccine is no longer used in the United States due to safety concerns. However, in 2023, approximately 108 million children globally received the vaccine, with a significant portion of these vaccinations occurring in African countries.

I could not find any information to corroborate Kennedy's claim that 1 in 300 children were severely injured from the DTP vaccine. (This doesn't automatically render it untrue; I was simply unable to confirm.) We *do* know that, when used in the United States, the DTP vaccine was associated with a risk of serious adverse events, such as high fever, seizures, and hypotonic-hyporesponsive episodes, estimated to occur in about 1 in 1,000 to 1 in 1,750 doses. Concerns over these risks, along with rare but severe neurological events, were the subject of multiple lawsuits and ultimately led to the DTP vaccine's removal and replacement with the DTaP vaccine in the United States and many other countries.

The funding for these global immunization programs primarily comes from international organizations, including Gavi and the Vaccine Alliance, which provide financial support to low-income countries to ensure widespread vaccine coverage.

A significant portion of the funding for DTP and other vaccines administered in Africa indirectly flows from the Bill & Melinda Gates Foundation. Since Gavi's inception, the Gates Foundation has contributed billions of dollars to it, helping fund vaccine distribution infrastructure and related health-care initiatives across Africa and other lower-income regions. This funding allows countries to access and administer vaccines at little to no cost, improving global immunization rates and targeting diseases such as diphtheria, tetanus, and pertussis.

In 2017, Danish researchers Søren Wengel Mogensen et al. conducted a retrospective study examining the mortality effects of the DTP and oral polio vaccines in infants. The study was part of the Bandim Health Project—a health and demographic surveillance system that works with population-based health research in Guinea-Bissau, West Africa, where children are routinely given the DTP vaccine. The study found that children who received DTP (+/- OPV) had a *fivefold higher mortality hazard ratio (HR)* compared to DTP unvaccinated peers, with the increased deaths primarily due to infections unrelated to diphtheria, tetanus, or pertussis. These findings suggest potential, nonspecific effects related to the DTP vaccine that may negatively impact overall immunity, with an even higher hazard ratio observed in girls.

Corroborating this finding is a meta-analysis by Peter Aaby et al., which suggested that DTP-vaccinated female children had approximately double the mortality rate of children who were not vaccinated with DTP. Another meta-analysis, this one from 2018, concluded, "Although having better nutritional status and being protected against three infections, 6–35 months old DTP-vaccinated children tended to have higher mortality than DTP-unvaccinated children. All studies of the introduction of DTP have found increased overall mortality."

Kennedy's statement was, therefore, largely correct. If I were to nitpick at all (and in the interest of accuracy, I most definitely will), Kennedy refers to the mortality rates observed in these studies as long-term consequences.

In the Bandim Health Project's Guinea-Bissau study, researchers observed a fivefold increase in mortality among infants aged three to five months who received the DTP vaccine compared to those who had not yet been vaccinated. This increased mortality risk was predominantly noted during the period between the first and second weighing sessions, which were conducted every three months. Accordingly, the elevated risk was assessed over a span of approximately three months after the initial DTP vaccination. I would not consider three months long-term, *per se*. Kennedy's point is otherwise founded.

The studies conducted by the Bandim Health Project underscore both: the need for postmarket research that more closely focuses on the long-term and nonspecific effects of vaccines not observed during prelicense trials, *and* research that is not funded by the vaccine manufacturers.

Vaccines like DTP have been shown to be effective in reducing the targeted diseases—diphtheria, tetanus, and pertussis. No doubt, the DTP vaccine saves lives. But if some vaccinated children truly face a higher mortality rate from unrelated infections or experience a host of other immune dysfunctions, then this raises significant questions about the ancillary effects of the DTP (and other vaccines) on the immune system. If there are at least theoretical mechanisms through which vaccines could cause long-term adverse consequences, then the scientific community may wish to reevaluate its stance on biological plausibility.

The findings of these Bandim Health Project studies force us to contemplate the benefits of disease protection in conjunction with the potential broader adverse consequences. Reducing this issue to anti-vax or pro-vax irresponsibly ignores (or perhaps deflects) from the very palpable and critical public health implications integral to this debate. Obviating diseases, such as diphtheria, is a remarkable achievement. If the consequence is a higher susceptibility to other infections, that risk must be weighed carefully against the benefit. Public health policies demand a comprehensive risk-benefit analysis that cannot be performed without accounting for all possible short- and long-term effects of vaccines. And without studies, such analysis is impossible.

Although commonly dismissed as "anti-vax" or "conspiracy theorists," those advocating for more rigorous long-term vaccine safety testing believe in science so much they actually demand more of it. These people generally agree that vaccines have vastly improved our ability to prevent debilitating and fatal diseases. They do not deny that the rate of morbidity and mortality is a fraction of what it once was. Nevertheless, they are alarmed by the potential slew of unexplored, potential adverse vaccine consequences and the absence of prospective clinical trials to adequately research them. These people are understandably skeptical when vaccine inserts tell them minor and severe side effects are possible, while the scientific community concurrently tells them that long-term side effects are not biologically plausible. These so-called anti-vax conspiracy theorists are trying to understand how the scientific community can emphatically claim long-term consequences are biologically implausible when the vaccine inserts plainly state vaccines have not been studied for carcinogenesis, mutagenesis, or impairment of fertility. What are these if not biologically plausible long-term consequences? We cannot find what we do not look for. More research, conducted in the most efficacious manner, translates to greater safety outcomes. Our efforts should be focused *not* on ignoring adverse consequences but on minimizing them.

There is a pressing need for more comprehensive studies monitoring long-term health implications across different populations and demographics, especially in communities where access to health care is limited and alternative diseases consequent to vaccination can pose serious risks. So long as we don't have all the answers, this conversation must be approached thoughtfully, with transparency and humility. Not only is this our scientific imperative, it is a moral one.

ROBERT F. KENNEDY JR. VS. ESTABLISHED MEDICAL AUTHORITY: NAVIGATING VACCINE DEBATES

RFK is saying one thing and one thing only about vaccines: that they should be studied like any other pharmaceutical product.

—CALLEY MEANS, HEALTH ADVOCATE AND COAUTHOR OF NYT BEST-SELLING *GOOD ENERGY*

No one is saying to ban vaccines at all. I'm simply saying, don't we want really rigorous testing?

—JILLIAN MICHAELS, RENOWNED FITNESS EXPERT

Whereas a decade ago, Jenny McCarthy was synonymous with the term "anti-vax," more recently, that illustrious torch has been passed to Robert F. Kennedy Jr., who now holds the coveted title. The playbook clearly instructs: Defame, ostracize, gaslight.

Today, it seems that anyone who questions vaccine narratives is automatically deemed a congregant of the "Church of Kennedy." While Kennedy is not the focus of this book, I would be remiss if I did not mention him . . . for obvious reasons. Kennedy has repeatedly sworn he is not anti-vax. Despite this, he has unintentionally become a figurehead of the anti-vax movement. In 2025, Kennedy was appointed to lead the Department of Health and Human Services. In recent memory, I cannot recall a more polarizing figure in the realm of health and medicine.

A simple internet search quickly reveals that Kennedy's remarkable accomplishments as an environmental attorney and activist are grossly overshadowed by claims that he is both "anti-vax" and a "conspiracy theorist." In 2024, the media fabricated the *false* claim that, upon his appointment as secretary of the Department of Health and Human Services, Kennedy planned to revoke the polio vaccine. In a 2024 interview on News Nation, Kennedy stated:

> I've never been anti-vaccine and I've said that hundreds and hundreds of times. Because that is a way of silencing me. Using that pejorative is a way of silencing or marginalizing me. My position on vaccines, I think that virtually every American

would agree with my stance on vaccines, which is that vaccines should be tested like other medicines. They should be safety tested.

Indeed, designating those who question vaccine efficacy or safety as anti-vax and conspiracy theorists is a masterful way to discredit them. The modern-day equivalent of the scarlet letter, such pejoratives (1) deter others from questioning, lest they risk public and even professional remuneration; (2) undermine the speaker's credibility by dismissing him or her as fringe; and (3) prove an effective intimidation strategy that carries with it a potential social stigma. Anyone who believes in or repeats the supposed anti-vax conspiracy theory is, by extension, a "crackpot."

However, dismissing someone as anti-vax is problematic for several glaring reasons: It ignores nuance by lumping together militant nonvaccinators with those merely advocating for improved safety testing or beneficial policy changes; and it stifles debate. When asking questions is regarded as inherently dangerous, we quash legitimate scientific inquiry and public discourse (which, of course, may be the point). Furthermore, such labels engender polarization; branding one an anti-vaxer earmarks him or her apathetic to the greater good. In reality, the converse may be true: One who campaigns for improved safety testing *at the expense of his or her reputation* actually champions the greater good. And by grouping legitimate concerns in the same category as conspiracy theory, we run the risk of overlooking genuine public health threats.

Kennedy, who has tirelessly repeated he is not anti-vax, is now (inadvertently) emblematic of the anti-vax movement. At the risk of inviting accusations that this book is in defense of Kennedy, I will point out that, in my opinion, based on my understanding of his position, Kennedy is *not* anti-vaccine but pro-safety and pro-transparency. In 2022, I appeared as a guest on his podcast. Although we did not discuss vaccines in any capacity, I found Kennedy to be intelligent, kind, and deeply committed to children's health. One might disagree with his specific demands or interpretations of the data. The call for more safety testing is not invariably anti-science—it is *pro* science and anti scientific absolutism.

Anyone who has taken the time to listen to Kennedy speak (as opposed to relying on sensationalistic and deliberately misleading media headlines or cherry-picked sound bites) *understands* that he is a proponent of more robust, long-term, and inert placebo-controlled safety trials. He does not advocate for the abolition of vaccines. In alignment with scientific principles, he believes that the current testing protocols are inadequate and that to build public trust, vaccines should meet higher safety standards. On countless occasions, Kennedy has explicitly stated that vaccines can be effective and beneficial and that he and his family are vaccinated—though you're unlikely to hear *these* sound bites on any of the major networks, the same networks that receive billions of dollars annually from pharmaceutical advertisements.

To better comprehend the reasons Kennedy is both important to public health and threatening to vaccine manufacturers, we must understand that his position is based on the premises that (1) vaccines are not tested against *inert* placebo and (2) no prospective long-term vaccine studies exist (meaning, studies that follow a group of individuals over a significant period of time, to regularly collect data and evaluate the way certain factors may influence the development of a particular outcome).

In May 2017, Kennedy invited the founder of the Informed Consent Action Network (ICAN), Del Bigtree, prominent vaccine litigation attorney, Aaron Siri, and cofounder of SafeMinds autism research organization, Lyn Redwood, RN, MSN, to a meeting with immunologist and former director of the National Institute of Allergy and Infectious Diseases (NIAID), Anthony Fauci, MD, geneticist and former director of the National Institutes of Health (NIH), Francis Collins, MD, MS, PhD, and several other public health officials at the executive office of the NIH. For many years prior, Kennedy continuously pointed out that the Department of Health and Human Services (HHS) neglected not only to conduct large-scale vaccinated versus unvaccinated research but also to test the vaccines on the childhood schedule against *inert* placebos. During this meeting, Kennedy directly asked Fauci and Collins for evidence of true placebo-controlled studies— using *inert* placebos. (As you may recall, true inert placebos include sugar pills, salt water, and water.) Neither Fauci nor Collins could produce such studies, suggesting that the HHS might not be fulfilling the obligations imposed upon it under 42 USC § 300aa-27. This legislation requires the HHS to ensure vaccine safety and to conduct ongoing improvements to the vaccine program.

Bigtree submitted a series of questions to HHS, to which, on January 18, 2018, the agency replied. Among other questions, Bigtree asked: "Please explain how HHS justifies licensing any pediatric vaccine without first conducting a long-term clinical trial in which the rate of adverse reactions is compared between the subject group and a control group receiving an inert placebo?"

The HHS responded:

> Inert placebo controls are not required to understand the safety profile of a new vaccine, and are thus not required. In some cases, inclusion of placebo control groups is considered unethical. Even in the absence of a placebo, control groups can be useful in evaluating whether the incidence of a specific observed adverse event exceeds that which would be expected without administration of the new vaccine. Serious adverse events are always carefully evaluated by the FDA to determine potential association with vaccination regardless of their rate of incidence in the control group. In cases where an active control is used, the adverse event profile of that control group is usually known and the findings of the study are reviewed in the context of that knowledge.

Without providing any scientific justification, the HHS, in essence, informed Bigtree that inert placebo-controlled studies are not required for vaccines.

Approximately six years later, Kennedy was interviewed by Elizabeth Vargas on News Nation. The relevant portion of the interview is transcribed below:

> KENNEDY: I don't want to get rid of vaccines. If you want to take a vaccine you should be able to do it and we need good science and that's all I've asked for.
>
> VARGAS: So what do you say to people, I mean it sounds like you're saying that every scientist, every government, our government, governments around the world, and doctors like Dr. Butts are all lying about vaccines.
>
> KENNEDY: I never said anything like that.

VARGAS: The AMA, the American Academy of Pediatrics, and the FDA says, and in fact on its website you can clearly see, they go through three stages of FDA testing against double-blind placebos. They already do that testing for vaccines.

KENNEDY: Elizabeth you can say that.

VARGAS: I'm not saying that the FDA is saying that.

KENEDY: No, the FDA is not saying that. They will not tell you that there's any vaccine that has ever undergone a long term placebo-controlled trial prior to licensure.

Kennedy is correct. The FDA's website makes no mention of *long-term*, inert, placebo-controlled trials . . . at least not that I was able to find. Rather, it states:

Vaccines, as with all products regulated by FDA, undergo a rigorous review of laboratory and clinical data to ensure the safety, efficacy, purity and potency of these products. Vaccines approved for marketing may also be required to undergo additional studies to further evaluate the vaccine and often to address specific questions about the vaccine's safety, effectiveness or possible side effects.

The apparent disconnect lies in the discrepancy between the scientific community's and Kennedy's respective definitions and interpretations of the terms "long-term" and "placebo-controlled." In this interview, it is as if Kennedy was speaking French, and Vargas, who was speaking German, incorrectly attributed meaning to Kennedy's words. We cannot engage in respectful vaccine discourse when we unwaveringly cling to our positions. Preoccupied with playing "gotcha," Vargas refused to listen to the specific verbiage Kennedy used.

To the best of my knowledge and research, Kennedy correctly points out that there have been no *inert*, placebo-controlled trials prior to vaccine licensure for the standard and current iterations of vaccines on the pediatric schedule. The evidence demonstrates that placebo-controlled trials have occurred, but these do not use *inert* placebos. Kennedy is, of course, referring to the flawed "turtles all the way down" method of testing vaccines, whereby the comparison group receives an adjuvant or another vaccine. This masks the potential side effects that could be attributable to the ingredient itself, leading to skewed results and misinterpretation of safety data.

Kennedy's statements do, however, oversimplify the issues. He makes the blanket assertion that no placebo-controlled trials exist. In reality, such trials do exist. They just may not align with his specific expectations regarding duration or placebo type. This distinction is critical to comprehensively understanding and addressing vaccine safety concerns. Ultimately, Kennedy has identified possible flaws in the mechanisms currently utilized to determine vaccine safety and efficacy, demanding more stringent protocols to address potential public health consequences.

Science is rooted in inquiry. Science is mutable. Merely urging further safety testing is *not* anti-science. It *is* science. The medical community will, no doubt, point out that the call for further safety testing implies that vaccines are unsafe, which, in turn, promotes vaccine hesitancy. It may further argue that no additional testing is necessary when vaccines have already been proven safe. Sweeping justifiable safety concerns under the rug does not negate them. *The solution is not to silence those who push for more rigorous safety testing; it is to provide better safety testing.* In the face of emerging data, science asks questions it may not have previously considered, tests hypotheses, and revises conclusions based on new evidence. Thalidomide, Vioxx, and the DTP and rotavirus vaccines are a mere few among many examples that underscore this principle. Science requires the ongoing evaluation of the safety of medical interventions even after their approval, particularly when so many echo similar concerns around severe reactions. Demanding more rigorous testing reflects a commitment to evidence-based decision-making. Labeling anyone who questions vaccine safety as anti-vax deters the critical thinking and open inquiry upon which science is fundamentally based.

Oversimplifying an issue as complex as vaccines is dangerous. People are less likely to trust public health institutions when they feel their rational concerns are dismissed. The current approach precipitates a deeper distrust of the medical community. Moreover, labeling individuals as anti-vax could cause them to seek validation in spaces that may lack scientific rigor, deepening polarization.

Thoughtful critique improves vaccine design, safety, efficacy, testing protocols, and communication. This is achieved only by acknowledging valid concerns, as opposed to rejecting them. But how do we maintain trust in vaccines while simultaneously admitting that more rigorous safety testing may be appropriate? This question seemingly answers itself. Performing further safety testing *will* instill greater trust in vaccines. The medical community must recognize that questioning safety does not equate to opposition. We must willingly discuss all existing evidence and testing processes transparently, hear criticisms, and candidly admit the shortcomings in the data. In my opinion and based on my research, severe deficiencies and gaps do, in fact, exist. We must invite critical analysis and shared understanding, avoiding polarizing terms like "anti-vax" and "conspiracy theorist" that deter meaningful discourse. Kennedy beautifully said, "We have to love our children more than we hate each other." I could not agree more. Public health is advanced through constructive engagement, not suppression. We must come together for our children.

IS THERE A LINK BETWEEN VACCINES AND ASTHMA, ALLERGIES, AND ECZEMA?

You cannot see what you don't look for.

—DARREN HARDY

In researching this book, I reviewed and tried to make sense of the vast gamut of vaccine books, literature, and studies on both sides of the spectrum. Candidly, rather than provide me with the clarity I sought, they left me more confused. Whereas one source cherry-picks data to neatly fit a particular bias, another source cherry-picks alternate data to conform to a different bias. For instance, in his book, pediatrician and internationally recognized expert in the fields of virology and immunology, Paul Offit, MD, masterfully provides a comprehensive inventory of studies that show no link between vaccines and long-term chronic conditions such as asthma and allergies. In stark contrast (and what feels like entering the twilight zone), medical research journalist and Director of the Thinktwice Global Vaccine Institute, Neil Z. Miller, paints a completely antithetical picture, leaving me genuinely questioning whether Offit and Miller live in parallel universes. The arguments presented by each are equally compelling. Of course, their competing and even contradictory positions cannot both be concurrently true.

Like a vaccine Goldilocks, my mission was to uncover data that was neither "too hot" nor "too cold," but "just right"—the unfiltered truth, free from bias—to get to the bottom of the critical question: Do vaccines cause or contribute to chronic conditions? First, I looked at statistics and existing scientific research. I quickly realized that the extensive list of chronic diseases potentially attributable to vaccines rendered it impractical to cover them all. I chose, instead, to focus on three prevalent chronic conditions— asthma, allergies, and eczema—to lend some insight into the relationship between vaccines and chronic diseases.

Those who argue that vaccines cause a slew of long-term, adverse health consequences typically point to the increase in conditions such as eczema, allergies, and asthma over the last few decades.

In the past fifty years, eczema rates have tripled. In the 1960s, eczema affected approximately 5% of children in industrialized countries. Today it affects around 15–20% of children. In the United States, the rates of eczema in children rose from 7.9% in 1997 to 12.6% in 2018.

Over the past fifty years, asthma rates have significantly increased in the United States, from about 3% of children in the 1960s, to roughly 5.5% in 1996, to about 8.7% in 2022, reflecting nearly a tripling in prevalence. Globally, asthma has been on the rise, predominantly in urban and industrialized regions.

The incidences of allergic conditions, like food allergies and hay fever, are climbing as well. Up by 50% between 1997 and 2011, and again up by 50% between 2007 and 2021, allergic conditions among US children are becoming more commonplace. According to the CDC, in 2021, 27.2% of all children were diagnosed with one or more allergic conditions, with seasonal allergies accounting for 18.9% and food allergies accounting for 5.8% of all allergies. In England, food allergies in children under five increased from 1.2% in 2008 to 4% in 2018. In the 1950s, peanut allergies were almost unheard of. Now they affect about 2.5% of US children. In the United States, the prevalence of self-reported peanut or tree nut allergy in children more than tripled between 1997 and 2008.

The relationship between vaccines, allergies, and asthma has been the subject of extensive debate, with the majority of evidence finding no causal link between vaccination and the development of these conditions. Early concerns stemmed from smaller studies that suggested possible associations; these findings were often limited by confounding factors, such as genetic predispositions, environmental exposures, or parental health-seeking behaviors. A 2002 report from the IOM thoroughly reviewed the evidence and concluded that vaccines are not associated with the development of asthma or allergies.

More recent large-scale studies (among them, those using Scandinavian registries and US-based datasets) have reinforced these findings, showing no significant increase in risk. Furthermore, some evidence indicates that vaccines—namely, influenza vaccines—may actually have protective effects by preventing respiratory infections known to exacerbate asthma symptoms and potentially contributing to allergy sensitization.

From these studies, I next turned my attention to Offit's book *Vaccines and Your Family*. In the section conveniently entitled "Do Vaccines Cause Allergies or Asthma," Offit details a number of major studies, including, just by way of example, one that followed more than 18,000 children between 1991 and 1997 and another consisting of 600 children. Offit concluded: "Taken together, these studies show that vaccines do not cause allergies or asthma." There you have it. It doesn't get more emphatic than this.

If you stopped reading here, you would most certainly be left with the impression that the scientific consensus on this issue is that vaccines do not contribute to these chronic conditions. However, as we step into the twilight zone, Miller and Kennedy's (along with several other books and resources) paint a drastically different picture. We are inundated with a slew of cherry-picked—albeit not necessarily less legitimate—studies.

Conspicuously absent from Offit's book is a 2008 study published by McDonald et al. in the *Journal of Allergy and Clinical Immunology*, which examined the potential link between early vaccination with DTaP and the risk of developing asthma in children. The study found that children who received the DTaP vaccine earlier might be at a higher risk of developing asthma compared to those who were vaccinated later. The study further explored whether the timing of childhood DPT immunizations influenced the development of asthma by age seven. It analyzed a cohort of 11,531 children in Manitoba, born in 1995, using their complete immunization and health records. The results showed that delaying the first dose of whole-cell DPT by more than two months reduced the risk of asthma by half, while delays in all three doses further decreased the likelihood of asthma. The study concluded that a delay in the administration of DPT immunizations was negatively associated with asthma development, though the underlying mechanism requires further research.

Using data from the National Health and Nutrition Examination Survey, another study, this one published by E. L. Hurwitz et al., examined the DTP or tetanus vaccination, lifetime allergy history, and allergy symptoms in infants aged two months through adolescents aged sixteen years over the course of twelve months. The study found that the likelihood of having a history of asthma was twice as great among vaccinated subjects than among unvaccinated subjects. The odds of having had any allergy-related respiratory symptoms over the course of twelve months were 63% greater among vaccinated subjects than unvaccinated subjects. The associations between vaccination and subsequent allergies and symptoms were greatest among children five through ten years of age.

A 2023 study by Matthew Daley et al., published in *Acad Pediatrics*, looked at over 326,000 children. It found that about 4.4% of these children had eczema. They compared the amount of aluminum to which these children were exposed from vaccines. Children with eczema had slightly more aluminum exposure than those with no exposure. The study found that for every 1 mg increase in aluminum exposure, the risk of developing persistent asthma increased slightly both for children with and without eczema. (Notably, one of the coauthors of this study was Frank DeStefano. Keep his name in mind as we discuss him in connection with several autism studies in a coming chapter.)

A 2004 study, published in the *American Journal of Public Health*, examined the health records of 29,238 children between birth and eleven years of age. The study found that children vaccinated with DPPT (diphtheria, polio, pertussis, tetanus) versus children unvaccinated with DPPT were fourteen times more likely to develop asthma and nine times more likely to be diagnosed with eczema. The study further found that children vaccinated with MMR were 3.5 times more likely to develop asthma and 4.6 times more likely to develop eczema. After adjusting the results to account for the fact that unvaccinated children had fewer doctor visits and, therefore, theoretically fewer opportunities to be diagnosed, the authors concluded that vaccines were not a risk factor for allergic disease. While fewer visits could equate to fewer opportunities for diagnosis, it also suggests that the symptoms of asthma, allergies, or eczema, if sufficiently severe, would warrant a visit with the physician, which, in turn, would result in a diagnosis. Is it possible that these children who visited the doctor with less frequency were just healthier?

A 2005 study conducted by S. A. Bremner et al., published in *Archives of Disease in Childhood*, analyzed two large UK databases with health records of over 116,000 children to investigate whether the timing of DTP, MMR, and BCG vaccinations influences the risk of developing hay fever. The researchers concluded that immunization against DTP or MMR does not increase the risk of hay fever. Their findings *did* reveal notable timing-related differences. Children who received their third DTP shot after their first birthday had a 40% reduced risk of developing hay fever compared to those vaccinated by five months of age. Similarly, children who delayed their first MMR shot until after two years of age had a 38% reduced risk of hay fever compared to those vaccinated by fourteen months. In contrast, children who received a BCG vaccine before their second birthday had a significantly increased risk of developing hay fever compared to those who never received it or were vaccinated later. Adjustments for the frequency of health-care visits did not alter these results, underscoring the robustness of the findings. The authors stated: "The finding of a protective effect of late immunization was unexpected, but was consistent in the two databases; a powerful indication that the findings are not artifacts of a specific method of recording."

Yet another study, this one conducted in 2005 by Rachel Enriquez et al., which was published in the *Journal of Allergy and Clinical Immunology*, investigated the association between childhood vaccination and atopic diseases, analyzing survey responses from 1,177 children, including 515 who were never vaccinated, 423 who were partially vaccinated, and 239 who were fully vaccinated. The findings revealed a significant negative association between vaccination refusal and self-reported asthma, hay fever, and eczema, particularly among children without a family history of these conditions or without antibiotic exposure during infancy. For instance, parents of unvaccinated children were ten times less likely to report hay fever, and nonvaccinating parents were 2.5 times less likely to report eczema or wheezing.

Are you as perplexed as I am? I shared these several studies *not* to posit that Miller, Kennedy, and others like them are right but to point out that a counter-perspective to Offit, the CDC, and the IOM (among others) exists, and it is backed by legitimate research. Moreover, it illustrates the danger inherent to selecting research to accommodate one's bias. The studies shared by Miller, Kennedy, and others, while compelling evidence in support of their positions, conflict with the equally compelling studies shared by Offit, the CDC, and various prominent vaccine advocates. If someone read a singular book or referenced a singular source, he or she would be convinced of the author's position yet remain blissfully unaware of the counternarrative. How are concerned parents to make informed decisions when they are spoon-fed carefully curated, as opposed to *all* available information? As if this was not sufficiently confusing, the research appears to reinforce *both* positions. So what are we to think?

For now the scientific community agrees that vaccines are not associated with allergies, eczema, or asthma. Research has identified several factors that may contribute to these conditions. Similar to the way early exposure to allergens or irritants—such as pollen, pet dander, and dust mites—may cause allergies, asthma, and even eczema, genetic predisposition, too, plays a significant role in their development. Environmental pollutants, like tobacco smoke and air pollution, are also contributors. Additionally, dietary factors during early childhood, the use of antibiotics, and disruptions to the microbiome may influence the risk of developing these conditions. Finally, modern hygiene practices, which reduce exposure to beneficial microorganisms, have been proposed as a potential factor under the hygiene hypothesis, suggesting that less microbial exposure might lead to immune dysregulation and higher susceptibility to allergic diseases. Several studies have shown that children raised on farms tend to have lower rates of allergies and asthma compared to those in urban environments. This is believed to be due to early and regular exposure to diverse microbes found in farm soil, animals, and unprocessed foods, which help strengthen the immune system.

In fact, the majority of the most recent large-scale epidemiological studies have found no consistent link between vaccines and increased rates of allergies, asthma, or autoimmune diseases. One such example is a 2021 meta-analysis, published in the journal *Vaccine*, that looked at thirty-seven studies. It concluded that no vaccine regimens or single vaccines were associated with an increased likelihood of developing atopic dermatitis (eczema).

If making sense of the seemingly conflicting data feels as though you're back at that riveting (and frustrating) tennis match, you're not alone.

Chronic conditions are invariably on the rise. According to the current scientific consensus, these conditions are not attributed to vaccines. Yet we have not been offered any definitive alternate explanation for the rising rates of asthma, allergies, and eczema. The studies referenced above are published in reputable journals. Although some diverge from the pervasive scientific understanding, they provide valuable insights into the timing of vaccination and potential health consequences. For instance, some data suggest that delayed vaccination reduces the risk for certain conditions, such as asthma or hay fever. These are the types of questions we should continue to explore—not to frame vaccines as inherently good or bad, but to determine whether adjusting the timing of particular vaccines might reduce the risk of chronic conditions. Posing such questions results in a more balanced approach—still reducing the risk of infection from vaccine-preventable diseases while mitigating conditions potentially associated with them.

At this point, I can't help thinking that our understanding of the relationship between vaccines and risk is incomplete. If we are to advance our scientific knowledge *and* also foster public trust and safety in vaccination programs, humility and vaccine science must go hand in hand.

TOO MANY POKES?

There is no upper limit for the number of vaccines that can be administered during one visit. ACIP and AAP consistently recommend that all needed vaccines be administered during an office visit. Vaccination should not be deferred because multiple vaccines are needed.

—IMMUNIZE.ORG

We've all heard the adage "It's possible to have too much of a good thing." Though in the opinion of Immunize.org, a website developed in consultation with the CDC, "There is no upper limit for the number of vaccines that can be administered during one visit." According to a 2002 article authored by Offit and published in *Pediatrics*, "Each infant would have the theoretical capacity to respond to about 10,000 vaccines at any one time." In his 2003 book, *Vaccines: What You Should Know*, Offit professed, "The vaccines given in the first two years of life are literally a raindrop in the ocean of what infants' immune systems successfully encounter in their environment every day." It turns out that, unlike other good things, such as dessert and vacation, it is nearly impossible to have too many vaccines. But is this true? Is there a point at which too many vaccines can be administered at a singular visit or cumulatively spaced out over multiple visits? Parents grappling with the growing number of vaccines on the recommended schedule frequently ask precisely such questions.

On an episode of his podcast, *Dark Horse*, brilliant author, speaker, and professor of evolutionary biology, Bret Weinstein, stated:

> We are very likely to discover that vaccines have a place but that the technology by which they are produced is very important and we've made wrong turns.
>
> We've also made an error thinking that we should be vaccinating against any disease for which we can come up with a useful inoculation and we've also had our mechanisms for testing safety and effectiveness gamed by people with a perverse incentive because they're making money.
>
> My position. Antibiotics and vaccines are a precious technology that must be deployed very carefully for benefit to exceed harm and that the Willy-nilly use of antibiotics and vaccines will be recorded as a great error of medicine.

While this sentiment may (and no doubt will) be construed as anti-vax, in reality, it speaks to the growing concern over the increasing number of vaccines that continue to be added to the schedule.

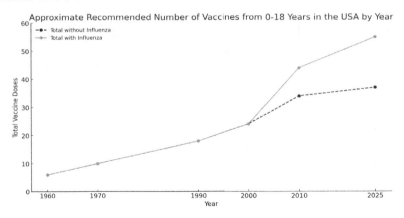

Approximate Recommended Number of Vaccines from 0-18 Years in the USA by Year

1960: 1 Smallpox, 1 Vitamin K, 4 DTP (6 total)

1970: 1 Smallpox, 1 Vitamin K, 4 DTP, 3 OPV, 1 MMR (10 total)

1990: 1 Vitamin K, 4 DTP, 4 Hib, 4 OPV/IPV, 3 Hep B, 2 MMR (18 total)

2000: 1 Vitamin K, 5 DTaP, 4 Hib, 4 IPV, 3 Hep B, 4 PCV, 2 MMR, 1 Var (24 total)

2010: 1 Vitamin K, 5 DTaP, 1 Tdap, 4 Hib, 4 IPV, 3 Hep B, 3 Rotavirus, 4 PCV, 2 MMR, 2 Var, 2 MCV, 3 HPV (34 total)

2025: 1 Vitamin K, 1 RSV, 5 DTaP, 1 Tdap, 4 Hib, 4 IPV, 3 Hep B, 3 Rotavirus, 4 PCV, 2 MMR, 2 Var, 2 MCV, 2 HPV, 3 CV19—primary series (37 total)

*Annual influenza recommendation began in 2008 for six month to eighteen years (two doses in first year)

**Total number of vaccinations is lower if combination vaccines are used (such as Pentacel-DTaP/Hib/IPV)

Currently, a six-month-old infant visiting his or her pediatrician during the winter season could receive all the following vaccines on the same day:

- Shot 1: *VAXELIS* (combines DTaP, Hib, IPV, HepB)
- Shot 2: *PCV* (pneumococcal)
- Shot 3: *Rotavirus*
- Shot 4: *RSV*
- Shot 5: *Influenza*
- Shot 6: *COVID-19*

Yes, you counted correctly: That is six vaccines in a single visit, one of which is a combination shot consisting of six antigens. These vaccines are designed to and, no doubt, *do* protect against serious illnesses. The concern lies in balancing protection with a child's immune response to so many simultaneous shots. Some parents and experts wonder whether spacing out vaccines could reduce the risk of side effects and better support children's developing immune systems.

We are repeatedly reassured that individual vaccines are rigorously tested and, therefore, safe. Yet we know that individual vaccines are often studied in isolation or in comparison to earlier versions of the same or similar vaccines. In some cases, clinical trials do test vaccines administered concomitantly with other vaccines typically given at the same time. To my knowledge, the entire vaccination schedule in its totality (including all doses and combinations administered as recommended) has never been rigorously studied, leaving unanswered questions about the cumulative effects of multiple vaccines given simultaneously or in quick succession.

Unless you are one of those unwaveringly clinging to your pitchfork, by now you (hopefully) know I pose such questions *not* to promote vaccine hesitancy but to demand accountability. How can we categorically declare something safe unless we test it in the way it is actually used? This is not to say administering multiple shots in a singular visit is unsafe or that administering one vaccine at a time is safer than multiple on the same day. In weighing the benefits against the risks, the current schedule may very well be the overall safest possible. We simply don't know . . . because we haven't studied it.

Further complicating the discussion is the fact that, from time to time, new vaccines are added to the schedule. Each new vaccine has the potential to change the equation in ways we do not fully comprehend. There are also multiple versions of the same vaccines, produced by different manufacturers. Are all vaccines equally safe in combination with one another? Is it truly a mix and match that deserves no thought or safety comparison testing? Physiological responses to vaccines may differ when multiple immunizations are successively administered in combination versus when they are spaced out. For instance, the combination of Daptacel and RECOMBIVAX HB may have a worse safety profile than the combination of Daptacel and ENGERIX-B. Perhaps adding MMR II to the mix increases the risk of febrile seizures. You would want to know whether the act of combining certain vaccines increased the risk of adverse events, right?

The safety of giving four or more vaccines in a single day, which is common practice under the current schedule, is a question that remains largely unexplored. If we are comfortable giving six vaccines in one day, where do we draw the line? What about ten vaccines? Or twenty? These numbers may seem relatively innocuous. But what if I told you that the CDC recommended fifty shots in a single visit?

I use this admittedly absurd hypothetical to provoke thought. Offit, however, did not think it was absurd when he discussed the theoretical capacity of an infant to respond to ten thousand vaccines at one time. According to a number of prominent vaccine educators, there is no upper limit of vaccines that can be administered in one visit. By this rationale, giving fifty vaccines during one visit may not be as absurd as common sense seemingly dictates. In the face of accelerating vaccine development, could we one day encounter schedules when dozens of shots are given at once? Is there a biological or practical limit to the number of vaccines the human body can process safely at one time? When we confidently make blanket statements without first performing adequate research, we are doing a great disservice to our children and not furthering science.

Since I will undoubtedly be accused of, among other nefarious things, proposing an alternate schedule, here's the part where I pause to make explicitly clear: I *am* not *advocating that anyone follows a slow or alternate schedule.* (To those men in dark suits lurking behind the tinted windows of their black vehicles, there it is.) In fact, and I reiterate, I am not suggesting or recommending anything. Any decision to deviate from the CDC or your country's standard public health devised schedule should be made only after careful discussion with *your* physician. This book is not a replacement for, nor does it constitute, medical advice.

Now that we've gotten that out of the way (again), let's look at the 2009 Shneyer study, which examined the rate of side effects in children receiving the MMR vaccine and Pentacel (DTaP-Hib-IPV) vaccine either simultaneously or on separate days. Conducted in a primary care clinic in Israel, the study followed 191 infants born between 2004 and 2005. It found that children vaccinated with MMR and Pentacel separately had significantly fewer reported minor and moderate side effects (40%) compared to those vaccinated simultaneously (57%). Side effects included fever, rash, irritability, and local reactions. The authors suggested reconsidering the policy of concomitant vaccinations to minimize adverse effects. They also note the need to balance such concerns with timely immunization.

This study is one of the few that investigated slower vaccination schedules compared to the traditional, accelerated schedule. While in no way dispositive, it highlighted the growing need for large-scale, controlled trials to compare health outcomes across different vaccination approaches. Studies of this nature would help determine whether spacing out vaccines or giving fewer shots at one time may reduce the likelihood of adverse events without significantly increasing the risk of disease.

IS THERE SUCH A THING AS TOO MANY ANTIGENS?

Too much of anything isn't good for anyone.

—RAY BRADBURY

The Shneyer study and our conversation thus far have focused predominantly on the number of pokes. However, we know that combination shots, which are regularly administered, contain more than a single antigen, which begs the question: Is there an upper limit of the number of antigens that should be given during a single visit or even over the course of multiple visits? Is it possible that bombarding the immune system with too many antigens could have adverse health implications, particularly as we continue to add new vaccines to the schedule?

According to the CDC, "When a child has a cold, he or she is exposed to up to 10 antigens, and exposure to strep throat is about 25 to 50 antigens. Each vaccine in the childhood vaccination schedule has between 1-69 antigens. A child who receives all the recommended vaccines in the 2018 childhood immunization schedule may have been exposed to up to 320 antigens through vaccination by the age of 2." But what bearing, if any, do these numbers have on our health?

Over the past few decades, advancements in vaccine science have rendered it possible to develop vaccines that require fewer antigens to protect against a broader range of diseases. Modern vaccines use more precise components, such as specific proteins or sugars from pathogens, rather than whole-cell formulations. This improved technology reduces the number of antigens needed while maintaining or even enhancing the immune response. Additionally, combination vaccines, such as DTaP and MMR, protect against multiple diseases, with fewer injections and antigens, simplifying the immunization process.

In the past thirty years, vaccines have evolved significantly, with the goal of becoming safer and more efficient. For instance, the older whole-cell pertussis vaccine (DTP) used three thousand antigens from killed bacteria and had higher rates of side effects, like fever and swelling. In contrast, today's acellular pertussis vaccine (DTaP) contains just two to five purified antigens, greatly reducing side effects but still providing protection. Similarly, the oral polio vaccine (OPV) once used a weakened live virus, which carried with it the risk—albeit rare—of vaccine-derived polio. As we addressed earlier, between 1980 and 1992, 109 cases of vaccine-associated polio were reported in the United States—an average of 8.4 cases per year. During this interval, 262 million doses of OPV were distributed. The overall risk of vaccine-associated polio was 1 in 2.4 million doses distributed. In contrast, the inactivated polio vaccine (IPV) now uses a killed virus, entirely eliminating the risk of vaccine-associated polio. These advancements demonstrate the way modern vaccines have been refined to maximize safety.

Research consistently shows that vaccines containing multiple antigens do not lead to an increased risk of side effects compared to a monovalent vaccine, one that only targets one specific strain or type of virus or bacterium. A study published in *Pediatrics* found that the safety profiles of multivalent vaccines administered to infants and children were comparable to single-antigen vaccines. Research in the *Journal of Infectious Diseases* demonstrated that a pentavalent vaccine (one that protects against five diseases) for diphtheria, tetanus, pertussis, hepatitis B, and Hib was both immunogenic and safe, with no heightened adverse events. A review in *Vaccine* also assessed clinical data and found no significant link between the number of antigens in a vaccine and increased reactogenicity, further confirming the safety of multivalent vaccines.

In support of this position, scientists contend that we are daily exposed to many antigens—whether through the food we eat or the air we breathe. They maintain that our bodies can handle a few disease antigens delivered through a vaccine. To me, this argument oversimplifies the issue—namely, we do not have definitive evidence to support the conclusion that a natural antigen, encountered through touch or ingestion, is equivalent to an antigen in a vaccine. Injecting an antigen bypasses the skin or mucosal barriers, the natural entry points of the immune system. This may alter the way the body responds to it. The claim that the immune system can handle multiple antigens simultaneously may be true. Or it may not be. In my opinion, we lack sufficient research to fully and adequately comprehend the differences between natural exposure to antigens versus injecting them.

Moreover, the ingredients in a vaccine—including adjuvants, preservatives, and other components—could potentially affect the way the immune system responds to the antigen. Adjuvants are literally designed to bolster an immune response. These added substances are not present in natural exposures and may influence the overall immune reaction in ways we don't completely understand. For instance, a bacterium that normally lives harmlessly on the skin can cause disease if introduced into the wrong part of the body. Similarly, injecting an antigen may not exactly mimic the immune response triggered by a natural exposure.

The notion that children can handle unlimited vaccines assumes they can handle unlimited antigens. Yet this has not been entirely proven. Even assuming it is true, this perspective overlooks the potential cumulative effects of the other vaccine components, such as preservatives and adjuvants, which most certainly have some upper limit for safety. We cannot declare the immune system capable of processing an unlimited number of vaccines without fully considering the complexity of the way vaccines interact with the body.

Unfortunately, to date, no comprehensive study has been conducted to evaluate the cumulative effects of the full vaccination schedule versus alternative approaches. This lack of data leaves many parents and practitioners with unanswered questions.

TOO MUCH VOLUME PER INJECTION LOCATION?

Although the research emphasizes the safety of administering numerous shots and multiple antigens within a single visit, it overlooks another critical inquiry: With the current number of vaccines on the recommended schedule, is it possible that we may be injecting in excess of the recommended volume per injection site?

For infants and young children, the recommended maximum volume per injection site (i.e., the thigh or deltoid muscle) is 1 mL. For older children and adults, the maximum volume per injection site can be higher—up to 2 mL, depending on the vaccine and the size of the muscle. This is based on the capacity of the muscle tissue to safely absorb the vaccine and avoid excessive discomfort or complications like muscle damage.

When multiple vaccines are given at the same visit, health-care providers often use different sites. For instance, to ensure comfort for infants and avoid exceeding the maximum volume in one muscle, vaccines may, respectively, be given in each leg. The 1 mL limit per leg in infants is a general guideline to promote safety, comfort, and effective absorption of the vaccine. However, the RSV vaccine alone may contain a volume of 1 mL. Given the number of vaccines recommended per visit, we may plausibly run out of legs before we can administer the full battery of vaccines at the recommended volume.

These details, while subtle, are critical and generally go unnoticed in vaccine discussions. During my training, I don't recall ever being taught about maximum volume recommendation per injection site. With the addition of more vaccines and increased volumes, it's easy to exceed the recommended limit during a single visit. This oversight could inadvertently heighten the risk of side effects. Our objective should always be to minimize these risks and to never overlook their possibility.

ARE WE DOING ENOUGH TO ADDRESS THESE CONCERNS?

As a pediatrician and a parent, I get it: Practical considerations support giving multiple vaccines during a single visit. Parents of newborns are already asked to, virtually monthly, make the harrowing trek to the pediatrician's office. This is no easy task when every moment of those first few months revolves around naps, feeding schedules, and yes, basic survival. Leaving the house for an hour may require a level of packing more ambitious than a two-week European vacation.

Assuming these parents of newborns overcome this momentous feat and make it to their scheduled appointment, there is the added financial component. For many, additional visits means more co-pays, which also equates to higher coverage costs for insurance or government-subsidized health care. Packing multiple vaccines into a single visit successfully addresses these logistical and financial issues, but not the unknowns surrounding cumulative vaccine safety. This leaves a gap in trust for many families who are expected to give increasingly more shots as new vaccines are added to the schedule.

Parents stand in an unenviable position. Many of them feel as though they're "damned if they do and damned if they don't." In what is the ultimate catch-22, parents want to protect their child against the debilitating, life-threatening, and vaccine-preventable diseases; these *same* parents simultaneously want to protect their child against the potential serious side effects that vaccines may and have been known to cause. The impetus for questioning vaccines is not rooted in some anti-science ideology but, rather, in a parent's primordial urge to protect his or her child.

Until more research is conducted, the questions remain: How many vaccines are too many, and how do we ensure that we strike the right balance for the health and safety of all children? As physicians, we want to believe we know all there is to know about vaccines. However, maybe, just maybe, we do have more to learn. Even the most well-intentioned among us might be surprised by what we find.

16

AUTISM AND VACCINES: THE SCIENCE IS NOT SETTLED

Current Science shows that no child is autistic as a result of vaccination —it is simply impossible.

—ARTHUR L. CAPLAN

IN THE FOREWORD TO PETER HOTEZ'S BOOK, *VACCINES DID NOT CAUSE RACHEL'S AUTISM* (CAPLAN IS ALSO THE PROFESSOR OF BIOETHICS, DEPARTMENT OF POPULATION HEALTH, AND DIRECTOR OF DIVISION OF MEDICAL ETHICS AT NEW YORK UNIVERSITY SCHOOL OF MEDICINE)

We have finally arrived at the moment you have all been waiting for . . . (cue suspenseful music): autism.

Autism—or autism spectrum disorder (ASD)—is a complex neurodevelopmental condition characterized by challenges with social interaction, communication, and repetitive behaviors. The symptoms and their severity vary widely from individual to individual. According to CDC estimates, in 2025, roughly 1 in 31 children in the United States was diagnosed with ASD—this, up from 1 in 36 in 2024 and 1 in 150 children diagnosed with ASD approximately twenty years earlier. According to the most recent CDC estimates, in 2025, 1 in 12.5 boys in California were diagnosed with ASD. All the more disconcerting is the increasing severity of the symptoms. The CDC revealed that nearly two-thirds of children diagnosed with autism had severe or borderline intellectual disabilities. Although the specific cause or causes remain unknown, it is believed that ASD stems from the complex interplay of genetic and environmental factors that influence early brain development, including parental age, exposure to toxins, and genetic variations.

We *do* know that autism is one of the most controversial topics in the vaccine universe, if not the most controversial. People are either convinced that vaccines cause autism or adamant they don't, and each side will die on his or her respective hill.

When I set out to write this book, I expected to find a wide breadth of studies that would resolve this debate once and for all. I envisioned myself gallantly riding in on a white steed, cloaked in shining stethoscope and lab coat, to present you with a bevy of high-quality, randomized, controlled studies proving definitively that there is no correlation between vaccines and autism. As much as I covet this image (and using the word *gallant* to describe myself), the information I will instead present is far different from what I anticipated. What I found shocked me, as I suspect it will shock you. My toddler possesses an impressive flair for hyperbole; I, on the other hand, am far more pragmatic. When I say this may be one of the most astounding revelations of my life, I sincerely mean it.

I won't belabor the point: After extensive, painstaking research, I have determined that *the science on autism and vaccines is . . . not settled. I cannot conclude that vaccines don't cause autism.* In fact, based on the data available to me, I cannot make *any* categorical conclusions on this topic, nor do I believe anyone can. For myriad and obvious reasons, the former sentences are extremely difficult and troubling to write (and not just because the double negatives render them grammatically confusing).

Danish theologian and the father of existentialism, Søren Kierkegaard, said, "There are two ways to be fooled. One is to believe what isn't true; the other is to refuse to believe what is true." *We have been told that the link between vaccines and autism has been thoroughly studied and disproved. We have also been told that the link between vaccines and autism has been debunked. Based on the research I was able to find, as best as I can tell, neither of these statements is true.* In reality, the research on the link between vaccines and autism is relatively narrow in scope. As you will learn, the existing research that has been performed is, in my opinion, of moderate quality at best. It predominantly focuses on the correlation between autism and the MMR vaccine or autism and thimerosal. Little, if any, of the research looks at the correlation between autism and other childhood vaccines or other individual ingredients.

Medical doctors, our government, and vaccine manufacturers have repeatedly and emphatically reassured us that there is *no* connection between vaccines and autism. To suggest otherwise would automatically classify one a "conspiracy theorist"—or far worse, [insert your favorite pejorative here]. I scrupulously searched for any information that would disprove my findings.

I thought, *I must be missing something.*

Maybe I still am. I engaged in a level of self-doubt rivaled only by George McFly in *Back to the Future . . . before* he became cool and stood up to Biff. This isn't fearmongering. This is the preeminent research, readily available to anyone willing to look it up—and you *should.*

Earlier I explained that my epidemiological background perhaps best positions me to author this book. My training is deeply grounded in research. I know what to look for and the way to look for it; I know how most studies are conducted; I know the way to process data. I have authored articles in leading medical journals, including *Pediatrics, BMJ,* and *Obesity Facts.* I even published a meta-analysis literature review paper in the *Clinical Journal of Sports Medicine.* I am no stranger to this world but, rather, very much a part of it.

I approached this book—and this chapter in particular—from an epidemiological perspective. Welcome to Epidemiology 101: To definitively conclude that X does or does not cause Y (i.e., glucose control causes a reduction in long-term diabetes complications), an epidemiologist must draw on a *vast* body of research—ideally, randomized control trials that involve large populations. Such studies must consistently show the *same* results. An epidemiologist can scientifically determine causality only when he or she meets this extremely high burden of proof.

Studies that consist of small sample sizes, retrospective research, or prospective cohort studies, can lend insight into a strong correlation between X and Y. By providing increasing information and discussing a deeper understanding of biological plausibility, such studies may logically lead us toward a conclusion, though they do not generally allow us to decisively state a causative conclusion without further appropriate research.

Accordingly, if I were a researcher tasked with publishing a review of the scientific literature on the link between vaccines and autism, I *could not conclude anything* until I *first* looked at the double-blind, long-term, large population, controlled trials between vaccinated and unvaccinated children and then assessed the rates of autism in each. If my aim was to prove causation—to categorically conclude whether a link between vaccines and autism exists—I would conduct every conceivable randomized and nonrandomized clinical control trial. To demonstrate a *strong* association and correlation, I would review large-scale prospective studies, or alternatively, I would look to large-scale retrospective studies. I would scour any large dataset and compare vaccinated children to partially vaccinated children, to unvaccinated children. I would research and compare each individual vaccine, a combination of various vaccines, along with the full battery of vaccines on the schedule. I would run numerous studies and expect each to produce the *same* result. Only *then* would I be in the position to conclude one way or another with a high degree of confidence.

As we established, vaccines are the standard of care. Consequently, running randomized and blinded control trials that compare vaccinated and unvaccinated children is likely improbable, although, as I previously noted, voluntary participation could adequately address the ethical constraints. Assuming I was unable to study vaccinated and unvaccinated children in accordance with "gold standard" methods, I would perform large-scale studies that, ideally, look prospectively, but if not, then retrospectively, at autistic children to ascertain (1) whether these children received vaccines, (2) when they received them, and (3) how many they received. From what I can tell, no prospective or retrospective studies exist comparing the current list of vaccines on the CDC schedule against fully unvaccinated children. *There are no studies that explore the relationship between autism and all childhood vaccines administered concomitantly as opposed to individually.*

Further muddying the waters is the fact that, over the past several years, new vaccines have been added to the schedule. Given they were just recently introduced, we cannot draw any conclusions regarding their long-term implications. We have no idea whether they may contribute to autism many years down the road. This is not to say that they do. We simply don't know. Causation or even correlation between these newer vaccines and autism would *first* need to be studied.

The existing research on vaccines and autism primarily looks at the link between the MMR vaccine and autism and thimerosal and autism. These studies mainly compare children who received the MMR vaccine or thimerosal to children who received *other* vaccines on the schedule, as opposed to comparing them to unvaccinated children. Unless there's a secret stash of vaccine autism research hidden away somewhere, that's it!

The focus on the MMR vaccine is most likely attributable to a now-retracted 1998 paper, published by Andrew Wakefield et al. in *The Lancet*.

Wakefield's research showed a possible link between the MMR vaccine and autism. The study was later retracted due to alleged ethical violations, undisclosed financial conflicts of interest, and fraudulent data. As a result of this study, MMR vaccination rates precipitously dropped. Subsequently, the research heavily concentrated on debunking Wakefield's findings, leaving little research on any other vaccines.

Thereafter, concerns around mercury emerged. Thimerosal was implicated as the likely cause of autism. Research naturally turned to discrediting the claim that thimerosal caused autism. Despite having never been proven to cause autism, thimerosal was precautionarily removed from the regular childhood vaccines on the schedule.

To explain the way I arrived at these astonishing findings, I will walk you through my methodical process. My epidemiological background initially led me to a meta-analysis review article and all its referenced articles. A "meta-analysis" is a fancy term researchers use to say: "We examined data from a number of independent studies of the same subject, in order to determine overall trends." An ideal starting point, a meta-analysis explores a given question by reviewing only those studies the authors deem the best available and most appropriate on the topic. In short, the authors perform the quality control.

In the 2014 meta-analysis "Vaccines Are Not Associated with Autism: An Evidence-Based Meta-Analysis of Case Control and Cohort Studies," by Luke E. Taylor et al., the authors looked at data from five case control and five retrospective cohort studies to determine whether vaccines are linked to an increased risk of autism spectrum disorders. The meta-analysis details from the 2014 Taylor study may not be of tremendous interest to you. Nevertheless, in my commitment to thoroughly presenting all information, I will enumerate them for you:

First, the meta-analysis looked at a 2002 study entitled "A Population-Based Study of Measles, Mumps, and Rubella Vaccination and Autism," conducted by Kreesten Madsen, MD, et al. and published in the *New England Journal of Medicine*. This Danish retrospective cohort study of over 500,000 children found no increased risk of autism among children vaccinated with MMR compared to those not vaccinated with MMR.

Next, it looked at a 2003 study, published in *JAMA*, by Anders Hviid et al., which evaluated the association between thimerosal-containing vaccines and non-thimerosal-containing vaccines and autism, finding no increased risk.

A 2003 retrospective-cohort study by Thomas Verstraeten et al., published in *Pediatrics*, found no consistent association between thimerosal-containing vaccines and neurodevelopmental disorders, including autism.

A 2004 study by Nick Andrews et al., published in *Pediatrics*, was a retrospective cohort study conducted in the United Kingdom that assessed thimerosal exposure and developmental disorders, including autism. It found no evidence of a causal association.

A 2004 study published in *The Lancet* by Liam Smeeth et al. found no association between MMR vaccination and an increased risk of pervasive developmental disorders, including autism.

A 2004 US case-controlled study by Frank DeStefano, MD, et al., published in *Pediatrics*, found no difference in the age of MMR vaccination between children with autism and those without, suggesting no association.

A study out of Japan—this one, a retrospective cohort study from 2007—was conducted by Tokio Uchiyama et al. Published in the *Journal of Autism and Developmental Disorders*, it found no significant difference in the incidence of developing regressive phenotype of autism spectrum disorders between children vaccinated with the MMR vaccine and those who were not.

A 2010 study by Dorota Mrozek-Budzyn et al. found no association between MMR vaccination and autism.

A 2010 case-control study conducted by Cristofer S. Price et al., published in *Pediatrics*, found no association between prenatal and infant exposure to thimerosal-containing vaccines and immunoglobulins and the risk of autism spectrum disorder.

Finally, a 2012 case-control study, this one conducted by Yota Uno et al. in Japan, published in *Vaccine*, found no association between the combined MMR vaccination and the incidence of autism spectrum disorders in Japan.

Are we having a good time yet? Yes, going through the meta-analysis isn't all that exciting. Some (okay, most) may even call it tedious. But it's important. The studies examined in the 2014 Taylor meta-analysis focus chiefly on:
1. the link between the MMR vaccination and autism,
2. the impact of thimerosal exposure from vaccines on autism rates, and
3. the timing of vaccination and autism diagnosis.

This meta-analysis reveals several key takeaways. With the exception of the MMR vaccine, there appear to be no studies on the link between *other* vaccines and autism; with the exception of the impact of thimerosal exposure, there appear to be no studies on the impact other adjuvants or ingredients may have on autism rates. This is particularly interesting given that thimerosal has been removed from single-dose vaccines in the United States for two decades. None of these studies compare fully vaccinated children to unvaccinated children. Instead, they primarily evaluate the receipt of specific vaccines (i.e., MMR) or ingredients (i.e., thimerosal) and the autism rates in children who received them versus those who did not. As we have already addressed the limitations associated with conducting research this way, I will not elaborate on the shortcomings intrinsic to these findings.

Unsatisfied by the paltry results of my search thus far, I turned to two of the most acclaimed and well-respected studies for answers: the 2002 Madsen and the 2013 DeStefano studies.

The first of these studies—"A Population-Based Study of Measles, Mumps, and Rubella Vaccination and Autism"— was mentioned in the 2014 Taylor meta-analysis and published in *The New England Journal of Medicine* in 2002. The author, Kreesten Madsen, MD, and his colleagues conducted a comprehensive retrospective population-based cohort study in Denmark to investigate the potential association between the MMR vaccine and autism. The Madsen study, which totaled 537,303 participants, encompassed all children born in Denmark from January 1991 through December 1998. Vaccination data were obtained from the Danish National Board of Health, and autism diagnoses were sourced from the Danish Central Register.

The researchers compared the incidence of autism and other autism spectrum disorders between those children who were vaccinated with the MMR vaccine and those who were not. The study identified 316 children with a diagnosis of autistic disorder and 422 with a diagnosis of other autistic-spectrum disorders. The study further determined there was no association between the age at the time of vaccination, the time since vaccination or the date of vaccination, and the development of the autistic disorder.

Many institutions—among them, the CDC, WHO, and AAP—reference this study when discrediting claims of a link between *all* vaccines and autism—albeit, this study was clearly specific to the MMR vaccine and *not* a comparison of *all* vaccines. Most children in both the MMR vaccinated and unvaccinated groups still received the other childhood vaccines such as DTaP and polio.

In 1995, the Institute of Medicine (IOM) created the Vaccine Safety Forum to examine critical issues relevant to the safety of vaccines used in the United States and to discuss methods for improving vaccine safety and vaccination programs. The Madsen Study was so exalted that the IOM discussed it at length in chapter two of its 2011 report. In fact, the Madsen Study was *one of only five* vaccine-autism studies that met the quality threshold to be included in the IOM's report that year. You get the point. This seminal study is considered among the most reliable and compelling of its kind.

The Madsen study is heavily cited not just because it was published in the *New England Journal of Medicine*, a leading medical journal, but because it examined a large sample of children. A closer exploration curiously reveals that, although the records of over 500,000 children were looked at, *only a small portion of those records were used.* Specifically, the study looked at a mere 263 children of the total 440,655 who were vaccinated with MMR vaccine. It looked at just 53 children of the total 96,648 who were unvaccinated. The number 500,000 appears impressive in the media; the reality is, this study focused on just a small subset of children—hardly enough to make any definitive conclusions.

Furthermore, the children in the Madsen study still received their other vaccines. This study was not controlled. It was not prospective. While the subject of this study was the MMR (and not other vaccines) and despite that it claimed to account for additional confounders, this study is often (incorrectly) cited as evidence of no link between *any* vaccines and autism. Is it possible that there may have been a link between any of the other vaccines administered and autism or other autism spectrum disorders? We simply don't know. At best, this study is moderately good evidence against a link between MMR and autism. It did not explore other vaccines or their components in any way, so we cannot, nor do the authors conclude that other vaccines don't cause autism. The authors simply purport: "This study provides strong evidence against the hypothesis that MMR vaccination causes autism."

The other eminent study, the DeStefano study, published in the *Journal of Pediatrics*, was conducted in 2013 and is titled "Increasing Exposure to Antibody-Stimulating Proteins and Polysaccharides in Vaccines Is

Not Associated with Risk of Autism." The study evaluated whether the cumulative exposure to antigens from vaccines during the first two years of life is associated with the risk of developing autism spectrum disorder (ASD). The findings indicated no increased risk of ASD with higher antigen exposure, supporting the safety of the recommended immunization schedule. Analyzing data from 256 children with ASD and 752 children without ASD, the study assessed the total antigen exposure each child received through vaccinations.

This study has been widely used in the media to debunk the notion that too many vaccines cause autism. The nuance in the language here is noteworthy: The DeStefano study did not focus on the number of vaccines given; rather, it looked at the *number of antigens* in children with and without ASD.

The DeStefano study consisted mainly of children vaccinated according to the recommended immunization schedule during the 1990s, when both the DTP and DTaP vaccines were in use. Because the presence of antigens in the DTP vaccine are significantly higher than the presence of antigens in the DTaP vaccine (approximately 3,000 in DTP to DTaP 2-5), the antigen exposures among the vaccinated children varied. The higher antigen count was attributable largely to the DTP vaccine. Most or all the children in the study still received their other vaccines. Since a majority of children were vaccinated, the comparison was among vaccinated children with different levels of antigen exposure, *not between* vaccinated and unvaccinated children.

Narrow in its scope, this study virtually exclusively focused on antigens and ASD. But vaccines contain numerous other components, beyond antigens, that could potentially contribute to ASD. This study provides evidence that higher antigen exposure is not associated with an increased risk of ASD *within a vaccinated population*. Though not the intended focus of the study, it perhaps even shows that, within a vaccinated population, there is no increased risk of ASD in children who receive the DTP vaccine versus the DTaP vaccine. However, the study fundamentally fails to address several key issues—namely, the potential effects of other vaccine components, the comparison between vaccinated and completely unvaccinated children, and whether a specific antigen from one of the other administered vaccines increased the risk of ASD.

271

My expedition into the world of vaccine-autism research was taking me down an unexpected path. Where were all the studies that show vaccines don't cause autism? This couldn't be it. What once seemed like an effortless assignment morphed into a serious investigation. My search led me to several bellwether studies, frequently referenced in vaccine-autism research:

In 2019, Anders Hviid et al. published a study in the *Annals of Internal Medicine*, entitled "Measles, Mumps, Rubella Vaccination and Autism: A Nationwide Cohort Study." Hviid and his fellow researchers conducted a comprehensive nationwide cohort study in Denmark to investigate the potential association between the MMR vaccine and autism. The study included 657,461 children born between 1999 and 2010, with follow-up extending through August 2013. The findings revealed no increased risk of autism associated with the MMR vaccine.

The study concluded:

> MMR vaccination does not increase the risk for autism, does not trigger autism in susceptible children, and is not associated with clustering of autism cases after vaccination. These results provide evidence supporting the safety of the MMR vaccine concerning autism risk.

While this is yet another excellent study on the MMR vaccine and its correlation to autism—or lack thereof—the study fails to address *all vaccines* and autism.

What I found next left me in utter disbelief: I read a 2014 review study on vaccine safety, in *Pediatrics*, "Safety of Vaccines Used for Routine Immunization of US Children: A Systematic Review," authored by Margaret Maglione et al. In the article, the word *autism* is repeated *nine* times. The first mention of *autism* can be found in the abstract:

> There is strong evidence that MMR vaccine is not associated with autism.

Autism is mentioned for the second time in the intro section:

> In addition, although multiple large studies have confirmed the lack of association between MMR and autism, parental worries about the safety of vaccines persist.

It appears for the third time in relation to the IOM report:

> They found the evidence 'favors rejection' of a causal relationship between MMR and autism.

Autism is again repeated twice in reference to the 2012 Uno study (noted earlier in this chapter). Finally, it pops up twice in the conclusion, where the authors state:

> Our findings support the following IOM results . . . MMR vaccine is not associated with autism.

For those with arithmetic skills similar to mine, that was only seven mentions. So what about the other two? The Maglione study goes on to cite a 2010 Gallagher and Goodman secondary analysis of the National Health Interview Survey conducted on 7,074 boys born prior to 1999, in which vaccination status and health outcomes were reported by parents. This survey showed:

> The results were *significant for the risk of autism in children who received their first dose of hepatitis B vaccine during the first month of life* (Odds Ratio 3.00, 95% Confidence Interval 1.11-8.13), compared with those who received the vaccination after the first month of life or not at all.

Yes, you read that correctly . . . although I wasn't sure I had. Earlier, I shared that I am not prone to hyperbole. So when I say my jaw almost hit the floor, you can be assured I was genuinely astounded. Did I miss something? I read and reread (and reread it again). Presumably, in authoring this review, the ten researchers involved in it fastidiously pored over all the available literature on autism and vaccine-adverse events. The study was submitted to *Pediatrics*, one of the most highly respected journals in the field of pediatrics, where it was scrutinized by an editorial team.

Ultimately, the authors concluded: "We found evidence that some vaccines are associated with serious AEs [adverse events]; however, these events are extremely rare and must be weighed against the protective benefits that vaccines provide." As the conclusion appears to suggest, the authors of this paper seemingly believe the protections vaccines offer outweigh their risks. I feel comfortable assuming the report's authors do not fall into the anti-vax or vaccine-hesitant camps. The authors presented little research on autism, and the first (albeit brief) seven mentions of autism virtually exclusively focus on it in connection to the MMR vaccine. Of all the compelling studies they reviewed, these researchers deemed the 2010 Gallagher and Goodman study of sufficiently high quality to include in their report. And *this* study actually showed a *significant* risk for autism in children who received their first dose of hepatitis B vaccine during the first month of life compared with those who received it after the first month of life or not at all! What the f@$k is going on here? Is the science settled, or isn't it?

Another dead end. I had to look elsewhere. I needed to find the studies that had been hailed as the "gold standard" I was told about my entire medical training and career. As I collected my awestruck jaw from the floor, I next turned to the IOM reports, which are the reports generated by the IOM's Vaccine Safety Forum that examine critical issues relevant to the safety of vaccines used in the United States and address methods for improving the safety of vaccines and vaccination programs. In its 2011 report, the IOM concluded that the evidence favors rejection of a causal relationship between the MMR vaccine and autism. The report also mentioned another vaccine: DTaP. Conclusion 10.6 of the report states: "The evidence is inadequate to accept or reject a causal relationship between diphtheria toxoid, tetanus toxoid or acellular pertussis-containing vaccine and autism."

In its 2013 report, the IOM revealed that the federally recommended birth to six-year-old child vaccine schedule had *not* been fully scientifically evaluated and there was *not enough scientific evidence* for physician committees to determine if the childhood vaccine schedule is or is not associated with the development of the following brain and immune system disorders prevalent among children today:

- Asthma
- Atopy
- Allergy
- Autoimmunity
- *Autism*
- Learning disorders
- Communication disorders
- Developmental disorders
- Intellectual disability

- Attention deficit disorder
- Disruptive behavior disorder
- Tics and Tourette's syndrome
- Seizures
- Febrile seizures
- Epilepsy

This was getting bizarre. In its section on autism, the 2013 IOM report stated:

> The initial literature search identified 32 papers on the relationship between immunizations or vaccines and pervasive developmental disorder (PDD), which includes the diagnoses autistic spectrum disorder, autism, and Asperger's syndrome. After an initial review, a team of two IOM committee members determined that 12 papers focused on some aspect of the immunization schedule. Three of the papers either addressed only one vaccine or had methodological limitations. The other nine studies examined the association between thimerosal and autism and other neurodevelopmental problems. Five of the studies had serious methodological limitations and were not helpful with examination of the association between thimerosal and vaccines. Each of the other four papers might help with a study of the schedule.

This section concluded:

> In summary, the evidence of an association between autism and the overall immunization schedule is limited both in quantity and in quality and does not suggest a causal association. The committee found the literature to be most useful in suggesting study designs that might be adapted and extended for the committee's core task of suggesting further research.

There goes my jaw again. Should I see a mandibular specialist? This could not be correct. It's impossible. After taking some time to process the 2013 IOM report, I decided to hold off on that appointment with the oral surgeon and, instead, bought Peter Hotez's book *Vaccines Did Not Cause Rachel's Autism*.

Peter Hotez, MD, PhD, is the Texas Children's Hospital endowed chair in tropical pediatrics and the codirector of Texas Children's Hospital Center for Vaccine Development at Baylor College of Medicine. He is one of the foremost vaccinologists in the world. In his heartfelt and moving book, Hotez approaches the vaccine discussion by sharing his personal family struggles with his daughter, Rachel, who is diagnosed with autism. Hotez reveals both the tribulations and the love that the parents of an autistic child experience.

As the title promised, *Vaccines Did Not Cause Rachel's Autism* was surely the answer. I read it from cover to cover. Chapter eight is entitled, "Vaccines Don't Cause Autism: The Scientific Evidence." Yes! The unambiguous proclamation I was looking for—*the vaccine holy grail*, I thought. I voraciously pored over chapter eight. In it, Hotez discusses his own *PLOS* journal discussion article, a 2013 AAP article and citations to Madsen, Smeeth, Jain, Uno, Taylor, and Hviid (all of which I referenced earlier). He further mentioned a few studies on thimerosal, peripheral blood, increasing rates of autism in California, evolution of adjuvants, and several CDC websites. That's it.

I did look up the 2013 AAP article. I was taken to the updated web page on healthychildren.org. The web page references several more recent studies. The majority of the studies predate 2014 and review the existing literature (which I have also already cited in this chapter). The studies focus on the MMR vaccine or thimerosal, and again, none make any sort of comparison against unvaccinated children.

Unfortunately, *Vaccines Did Not Cause Rachel's Autism* was not the bonanza I expected. Rather, it was another dead end. I felt much like Princess Leah—except, my only hope was not Obi-Wan but the great Paul Offit. One of the most knowledgeable experts on the topic, Offit would, no doubt, be crowned "King of Vaccines" . . . if the position existed. So naturally, I purchased his most recent book, *Vaccines and Your Family*. Admittedly, I have the utmost respect for Offit. I was genuinely curious to learn his perspective. Of the vast body of vaccine literature I have encountered, *Vaccines and Your Family* is one of the most well-written books on the subject, especially if one seeks a thorough and articulate explanation of the CDC/AAP viewpoint. Among the six-foot-tall (and increasingly growing) tower of vaccine-related books I have read, Offit's, by far, is the best at presenting the mainstream perspective with intelligence and clarity.

However (and yes, there is a "however"), the narrative was sadly familiar. As I dug deeper into the book, specifically into the chapter addressing the question, "Do vaccines cause autism?" (which can be found on page 42 of my edition), I encountered more of the same. Between pages 44 and 47, Offit lists his references, conveniently dividing them into sections: studies on the MMR vaccine (pages 44–45), studies on thimerosal (pages 46–47), and one additional study by Smith (2010) under the section he calls "too many vaccines too early." Conspicuously absent from *Vaccines and Your Family* is a single reference to *any* other data or studies addressing hepatitis B, DTaP, Hib, IPV, PCV, rotavirus, RSV, influenza, Vitamin K, hepatitis A, varicella, or any combinations of these vaccines in relation to autism in children.

This struck me as odd—nay, astounding. If such studies existed, surely, someone as thorough and accomplished as Offit—head of the Vaccine Education Center at Children's Hospital of Philadelphia and one of, if not, the most prominent vaccinologists—would have mentioned them. He would have proudly and exhaustively recited the data or clinical trials supporting the safety of these vaccines in relation to autism because, of course, his brilliance and dedication to his field are unquestionable. The dearth of additional references calls into question the depth and scope of available research on the other childhood vaccines on the CDC schedule and their relationship to autism.

Where are the recent studies, you ask? Where are the studies on all the other vaccines? Where are the studies on the new vaccines and autism? Where are the studies on the adjuvants we currently use, as opposed to the one that has been mostly phased out?

In a recent interview, I used the word *autism*. The interview, which was posted on social media, was quickly identified by so-called fact-checkers as lacking "context." The post was permanently flagged and branded with a banner that reads, "See context added to this post"—inviting the poor, unsuspecting masses to click and view the *real*, unadulterated "science."

I wondered whether the information for which I had so desperately been searching was hiding right there in that banner. Perhaps those fact-checkers knew something that I, Offit, and Hotez didn't. Of course, I clicked on the banner, only to learn that the scientific consensus is that vaccines do not cause autism and that this has been proven. This wasn't some earth-shattering revelation. There was no new evidence. These fact-checkers were relying on the same old studies.

Apparently, the "context" missing from my post was as follows:

> Health Feedback would like you to know that, "Popular claim #1: Unvaccinated children have lower rates of autism than vaccinated children" is untrue.

I have *never* made the claim that "unvaccinated children have lower rates of autism than vaccinated children." Nowhere in this book have I purported any such thing, nor did I so much as insinuate it in the flagged post.

Next, these fact-checkers proudly asserted:

> A recurring claim is that the prevalence of autism is lower among the unvaccinated population . . . most of the studies investigating the alleged link between vaccines and autism didn't include a fully unvaccinated group. This allowed some to argue that it was possible that children who received no vaccines at all were less likely to develop autism than children who received any vaccine, and that such studies didn't allow researchers to identify such a difference.

Who are these fact-checkers, and how do I thank them for suggesting (even if unintentionally) ways to improve vaccine safety testing? You're right, fact-checkers. You will not find the answer if you do not study it. It seems that the additional context these fact-checkers felt so compelled to provide actually highlights the fundamental flaws in the way the research is currently conducted.

Comparing vaccinated individuals against other vaccinated individuals to determine whether vaccines cause autism is akin to studying the risk of anaphylaxis from salted peanuts and comparing only those who eat the salt to those who do not. When—not surprisingly—researchers find there is no increased risk of allergic reaction in those who eat the salt versus those who do not, the claim that there is no increased risk of allergic reaction from eating a salted peanut is obviously misleading. Needless to say, researchers would have to study the peanut itself.

The fact-checkers did cite several additional studies that I have not yet referenced. To provide you with all the context, I will list these studies for you. A 2013 study by Shahed Iqbal et al. (on which DeStefano was a coauthor) found no adverse associations between antigens received through vaccines in the first two years of life and neuropsychological outcomes in later childhood. This study, similar to the 2013 DeStefano study, focused on the link between the number of antigens and autism.

Another study compared children who received at least ten vaccines and children who received fewer than six vaccines within the first seven months of life. While the authors *did not look at autism diagnosis,* they found that the children within the most vaccinated group performed similarly or better in several neuropsychological tests, which assessed speech and languages, memory, behavior regulation, and tics.

We are asked to silently accept the unfounded conclusion that vaccines don't cause autism because they haven't been proven to cause autism. Plummeting deeper down this bizarre rabbit hole and still determined to find that research I've always been taught exists, I performed further PubMed searches. Nothing else substantial came up. To be precise, my November 11, 2024, PubMed search of vaccines and autism yielded the following results, in this order:

1. The Taylor meta-analysis (covered that)
2. The Hviid study (check)
3. The DeStefano study (yep)
4. A discussion article by Gabis
5. An article by Erdogan discussing COVID-19 vaccines inducing autism-like behaviors
6. An article by Godlee claiming that Wakefield's papers were fraudulent (no surprise here)
7. A discussion article by Gerber and Offit, "Vaccines and Autism: A Tale of Shifting Hypotheses" (read it)
8. The Madsen 2002 *NEJM* study (we covered that in depth)
9. Another study by Taylor from 1999 on the MMR vaccine and autism
10. Another article by DeStefano, this time a discussion article, "Vaccines and Autism: Evidence Does Not Support a Causal Association" (yes, yes, yes, we get it)
11. A 2011 study by Delong (which, interestingly, I did not expect to find in the top twenty), published in the *Journal Toxicology and Environmental Health*, discussing *a positive association between autism and vaccine uptake.* The authors stated: "A positive and statistically significant relationship was found: *The higher the proportion of children receiving recommended vaccinations, the higher was the prevalence of Autism*

or Speech Language impairment." The study concluded, "Although mercury has been removed from many vaccines, other culprits may link vaccines to autism. Further study into the relationship between vaccines and autism is warranted." (Hmmmm, okay . . . major head scratch)

12. A discussion article by Taylor from 2006 (uh-huh)

I'll stop there. The point is, if another significant article on the topic existed, it would most likely pop up in the search. It did not. Don't take my word for it though. Go to PubMed and search "vaccines and autism." If your results differ from mine, I invite you to contact me and show me where I got it wrong. I will humbly amend this chapter for reprint.

In summary, my search generated a number of articles on thimerosal and multiple *discussion-based* studies, mostly delineating the reasons vaccines are not related to autism. But where are the actual *studies* medicine has repeatedly assured us exist? Where are the clinical control trials? Where are the prospective studies on the vaccinated versus the unvaccinated? Where are the retrospective studies looking at fully unvaccinated kids? Where are the studies looking at large groups of autistic children that describe whether they were vaccinated and, if so, the number of vaccines each received, along with any noted differences between them and other children? Where are the studies that evaluate vaccines (other than the MMR) and autism? In the first year of life, a child receives many vaccines. The MMR is not one of them. In fact, in the United States, a child does not receive the MMR vaccine until he or she is at least one year old. How can we make any categorical statement about *all* vaccines when the focus of research has been predominantly on the MMR vaccine?

I do not deny there is a moderately wide body of research exclusively on the MMR vaccine. These studies, which are limited in their scope, tend to show that, among the children who received their other childhood vaccines, there is no increased risk of autism between those who received the MMR vaccine and those who did not. We don't have any randomized control trials on MMR and autism. Even among those studies touted as the most preeminent and frequently used to counter claims that vaccines may cause autism, we seemingly have good reason to question some of the findings.

Earlier we discussed one of the most purportedly notable studies in the field, the 2002 Madsen study. The authors of this study are Kreesten

Meldgaard Madsen, Anders Hviid, Mogens Vestergaard, Diana Schendel, Jan Wohlfahrt, Poul Thorsen, Jørn Olsen, and Mads Melbye.

Poul Thorsen, MD is the coauthor of several significant studies analyzing the relationship between vaccines and autism, including, among them, the 2002 Madsen Study. In 2011, Thorsen was indicted in the United States on charges of wire fraud and money laundering.

The indictment claims that between 2004 and 2010, Thorsen allegedly diverted for his personal use over one million dollars in grant money awarded by the CDC for his autism research. He is accused of submitting fraudulent invoices and diverting funds intended for research into his personal accounts.

As a result of these charges, Thorsen was placed on the Office of Inspector General's (OIG) "Most Wanted Fugitives" list. Per the US Department of Health and Human Services, Thorsen remains at large and is wanted.

Of course, Thorsen was merely one of many authors of the Madsen study. The apparent conflict of interest stemming from the allegations against Thorsen does not necessarily invalidate the research. It does raise an eyebrow, right?

As for the 2013 DeStefano study, the lead author, Frank DeStefano, MD, headed the CDC Immunization Safety Office and remains a prominent figure in vaccine safety at the CDC. In 2004, he was appointed acting chief of the Immunization Safety Branch of the National Immunization Program, now known as the National Center for Immunization and Respiratory Diseases. DeStefano has also served as the director of the Immunization Safety Office at the CDC.

At the time of publication, two-thirds of the study's authors were employees of the CDC. The study was funded by a contract from the CDC and Prevention to America's Health Insurance Plans (AHIP) and by subcontracts from AHIP to Abt Associates Inc. The researchers contended that the "findings and conclusions in this study are those of the authors and do not necessarily represent the official position of the CDC."

Despite their obvious affiliation with the agency that not only cofunded the study but by which a majority of the study's authors were employed, the authors declared *no conflicts of interest*. Again, this does not nullify the findings, though, in my opinion, this may not entirely qualify as "no conflict of interest."

In 2004, DeStefano conducted a study also examining the relationship between the MMR vaccine and autism. Published in *Pediatrics*, the study was coauthored by senior CDC scientist William W. Thompson, PhD. A decade later, Thompson publicly expressed concerns over the study's handling of data concerning African American children. In a statement released on August 27, 2014, Thompson revealed: "I regret that my coauthors and I omitted statistically significant information in our 2004 article published in the journal *Pediatrics*. *The omitted data suggested that African American males who received the MMR vaccine before age thirty-six months were at increased risk for autism.*" Thompson further indicated that some of the decisions regarding which findings to report were made *after* data collection. Ultimately, he felt that the final study protocol was not followed. He emphasized his belief in the overall benefits of vaccines while voicing his misgivings around the omission of relevant findings for specific subgroups.

You may also recall the 2019 Hviid study. Posing another potential conflict of interest, the primary funding sources for his study were the pharmaceutical company Novo Nordisk Foundation and the Danish Ministry of Health. (This is analogous to Pfizer and the CDC funding a US vaccine study, the outcome of which has tremendous public health implications.)

To be clear, I do believe the CDC should fund vaccine studies. However, we cannot ignore the unassailable fact that a CDC-funded vaccine study or vaccine research conducted by a CDC employee is inherently biased. If a noted anti-vaxer published a study linking vaccines to autism or other side effects, the headline would invariably read: "Anti-Vax Conspiracy-Theorist Published Research Showing X." We are human; we all have our biases. Realistically, how long do you think the head of the Immunization Safety Branch of the CDC would keep the position if he or she began presenting research showing that vaccines caused significant harm? You see the potential conflict of interest here, right? The CEO of a sugar company will never reveal that excessive sugar consumption is known to cause a bevy of health issues. A glyphosate salesman is unlikely to begin his presentation by sharing that the product has been linked to cancer. In the context of vaccines and autism, bias, specifically the source of and impetus for that bias, is significant.

Again, I found myself at another impasse, struggling to find my way through the mighty vaccine labyrinth but, instead, encountering one dead end after the next. In a last-ditch effort to restore glory to my name (or at the very least, not walk away with my tail between my legs), I searched a different way. I typed the words "autism etiology" into PubMed. What popped up? A long list of studies that looked into genetics and environment, none of which really covered vaccines. I searched "autism etiology and vaccines." The results were virtually identical to those yielded by "autism etiology."

I even looked to the Amish for answers. Due to their unique lifestyle and low reported prevalence of autism, the Amish are often part of the autism discussion. Some early reports claimed that autism rates were significantly lower in the Amish population, potentially linking its lack of routine vaccination to these reduced rates. There are fewer reports of autism among the Amish. Yet this may be related to various factors, including less access to health care, limited use of diagnostic tools, and the overall smaller population size. In a study of the Amish community, Frank Noonan, MD, noted that, while autism was rare, cases did exist among *both* vaccinated and unvaccinated children. The ostensibly lower rates of autism may be attributable to other factors: The Amish lifestyle, such as reduced exposure to environmental toxins, pesticides, processed foods, and screen time, is significantly different from mainstream society.

The research on autism rates within the Amish is not comprehensive, and most of the claims stem from anecdotal reports or smaller studies. There has been no large-scale, peer-reviewed study conclusively proving that lower vaccination rates are responsible for lower autism rates among the Amish . . . someone *should* do that research.

So maybe it's not my jaw that's the problem here. That fantasy where I heroically ride in on white steed and proclaim that there is no link between vaccines and autism has been dashed. Rather, I've landed myself in the unenviable position of . . . well, "villain." The ostensible mantra of the medical consortium is, "If you're not with us, you're against us."

But I'm *not* against medicine. I am against half-truths and outright lies by the people we trust with the health and safety of our children. When I was in residency, I would have eagerly joined the cohort of doctors clamoring for the opportunity to stomp out perceived vaccine misinformation and disinformation. Now I question the apparent witch hunt around studies that pose legitimate scientific inquiries.

Upon further investigation, it seems to me that Wakefield's studies were, indeed, fraudulent and, therefore, correctly debunked; I cannot say the same for the countless other discredited studies. I will not get into the details of such studies, because . . . well, medicine has obviously discredited them. The problem with discrediting inquiry that runs counter to scientific gospel is that it leaves us wondering whether it was discredited for its lack of quality or because it deviated from the sanctioned narrative. I can't help but wonder whether the effort to debunk such studies is indicative of some concerted effort to silence anyone who draws attention to the flaws in the existing evidence. (If I hadn't already been dubbed a "tinfoil-hat-wearing conspiracy theorist," this latter sentence should have successfully sealed the deal).

Though I am pleased to report my jaw remains intact, the rest of me stands before you completely baffled. In a letter sent by the Informed Consent Action Network (ICAN), an organization that advocates for informed consent regarding health interventions, to the US Department of Health and Human Services (HHS), ICAN requested clarification from the HHS regarding the scientific studies supporting the claim that "vaccines do not cause autism." This exchange occurred in the context of discussions about vaccine safety, particularly related to claims of a connection between vaccines and ASD. The ICAN letter read:

> Please confirm that HHS shall forthwith remove the claim that "Vaccines Do Not Cause Autism" from the CDC website, or alternatively, please identify the specific studies on which HHS bases its blanket claim that no vaccines cause autism?

In its January 19, 2018 response, the HHS wrote:

> Vaccines are held to strict standards of safety. Many studies have looked at whether there is a relationship between vaccines and autism spectrum disorder (ASD). These studies continue to show that vaccines do not cause ASD.

It seems we are being asked to accept the circuitous argument that vaccines don't cause autism because vaccines don't cause autism. Where exactly are those studies that show there is no relationship between *all* vaccines and ASD?

In the 2009 and 2010 Omnibus Autism Proceedings, which I previously referenced in connection with the legal history of vaccines, the US Court of Federal Claims evaluated over 5,000 claims alleging that vaccines, specifically the MMR and thimerosal-containing vaccines, caused autism. To manage these cases efficiently, the court selected six test cases, each examining one of the following three issues:

1. Whether the *combination* of the MMR and thimerosal-containing vaccines could cause autism. In 2009, the Special Masters concluded that the evidence did not support this claim.
2. Whether vaccines containing thimerosal could *independently* cause autism. The Special Masters found no credible evidence supporting this hypothesis.
3. Whether the MMR vaccine alone, without consideration of thimerosal, could lead to autism. Again, the Special Masters determined there was no causal link.

In the 2010 Omnibus decision, *Snyder v. Secretary of Health and Human Services*, Special Master Denise Vowell held: "Petitioners have failed to demonstrate that thimerosal-containing vaccines can contribute to causing immune dysfunction, or that the MMR vaccine can cause autism or autistic spectrum disorders." The Special Masters overseeing these respective Omnibus cases found that the scientific and medical evidence did not support the claims that the MMR vaccine, thimerosal-containing vaccines or a combination of both, caused autism.

Nowhere in the Omnibus proceedings did the court conclude that vaccines do not cause autism; rather, the court determined that, based on the legal standard of proof, the evidence presented did not demonstrate a causal link between the MMR vaccine and thimerosal-containing vaccines and autism. The court did not make any findings regarding *all* vaccines. The rulings were *specific* to one singular vaccine, MMR, and one singular ingredient, thimerosal. This distinction is, of course, crucial. The court's finding—that the MMR vaccine and thimerosal had not been proven to cause autism—is accurate. However, this is only part of the story. To truly answer a question, one must thoroughly investigate it. Without proper research, definitive conclusions cannot be drawn.

Consider historical examples: Smoking doesn't cause lung cancer, lead isn't neurotoxic, glyphosate is not carcinogenic, opioids are not addictive. These were widely accepted beliefs . . . until they weren't. Decades ago, these claims stood unchallenged because the necessary research had not yet been conducted. Once unmistakable patterns were identified, studies were performed, new evidence emerged, and these "truths" were reevaluated, often alongside significant legal and financial consequences.

A court's role is to assess available evidence under a defined standard of proof. Decades ago, a court would have declined to find that smoking causes or even contributes to lung cancer, a legally correct conclusion based on the evidence at the time. Once proper studies were completed, the narrative and public opinion shifted. The same principle applies here. Until rigorous, unbiased research on *all* vaccines and autism is conducted, we cannot make definitive claims regarding what vaccines do or do not cause.

On August 25, 2020, leading vaccinologist and professor of pediatrics at Vanderbilt, Kathryn Edwards, MD, was deposed by Attorney Aaron Siri. Edwards' list of credentials is quite impressive. In 1980, she joined the Vanderbilt Vaccine Program and has since led numerous critical vaccine studies. The following is an excerpt from the deposition transcript:

SIRI: Did the clinical trials relied upon to license the vaccines, many of which are still on the market today, were they designed to rule out that the vaccine causes autism?

EDWARDS: No. You badgered me into answering the question the way you want me to, but I think that that's probably the answer.

SIRI: In the expert disclosures for this case, it asserts that, among other things, you will testify that quote, "the issue of whether vaccines cause autism has been thoroughly researched and rejected." End Quote. It's your testimony that MMR vaccine cannot cause autism, that's correct?

EDWARDS: That's correct.

SIRI: It's your testimony that Hep B cannot cause autism?

EDWARDS: That's correct.

SIRI: It's your testimony that IPOL cannot cause autism?

EDWARDS: Yes.

SIRI: It's your testimony that Hib vaccine cannot cause autism?

EDWARDS: Yes.

SIRI: Your testimony that varicella vaccine cannot cause autism?

EDWARDS: Yes

SIRI: It's your testimony that Prevnar vaccine cannot cause autism?

EDWARDS: Yes.

SIRI: It's your testimony DTaP vaccine cannot cause autism?

EDWARDS: Yes.

SIRI: And you have a study that supports that DTaP doesn't cause autism?

EDWARDS: I do not have a study that DTaP causes autism. So I don't have either.

SIRI: Do you have any study one way or another on whether IPOL causes autism?

EDWARDS: No. I do not, sir.

SIRI: Do you have any study one way or another of whether ENGERIX-B causes autism?

EDWARDS: I do not have any evidence that it causes autism nor that it does not.

SIRI: And what about Hib titers vaccine. Any evidence one way or another whether it causes autism?

EDWARDS: No.

SIRI: And what about Prevnar vaccine? Any evidence one way or another?

EDWARDS: No, sir.

SIRI: And how about varicella vaccine?

EDWARDS: No, sir. No studies that say it does or no studies that say it doesn't.

Edwards confidently testified that vaccines do not cause autism. She simultaneously testified that there is no evidence that vaccines don't cause autism. (Joel screams internally.) Am I the only one astonished by this egregious disconnect?

At this point, you're probably frustrated. I know I am. You've just read through a lengthy and fairly complicated chapter (which commenced with suspenseful music, no less!) on one of the most eagerly anticipated subjects. And here we are, left with more questions than answers. Based on the research I have uncovered, I do not believe anyone can unequivocally conclude that vaccines do or do not cause autism.

In the end, one might make the case that the preponderance of research thus far leans in the direction that the MMR vaccine alone does not cause autism in vaccinated children. One could also reasonably claim that thimerosal in vaccines does not cause autism in vaccinated children, especially since it has been mostly phased out of vaccines, yet autism rates continue to rise. Even in the context of the MMR vaccine and thimerosal, there is little to (seemingly) no research comparing unvaccinated children to vaccinated ones. In the Maglione review article, other than the MMR vaccine, early hepatitis B vaccination is the only other mentioned in relation to autism, and it shows a three-times-odds ratio of *increased* autism.

Hotez attributes autism to differences in the brain—a certainly viable theory. Maybe autism is the result of an *in utero* insult. Perhaps it is the consequence of environmental exposures. However, nothing has definitively proven to me that vaccination cannot trigger the type of inflammation that ultimately damages or affects the brain, leading to the very changes contemplated by Hotez. I concede, this is mere speculation. Autism may have zero correlation to vaccines. Or vaccines could be a trigger in genetically susceptible children, lighting the proverbial match that stimulates a cascade.

I most certainly do not purport to ascribe a specific cause to autism. The disheartening fact remains, I don't know what causes it. Nobody does. Sure, there are lots of theories—some more sound or far-fetched than others. Vaccines are one theory. For now they remain merely that—a theory.

I *do* know that the rates of autism continue to increase. In California where I live, the rate of autism has skyrocketed to one in every twenty-two children, which is among the highest rates of autism in the world. Many are quick to credit "better diagnosis." Although increased awareness, improved testing, and diagnostic advances are certainly, in part, responsible for higher autism rates, these factors alone do not explain the meteoric rise in cases. Whatever the cause, we should resolutely refuse to overlook any potential risk factor, no matter how uncomfortable the results we uncover may be. I am left certain of only one thing: Vaccines should not be categorically ruled out because the science is *not* settled. We must get away from the circular thinking that vaccines are unrelated to autism because studies have not conclusively proven them to be a cause.

There is a viable solution. I propose that impartial researchers conduct prospective trials tracking children over at least a decade, to compare groups based on their vaccination choices: those who opted not to vaccinate, those who followed a delayed schedule, and those who adhered to the standard schedule. Because health-care visits often introduce confounding variables in vaccine research, the subjects of this study must be independently evaluated for autism every three to five years. The assumption that more frequent visits lead to more diagnoses does not account for the possibility that healthier children may not need to see a doctor as frequently. Therefore, the absence of a diagnosis at a doctor's visit does not necessarily indicate a missed autism diagnosis; it could simply mean the child was healthy and did not require a visit. These independent evaluations at regular intervals will obviate the number of health-care visits as a confounding variable.

Given that those who do not vaccinate may lead different lifestyles, this proposed study may prove less than perfect. At the very least, though, it would allow us to ascertain, at the five- and ten-year marks, whether an unvaccinated lifestyle influences autism diagnoses. This approach could provide clearer insights into the relationship between vaccination schedules and autism prevalence. In ten years' time, it would leave us with a far better understanding of whether there is any link between vaccines and autism. Don't our children deserve this?

I want to end this difficult chapter with a transcription of Brenda's story. Her story brings tears to my eyes, serving as a poetic reminder of the disconnect between scientific egoism and what is the palpable reality for so many parents. Medicine seems to have forgotten that it is inexorably intertwined with the human condition. We physicians are bestowed with the great honor and responsibility of caring for the sick, the vulnerable, and the healthy, who trust us not to adversely impact their well-being. Prioritizing dogma and rhetoric over patient welfare comes at too high a cost. Sadly, humility is one of the principles of the Hippocratic Oath that often goes overlooked. We must listen to moms and dads with empathy and compassion, parents who eagerly bring their children to the pediatrician's office to vaccinate and protect their children from potentially debilitating or fatal diseases, moms and dads *without* ulterior motives. I will refrain from offering any commentary on this excerpt. Instead, I leave it to you to draw your own conclusions:

We have beautiful triplets, we had two boys and a girl.

So we were going in on June 25th 2007. We [the triplets] were nine months and four days. We were to get the pneumococcal vaccine and we went in for a 10 a.m. appointment. They did Claire first and she got a really big red mark almost immediately on her legs, started screaming but that screaming kind of never really went away.

By noon we watched Claire, the only way we could describe it was her soul was sucked out of her body. She was literally the shell of a little person that we used to know. Her personality gone. All her reflex reflexes were gone, is what I've noticed. I'm an educational audiologist. So she stopped blinking, she stopped coughing, sneezing, yawning. Suck reflex was just gone. Everything was gone. She had a hard time taking her little Bubba and she acted deaf and blind. You could go near her and there was nobody home. All she wanted to do was stare at the ceiling fan in our dining room and so that was noon and I knew what I was witnessing. I've worked with autistic children before.

At 2:00 that day we lost Richie. We watched our first boy shut down.

They had full blown eye contact. They knew each other. They held hands constantly. Everything was a big giggle fest and we watched him shut off and the same thing happened. All of his reflexes disappeared and he acted like he couldn't hear. Completely stopped responding to their name and even their favorite songs and music.

All eyes were on Robbie. We were like "come on little buddy, hang on." And you could see his smile disappear, but he was still looking at us, still responding to his name and by 5:00 that night we watched Robbie slip away.

We were in shock. Everybody, our nanny, my family, we have many friends that are doctors, speech pathologists, sister-in-law is an occupational therapist, we all knew what normal was. We had normal fully developing children that morning and we now have three severely injured children that night.

We called immediately to report it. We brought them into the doctor's office. They did not file the report. We find out later that there was no report of any injuries with this vaccine. We received a phone call a week-and-a-half after the shot saying it was recalled for sterilization issues, but we were not to find out until seven years later what that actual contamination is in the shot.

A friend of ours who was a doctor was able to look up the shot and did find out that a two-year-old died from the lot number we got and they didn't want that to be public knowledge. So it wasn't something I could find out, it was only something a doctor was able to look up and still to this day it says no reported injuries to this vaccine.

There's absolutely no doubt in my mind that the vaccine was 100% the cause of them shutting off. We did nothing else that day. We did nothing before, nothing after it and all the neurologists we've seen since then, all the doctors we've seen, said it's just massive inflammatory response to, obviously, in this case, an environmental trigger.

We did see geneticists afterwards because some doctors pointed to us that it's genetic. And they said it was a one in four million chance that you would have two boys and a girl genetically shut off, all on the same day, within hours of each other.

It was 100% environmental and in our case, vaccine.

We were let go by our family practice because we were no longer going to continue vaccinating. So we were broken up with, in a nice breakup letter. (Transcribed excerpts from Brenda M. on michiganvaccineinjury.org)

17

SIDS LINK: A CENTURY OF CONTROVERSY

When a child loses his parent, they are called an orphan. When a spouse loses her or his partner, they are called a widow or widower. When parents lose their child, there isn't a word to describe them.

—RONALD REAGAN

You know that scene in Disney's 1937 version of *Snow White and the Seven Dwarves*, the one where Snow White runs through the haunted forest? The anthropomorphic branches claw at the hem of her dress; alligators menacingly chomp at her as she flounders out of a pond. No matter which way Snow White turns, she encounters one nightmare after another. Transitioning from our unsettling discussion of autism to a topic significantly more grim feels very much like stumbling through that terrifying forest. Far too horrific a thought to bear, even the name—Sudden Infant Death Syndrome (SIDS)—evokes a visceral response. And yet no discourse around vaccines would be complete without it.

SIDS is the unexplained death of a seemingly healthy baby less than a year old, usually during sleep. As they do with autism, people either adamantly insist vaccines cause SIDS or vehemently swear they do not. However, the subject is significantly more nuanced than either camp decisively proclaims it. The following tragic anecdote seems a fitting place to begin our conversation:

> On September 2, 2011, a healthy, happy, baby boy—J.B.—went to his Pediatrician's office for his four-month well child check-up. During the visit, he received all vaccines according to the CDC recommended schedule, including DTaP, IPV, PCV, Rotavirus and hepatitis B.

Later that evening, J.B. developed a fever and experienced restlessness. His parents administered Advil to manage the fever. The next morning, September 3, 2011, at approximately 4:00 a.m., due to a recurring fever, J.B. was given another dose of Advil. Later that day, J.B.'s father placed J.B. down for a nap. J.B. was laid on his back in his crib.

Shortly thereafter, J.B.'s mother found J.B. unresponsive on his right side. At 2:39 p.m., J.B.'s mother called 911 and initiated CPR. Emergency responders arrived promptly and transported J.B. to the hospital. Despite resuscitation efforts, J.B. was pronounced dead at 4:01 p.m.

The autopsy concluded that the cause of J.B.'s death was SIDS.

J.B.'s parents filed a petition under the Vaccine Injury Compensation Program (VICP), alleging that vaccinations caused their child's death. In the realm of vaccine injury litigation, J.B.'s case—*Boatmon v. Secretary of Health and Human Services*—is particularly notable. The Special Master initially ruled *in favor* of the J.B.'s parents, determining that the vaccines administered to J.B. substantially contributed to his death from SIDS. Upon review, the US Court of Federal Claims reversed the Special Master's decision, concluding that the evidence presented did not sufficiently establish a causal link between the vaccinations and J.B.'s death. This decision was later upheld by the US Court of Appeals for the Federal Circuit.

J.B.'s parents bore the burden of proof by presenting sound, reliable evidence demonstrating that vaccines were a substantial factor in causing their son's death. The US Court of Federal Claims reversed the Special Master's decision, holding that a temporal correlation between vaccination and SIDS alone is insufficient to establish causation without concrete evidence of the alleged underlying vulnerabilities or mechanisms. The court further found that the expert testimony lacked sufficient scientific backing to establish causation.

This heart-wrenching case reveals the complexities of this polarizing topic. For some, the timing and circumstances of J.B.'s death invariably lead to the conclusion that vaccines caused or contributed to J.B.'s untimely passing. For others, the counterargument is rooted in a broader understanding of SIDS—an inexplicably horrid condition, with no singular known cause. Vaccines are routinely administered, and SIDS occurs with certain frequency. Therefore, statistically speaking, some SIDS cases will inevitably coincide with vaccination without necessarily being caused by it. The case of J.B. forces us to grapple with these varying perspectives, highlighting the tension between correlation and causation under profoundly emotional circumstances.

In attempting to make sense of this topic, I first turned to an obvious starting point—the rates of SIDS. In 2022, 1,529 deaths in the United States were attributed to SIDS. This is equivalent to approximately four SIDS deaths each day. Children receive multiple rounds of vaccines in the first year. Inevitably, some cases of SIDS will occur on the same day or in close relation to vaccination.

Those who attribute autism or chronic diseases to vaccines conveniently note the corollary between the increased number of vaccines and increasing chronic disease rates. During the past few decades, the rate of SIDS has gone *down*. We know that the number of childhood vaccines on the CDC schedule has increased significantly. Therefore, if vaccines caused SIDS or there was a major relationship between them, the rate of SIDS should have correspondingly increased.

In the 1980s, the rate of SIDS in the United States was approximately 130 to 150 deaths per 100,000 live births, making it a leading cause of infant mortality in the postneonatal period (one month to one year). At the time, prone (stomach) sleeping was the norm for many infants, and public awareness of safe sleep practices was low.

In 1994, the AAP launched the Back to Sleep campaign, which suggested placing infants on their backs to sleep. Reflecting the success of this campaign, by the late 1990s, the SIDS rate drastically dropped by over 50%, to around 50 to 60 deaths per 100,000 live births. Between 1983 and 1990, the rate of SIDS decreased by an average of 1.6% per year; between 1990 and 1994, the rate of SIDS decreased by an average of 5.6% per year. Recent SIDS rates remain fairly stable, at approximately 35 to 38 deaths per 100,000 live births, although these rates vary depending on demographic and regional factors.

The earliest concerns about a link between vaccines and infant deaths emerged after the debut of the DPT vaccine in the early twentieth century. Shortly after the introduction of the DTP vaccine, physicians, primarily in Europe and North America, began documenting cases of sudden, unexplained infant deaths.

Consequently, pediatrician Robert Mendelsohn, MD, one of the most prominent critics of vaccine safety, hypothesized that many of the unexplained infant deaths—later termed SIDS—were attributable to routine vaccinations, specifically the pertussis (whooping cough) component of the DPT vaccine.

Mendelsohn was not alone in his beliefs. In the 1930s, physicians like Thorvald Madsen documented cases of infant deaths after DPT vaccination. Additional reports, such as those from Denmark, cited babies dying soon after vaccination from conditions like convulsions or respiratory distress. Pediatrician William C. Torch presented a study showing two-thirds of SIDS deaths occurred after DPT vaccination. This correlation between vaccination and timing of death (with clusters around two, four, and six months) drew attention but was often downplayed by health authorities.

Despite claims made by Mendelsohn, Madsen, Torch, and others, the recent research overwhelmingly shows that vaccines do *not* increase the risk of SIDS. Multiple studies from various countries and across different periods, a select few of which are enumerated below, have consistently found no causal link between vaccinations and SIDS:

A 1987 US study, authored by H. J. Hoffman et al., found no temporal association between DTP vaccination and SIDS. In fact, infants with SIDS were less likely to have been vaccinated.

A 2004 study by Eileen M. Eriksen et al. reviewed 360,000 US births and found no link between hepatitis B vaccine at birth and neonatal deaths, including SIDS.

A 2007 study, authored by M. M. T. Vennemann et al., looked at hexavalent vaccines in infants under one year. The study found no increased SIDS risk within fourteen days postimmunization; vaccinated infants were less likely to experience SIDS than unvaccinated ones.

A 2011 study by Giuseppe Traversa et al. investigated vaccination and sudden unexpected death in Italy during the first two years of life. This study found no increased risk of sudden unexpected death within seven or fourteen days postvaccination.

A 2018 study, authored by Y. Tony Yang and Jana Shaw, analyzed six years of vaccine uptake data in the United States and state-level SIDS reports.

They found no association between childhood vaccines and increased SIDS risk.

In contrast, a 1987 study by A. M. Walker et al. *did* find a temporal association between DTP vaccination and SIDS within three days of vaccination, with a 7.3 times higher incidence compared to the thirty days after vaccination.

The exact causes of SIDS remain elusive. However, the current scientific consensus suggests no causal link between vaccinations and an increased risk of SIDS. The extensive research, which has systematically reviewed the relationship between vaccinations and SIDS, was conducted and has shown that vaccines are unlikely the main cause of SIDS. Furthermore, we cannot overlook the inescapable fact that, even as the number of vaccines has increased, overall SIDS rates declined along with the implementation of safer sleep practices.

Still, the reasons behind SIDS are not fully understood. Considering all potential factors, including vaccines, remains imperative. The possibility that vaccines, a specific vaccine, or a component of a vaccine could contribute to a subset of SIDS cases cannot be entirely dismissed. At this time, the balance of evidence does not support vaccines as a significant factor in causing SIDS. Given the unequivocally serious nature of infant mortality, maintaining an open-minded approach to all potential contributing factors is critical. To ensure the health and safety of infants, parents and health-care providers must continue to engage in informed discussions and stay apprised of ongoing research.

As we move on from this heartbreaking topic and emerge from the haunted woods, I leave you with another story, one that I first heard in my pediatric training. The tenor of this anecdote differs slightly from that of the tragic tale I shared earlier yet is no less devastating.

> A two-month-old baby girl, let's call her Jenny, was scheduled for her routine wellness check-up. Her parents forgot and missed the appointment. The following day, hoping Jenny could still get the vaccines she should have received a day earlier, Jenny's mom, let's call her Anne, took Jenny to the pediatrician's office without an appointment. As cold and flu season was in full swing, the estimated wait time was between one to two hours. Preferring not to sit in a crowded waiting room with her young

baby for that long, Anne decided to go home and scheduled an appointment for the following week.

That afternoon, Anne put Jenny down for the usual nap. When, hours later, Anne checked on Jenny, she found Jenny limp and motionless. Panicked, Anne called 911. Jenny was pronounced dead at the scene. The cause of death could not be determined and was later ruled SIDS.

I offer this heartbreaking story to illustrate a crucial point about timing and perception. Had Jenny received her vaccines that morning, no amount of research or data would have likely convinced her grieving mother—or, for that matter, many of us—that Jenny's death was unrelated to vaccines. Anne would have almost certainly blamed vaccines because human nature has an aversion to question marks. In the wake of tragedy, to make sense of an incomprehensible situation, we search for answers. Candidly, had Jenny received her vaccines that morning, I, too, might have wondered whether Jenny's death was attributable to vaccines. But in this case, no vaccines were given. Thus, they were clearly not a factor in her passing.

While, sadly, the reason for SIDS remains a mystery, for now, the evidence largely suggests that vaccines are not one of its main causes.

18

BRIDGING THE DIVIDE—THE NEXT BIG STEPS FOR VACCINE POLICY AND PUBLIC TRUST

You're following where your interest takes you, and your curiosity takes you. And that's not something you can pre-plan. It's something that happens in the moment. So imagine that you're focused on your goal of having the most interesting conversation possible and communicating to the broadest number of people. That's the overarching goal. A spirit arises within you that leads you on a pathway. That's an investigation into the truth. That's part of that calling.

—JORDAN PETERSON

I never planned to write a book about vaccines. Far from it. No, this path wasn't some calculated scheme or strategic (or maybe a kamikaze) career move. It found me. An unsuspecting passenger driven through the meandering twists and turns of my life as a physician, husband, and father, I somehow arrived at this destination. It found me in the exam rooms of my practice, where concerned parents voiced their fears and frustrations about their children's health; it found me in conversations with mothers who, in their tireless search for answers, ultimately longed to be heard. Each of these moments, and others like them, planted an indelible seed that ultimately grew into the call to author this book.

Admittedly, I resisted the idea. Vaccines are among one of the most polarizing topics in modern times. I had always been keenly aware of the personal and professional repercussions that would invariably follow my decision to insert myself into the lion's den. So I quietly sat by on the sidelines, shamefully avoiding any mention of vaccines outside the sanctity of my office walls. However, the more I listened to parents, examined the research, and contemplated the gaps in our understanding, the more I knew I had a role to play in this discussion. My curiosity and commitment to truth led me *here*, because the pursuit of healthy children and informed choice demand it. This book isn't about taking sides or perpetuating division. To the contrary, it is about provoking thought and uncovering the answers that can and hopefully will bring those on diametrically opposing sides of the debate to a mutual understanding. Perhaps I may be overly naive and optimistic. Then again, I *am* Canadian.

As I researched and wrote this book, the last several lines of Robert Frost's poem "The Road Not Taken," repeatedly echoed through my mind:

> Two roads diverged in a wood, and I—
> I took the one less traveled by,
> And that has made all the difference.

Every step of the (perhaps less desirable) road I have chosen to travel has been guided by the spirit of compassion fundamental to my profession and the curiosity and commitment to truth that are indispensable to science. Although even a few years ago, I never could have fathomed writing this book, now I can't imagine not writing it. The conversations, the question marks, and the tears were the inexorable groundswell that led me here—that led *us* here. My hope is that this book serves as a healthy starting point, one that pushes us toward a united pathway forward, and that it makes all the difference.

A HYPOTHETICAL QUESTION ON VACCINE SAFETY AND PARENTAL CONCERNS

Earlier, I mentioned that my wife is an attorney. Specifically, she practices family law, which frequently requires her to settle cases through mediation, as opposed to litigation. She often shares that her most successful strategy in negotiation is to understand the other side's position and acknowledge it. This enables her to facilitate a peaceful resolution between two people who fundamentally disagree.

In much the same way, I view this book as a mediation between the pro and anti-vax camps; my role is to strike an equitable meeting of the minds forging a symbiotic pathway forward. I succeed in this admittedly formidable undertaking *not* by convincing both sides to agree with each other (I'm optimistic, not delusional) but by getting each to understand the other's position.

At this point, I hope we can all concede that a perfectly working vaccine is theoretically good. Regardless of what you think of vaccines, you must, at the very least, capitulate to the idea that, if effective, vaccines prevent debilitating diseases and even death; they promote herd immunity and protect the vulnerable; they minimize the strain that epidemics may place on the health-care system. The question is *not* whether most vaccines achieve their desired effect; the question is, at what cost do they do so? Do the risks outweigh the benefits? How many vaccines are too many? I am not asking the vaccine-hesitant or outright anti-vaxers to overlook these questions. I merely ask them to accept that, by and large, vaccines protect against the diseases they are designed to prevent.

Yet I *also* ask the pro-vax camp and the bulk of the medical community to recognize the other side's position. Perhaps, to do so, the pro-vax side of the negotiating table may find it helpful to consider the following hypothetical: Let's suppose that we live in a Bizzaro World universe in which, over the next forty years, the CDC conducts a prospective, double-blind, randomized trial that involves thousands of children. The study compares children who vaccinate in accordance with the CDC schedule, those who follow a slow schedule, and those who choose not to vaccinate. This study is rigorously designed. In short, it's the best possible study. This Bizarro World study hypothetically reveals that children who vaccinate on schedule, as recommended, have a significant increase in autoimmune conditions, all-cause mortality, and neurodevelopmental concerns.

In this purely fantastical study, researchers find the following:

- A three-times increased rate of autoimmune conditions in the vaccinated
- An eight times increased risk of neurodevelopmental disorders in the vaccinated
- A measurable and significant increase in overall chronic disease diagnoses, all-cause mortality, and/or serious infections unrelated to vaccine-preventable diseases
- A higher risk of serious, long-term, adverse consequences when the hepatitis B vaccine is given to a newborn than if it is given for the very first time at ten years old

- Children who only receive one vaccine per visit have a lower risk of short- and long-term adverse consequences than children who follow a regular schedule, without any significant increase of contracting a preventable disease
- Certain combinations of vaccines have an increased risk of serious side effects versus other combinations
- Children who delay vaccination until after two years of age have lower rates of allergies, asthma, and eczema

Right now, many of the vaccine-hesitant and anti-vax parents believe that, if vaccines were properly researched, the findings would yield results similar to those in this hypothetical Bizarro World study.

Many parents look to medical research to conclusively disprove perceived risks; they just feel that the current research doesn't adequately do this. These parents believe that vaccine research is being performed in a way that yields self-serving results. In short, you can't find what you don't look for. They are skeptical of the findings because many of the studies are being conducted by the very companies that profit massively from the product. These parents want easily accessible, high-quality, prospective studies comparing vaccinated and unvaccinated children that provide definitive data on long-term health outcomes.

Are we starting to understand the other side? What if a comprehensive study similar to the one in our Bizarro World existed and these hypothetical findings were real? If true, would the people on the pro-vax side of the negotiating table still insist upon mandating *recommended* vaccines? Would they still maintain that the current recommendations should be followed? How would they balance this information against the social contract?

Some would likely counter such questions by pointing out that none of the findings in this Bizarro World hypothetical are real and that the science shows vaccines, in the current recommended doses, are safe and effective. Technically, they would be right—though, if long-term studies comparing vaccinated and unvaccinated individuals have not been performed, how can we *emphatically* conclude that these hypothetical findings (or ones like them) are unfounded? *And therein lies the disconnect.*

Many vaccine-hesitant parents do not feel their concerns are being acknowledged. They distrust a system that, in their view, prioritizes profit and the continuous approval of new vaccines without addressing the long-term health impacts. They are reluctant to accept studies where the research is massaged in a way that, in their perception, produces desired results. These parents are frustrated that the absolutist "safe and effective" battle cry leaves no space for more nuanced conversations. Their confidence in the medical system has eroded not because they are necessarily against vaccines but because they do not feel their valid concerns are being heard or seen.

If the CDC conducted this Bizarro World hypothetical study and this same study *proved* that there is no significant increase in autoimmune conditions, all-cause mortality, or neurodevelopmental issues in children who are vaccinated as opposed to those who are not, then perhaps this would be the type of evidence that vaccine-hesitant parents would rely on to confidently proceed with vaccination. If vaccine-hesitant parents felt certain that every possible precaution has been taken to ensure safety, they might be more willing to follow the recommended schedule. Greater transparency, more rigorous long-term studies, and open acknowledgment of parental concerns would likely rebuild trust.

The militantly pro-vax and medical community do not need to agree with these vaccine-hesitant parents. They simply need to appreciate the reason vaccine-hesitant parents feel the way they do. It is not unreasonable.

Philosopher Georg Hegel's dialectic refers to a method of argument that uses contradiction between opposing sides to reach a new understanding. In essence, Hegel recognized that there is a *thesis* (representing the current viewpoint) and an *antithesis* (a challenge to the current viewpoint) that contradicts the thesis. Ultimately, the thesis and antithesis converge into a *synthesis*—a new truth that emerges from comparing and combining the merits of these contrasting ideas. Hegel believed that the dialectic method was the *"moving soul of scientific progression."* How very beautiful to think that the soul of scientific progress actually lies in the confluence of the pro-vax thesis and anti-vax antithesis--that the synthesis of these divisive perspectives is the spark that catalyzes a vaccine renaissance, in which personal choice and safety harmoniously coexist with public health considerations.

A NEW PATH FORWARD

*The secret of change is to focus all of your energy not
on fighting the old, but on building the new.*

—SOCRATES

Yes, idealism, platitudes, and fantasies that entail militant pro and anti-vaxers joining hands to sing *kumbaya* are all good and fine. But how do we implement changes in a way that strikes the necessary balance between freedom, accountability, safety, and confidence in vaccines? How do we dismantle the walls of fear and censorship and replace them with open dialogue, independent oversight, and bold actions that prioritize transparency and trust? Because my aim is not to rabble-rouse or merely poke holes in preconceived notions but to actually provide constructive solutions, I've come up with a road map, some practical steps to help us navigate this new frontier together:

1. Foster open dialogue
2. Empower vaccine-injured families
3. Host public debates
4. Ensure data transparency
5. Establish an independent vaccine commission
6. Launch large-scale studies
7. End social media censorship
8. Evolve vaccine messaging
9. Protect medical freedom
10. Respect personal choice

BREAKING THE SILENCE: VACCINES AS A PUBLIC DIALOGUE

First and foremost, we must remove the taboo around the word "vaccine." Every person should have the right to say "vaccine," even when the words "safe and effective" do not immediately follow or precede it. We must *stop* using divisive pejoratives and trendy buzzwords to dismiss anyone who dares say "vaccine" in a context that deviates from the scientific gospel. While we may not agree, respectful debate is the cornerstone of progress. We cannot engage in dialogue that is indispensable to a healthy future unless we can freely use the word *vaccine* without the threat or fear of reproach.

AMPLIFYING VOICES: LISTENING TO PARENTS AND VACCINE-INJURED FAMILIES

Nor can we continue to ignore and marginalize moms, dads, and families of vaccine-injured children. The government and scientists are understandably apprehensive; stories of vaccine injury could conceivably promote vaccine hesitancy. However, the appropriate response is *not* to silence and discredit these parents but to use their stories to guide and facilitate further safety research. Their experiences represent valuable data.

The parents of vaccine-injured children have no incentive to fabricate stories. They are *not* anti-vaxers. Rather, they are parents who *so* trusted medicine that they took their children to get vaccinated in accordance with the current recommendations. These parents weren't skeptical of vaccines; they were eager to offer their children the protections vaccines promised. By providing a platform for these parents to publicly share their stories— whether in hearings, debates, or media—policymakers and scientists can identify areas for improvement. This isn't about discrediting vaccines; it is about creating a system that minimizes risks and rebuilds trust.

OPEN DEBATES: ENGAGING THE BRIGHTEST MINDS

The discourse around vaccines is seemingly summarized by the paradoxical question "What is the sound of one hand clapping?" We validate those who agree with the scientific consensus while discrediting those whose opinions may diverge from it. Yet if we are to achieve not only the greatest efficacy but also safety outcomes, *all* voices must be heard.

One of the most effective ways to bridge the divide is to bring the smartest and most knowledgeable individuals from both sides of the debate into a public forum, akin to a town hall meeting. Imagine a conversation between figures like Robert F. Kennedy Jr. and Paul Offit, MD, where each is asked and answers tough questions in real time. Ideally, to reach diverse audiences, these conversations would take place on major media platforms, at top universities, and on alternative media outlets. Parents of vaccine-injured children would be invited to share their stories alongside experts who could explain the science.

A CALL FOR TRANSPARENCY: INDEPENDENT OVERSIGHT AND COMPREHENSIVE STUDIES

One of the biggest obstacles to public trust is the lack of perceived independence in vaccine oversight. This concern is easily addressed by establishing an independent vaccine committee to review vaccine safety, efficacy, and policy—free from bias, conflict of interest, or industry influence.

Additionally, comprehensive, large-scale studies that compare vaccinated and unvaccinated populations are long overdue. Although ethical concerns render randomized, controlled trials challenging, a prospective, nonblinded study could follow families who voluntarily choose not to vaccinate alongside those who do. Admittedly, such a study would come with certain confounding factors; it could still provide invaluable data that would further safety discussions while maintaining ethical boundaries. Moreover, all available large medical datasets, which include vaccination records and medical diagnoses, should be used to research questions pertaining to vaccines.

Finally, the FDA must set a higher bar for safety testing of new vaccines prior to allowing them on the market.

THE FEDERAL VACCINE COMMISSION: A PATH FORWARD

Taking independent oversight a step further, we must establish a federal vaccine commission to independently oversee vaccine policy, safety, and research. This body would have the authority to fund and oversee large-scale studies. The top priority of this commission would be the reexamination of all vaccine data.

Further, they should initiate a study similar to the Framingham Heart Study (FHS). Launched in 1948, the FHS has over fifteen thousand participants. The original goal of the FHS was to identify common factors or characteristics that contribute to cardiovascular disease. Over the years, the FHS has become a successful, multigenerational study that analyzes family patterns of cardiovascular and other diseases while gathering more genetic information from the two generations that followed the original study participants. Modeling vaccine research after the existing FHS framework, we can and must comprehensively explore long-term vaccine safety and the relationship between vaccines, chronic disease, and autism in a nonbiased and prospective environment. All data should be open access. The research needs to involve proponents *and* critics of vaccines to eliminate the potential for bias and ensure that every perspective has been carefully considered.

UNCENSORED DISCUSSIONS: ENDING THE SUPPRESSION OF VACCINE CONVERSATIONS

Censorship of vaccine discussions on social media and other platforms must end. Dismissing content that runs counter to the sanctioned narrative as misinformation or malinformation prevents open dialogue and fuels distrust. Open discussions, which, yes, include even those who question vaccine safety, should be encouraged, not suppressed. Vaccine science, like all science, thrives on debate, and silencing one side of the discussion only undermines public confidence.

SHIFTING THE NARRATIVE: FROM "SAFE AND EFFECTIVE" TO RISK-BENEFIT TRANSPARENCY

There is no denying that vaccines provide critical protection against serious diseases. But as with any medical intervention, they *do* carry risks. The words "safe and effective" are mechanically repeated like some incantation expected to spellbind the masses into blind compliance. Ironically, this mantra engenders the very skepticism it seeks to prevent. To restore public trust, the language around vaccines must shift. The known risks must be communicated along with the known benefits.

PROTECTING MEDICAL FREEDOM: SUPPORTING DOCTORS AND CHOICE

The current system, which in certain jurisdictions limits exemptions and subjects physicians to medical board review for exceeding arbitrary quotas, undermines the ability of doctors to practice individualized medicine. Doctors should not live in fear of losing their licenses for writing legitimate and medically indicated exemptions. Medicine is not one-size-fits-all.

Doctors should be free to provide care uniquely tailored to the individual needs of their patients without the threat of punitive repercussions.

Religious and personal belief exemptions and personal autonomy should be carefully balanced and contemplated within the broader framework of public health.

RESPECT PERSONAL CHOICE: BALANCING FREEDOM AND PUBLIC HEALTH

Even as we work to minimize risks to public health, freedom of choice must remain a pillar of public health policy. Whereas, for many parents, vaccine hesitancy is a knee-jerk response to current mandates, others fear that future policies might expand to require vaccinations for circumstances they find personally or ethically objectionable.

At its core, this is about the preservation of bodily autonomy and the fundamental right to make decisions about one's own health and the health of one's child without undue coercion. Vaccine mandates represent a deeper anxiety about losing control over personal decisions.

Acknowledging these concerns means prioritizing informed choice over compulsion and creating policies that emphasize dialogue, education, and trust. When individuals feel empowered to make decisions based on accurate information and personal values, they are more likely to engage constructively with public health initiatives.

No one should be forced to take a standard vaccine. Period. Ideally, in a free society, we should not impose mandates that restrict personal freedoms. To the extent they are absolutely necessary—as in the case of a severe public health crisis that presents a clear, immediate risk of widespread harm—such mandates should be exercised with extreme caution. They must be justified, rooted in solid science, and meet transparent and clearly delineated criteria to ensure they are reserved exclusively for extraordinary circumstances where public safety unequivocally outweighs personal autonomy. This stringent approach would preserve freedom while addressing dire public health threats. Furthermore, any extraordinary measure should be temporary, narrowly tailored, and subject to ongoing review to avoid overreach.

In addition, by reinstating personal and religious exemptions, we respect the diversity of beliefs and experiences that shape individual decisions about vaccines. Exemptions must be simultaneously balanced, contemplating safeguards to protect against preventable outbreaks. For instance, educational initiatives could accompany exemptions, ensuring that individuals understand both the risks and benefits of their choices—not as a punishment, but as a step toward informed decision-making. This approach preserves personal freedom while fostering accountability and community health.

Ultimately, building trust around vaccines requires policies that reflect respect for autonomy, robust safeguards for public health, and a commitment to transparency. A system that articulates when and why mandates might be necessary, while prioritizing choice in all other circumstances, creates a framework that protects public health and honors individual freedoms.

CONCLUSION

FLOWER POWER

Paradigm shifts don't happen instantly. It's the accumulation of evidence that finally discredits an old paradigm and allows eyes to open to new possibilities.

—GRAHAM HANCOCK

So here we are, the part where we awkwardly stare at *each other* as though to telepathically communicate the shared sentiment: "What the f@*k!" You might have read this book with the expectation that you would get straightforward answers. Instead, as you make your way through these final pages, you are left with even more questions, asking: "Yeah, but what should I do about vaccines for *my* child?" You're likely frustrated with me. I don't blame you. I'm frustrated too—not so much with myself but with the confusing messaging I had been spoon-fed and, for so long, naively swallowed.

You, like many others, want answers; you want me to tell you what to do.

Maybe you want my permission to follow a slow schedule or to agree that you shouldn't vaccinate at all. Maybe you want me to sternly wag my finger in the faces of the vaccine-hesitant and convince them to give their children all vaccines on the schedule, at the recommended times.

Sure, I could easily stand on my medical soapbox and sanctimoniously preach the "all vaccines are perfectly safe and effective" gospel. From the high and mighty comfort of my board-certified pulpit, I could sternly recommend that you follow the CDC schedule and, in the same breath, remind you that, according to CDC estimates, between 1994 and 2023, childhood vaccines prevented 1.1 million deaths, 508 million illnesses, and 32 million hospitalizations in the United States alone.

Or I could just as quickly tell you that you should never get a vaccine—albeit, that would be neither ethical nor honest. Just as no doctor should demand you vaccinate without question or exception, no doctor should stop you from vaccinating. These decisions are *yours* to make, based on what's right for *your* child.

Of course, the only vaccine schedule backed by extensive research is the one sanctioned by the CDC or the comparable public health authority in each country. This is the standard of care that the medical community is bound to recommend. This doesn't mean our conversations should end there. There is room for open dialogue and continued research.

Some will invariably chastise me for straddling both sides. They'll indignantly scoff, "Balance. What a cop-out!" Stalwart pro-vaxers will deem me a medical heretic, guilty of promoting vaccine hesitancy; ardent anti-vaxers will swear I am murdering babies. Of course, neither is true. I'm used to it though, and I have the "Troll Joel" folder in my phone to prove it. I am committed to authenticity and the thoughtful consideration of all valid perspectives. I am not beholden to a particular side—*solely* to the health of our children. I firmly believe hyperbole and extremism have no place in this conversation. No matter whether you perceive vaccines as bad, good, or somewhere in between, our mutual passion for this topic is fueled by our *common* desire for healthy children; we may just have different ideas on the way this is achieved.

When I embarked on the ambitious (or maybe impossible) journey of reconciling the vaccine paradox, I checked my ego at the door. Along every step of the way, I have been committed to truth—for a brighter future. John Lydgate famously said, "You can please some of the people all of the time, you can please all of the people some of the time, but you can't please all of the people all of the time." Indeed these words resonate with me.

The aim of this book is *not* to please everyone—or, for that matter, anyone. The purpose is to comprehensively present the information so that by the end of the book, you are in a better position than you were when you started—to provide you with a more confident grasp of the information needed to make informed choices that are best for *your* family.

The difficulty lies in the fact that you, like I, still have unanswered questions. Although I aimed to present the studies and data available to me in the most balanced fashion, the grim reality is there are so many remaining gaps in the research. For now, you will need to make the best decisions based on the information you *do* have. I *hope* that your frustration is tempered, even if only slightly, by your newfound understanding of this topic, gleaned from these pages; I *hope* that now you feel a little more equipped, a little more informed, and a little less alone as you make these important decisions; I *hope* you continue to ask the tough and important questions to push for more and better answers.

I don't have a crystal ball. I wish I did. I can't tell you whether your child will experience a severe vaccine reaction, whether your child will be hospitalized with a vaccine-preventable disease, or neither. You are a parent whose choices for his or her child are made with the deepest love and care. You are your child's fiercest advocate and protector, and you are *allowed* to trust your intuition and ask questions. While you may feel unsatisfied to finish this book without a concrete path forward, remember this: You already possess the most powerful tools needed to make decisions for your child—your instinct, love, and commitment to your child's well-being.

In my years as a pediatrician and a father, I have come to value one thing above all: listening to moms. The bond between a mother and her child is profoundly unique. Of course, no less special is the bond between a father and his child, which is beautiful in its own way. But on countless occasions, mothers have sincerely looked me in the eye and, with such unwavering conviction, insisted, "My child was thriving, full of life—and then something changed." I am acutely aware that science deals in hard data, and that anecdotal evidence is no replacement for it. Nevertheless, I firmly believe there is truth in these patterns that is simply too compelling to ignore.

In spite of such stories, science does not currently recognize any link between vaccines and conditions such as autism or chronic disease. However, as someone who hears stories like these directly from families with eerily similar experiences, I cannot outright dismiss the possibility that there is more to uncover. These parents aren't crazy. They aren't conspiracy theorists. Yet science, to date, has been unwilling to listen to them. We must acknowledge that these voices are an inextricable part of a larger conversation that needs to be had.

Ultimately, with respect to autism, my conclusion is, I am unsure. Sometimes, I question my sanity. My eyes and intuition lead me down a path that contravenes the "settled" science. While some may characterize Robert F. Kennedy's book *The Real Anthony Fauci,* Suzanne Humphries' book *Dissolving Illusions,* and Forrest Maready's book *The Moth in the Iron Lung,* "fringe," "faux-scientific alarmism," and of course, "conspiracy theory," the alternate histories of HIV/AIDS, smallpox and polio respectively presented in each of these works are compelling—so much so that they leave me questioning whether the history of disease taught to me in medical school was designed to inculcate a certain way of thinking, which appears to be unraveling before me.

The more I read (on *both* sides of the vaccine debate) and the more I learn, the more I am left with the sinking gut feeling that there is more to the vaccine debate than the *status quo* narrative asks us to believe. I cannot help but think that there may be a concerted effort to obscure the data and prevent us from connecting the dots. I concede, no double-blind, randomized, controlled, placebo trials have been performed on my gut to assess its efficacy. Nevertheless, opinion, rooted in a combination of intuition and educated thought, has its place in science. Perhaps this officially earns me the coveted title of conspiracy theorist. I must acknowledge that possibility.

History must also serve its didactic function, reminding us that we should be open to what we don't fully comprehend. Our understanding of health—of cause and effect, of the delicate balance in our bodies and our children's bodies—is constantly evolving. At one time, science resolutely defended opioids, assuring us they were not addictive. Despite the scientific data, doctors witnessed their patients succumb to opioid addiction. I am certain the scientific community would have dismissed any doctor who insinuated that opioids are addictive, just as, at one time, it would have dismissed any doctor who claimed there to be a link between cigarettes and lung cancer or heart disease. Maybe vaccines are the next big reversal in medicine, and you and I have front-row seats to the main event. Maybe not.

This book was never intended to prescribe a one-size-fits-all solution because, to me, in the context of medicine, "one-size-fits-all" is an oxymoron. We all come with our unique set of genetics that interact differently with our individual environments. What's right for one person may not be right for another. By framing the issues as either black or white, the pro and anti-vax camps oversimplify them. This has merely served to relegate the vaccine debate to a purgatory of futile rhetoric, where each side thinks that by screaming louder, it will win the argument. It's falling on deaf ears. There is validity to both the pro and anti-vax positions; neither side actually *hears* the other. As the grayscale gradient on the cover of this book reminds us, the reality lies not in the black nor the white, but somewhere in the nuanced and uncertain shades of gray in between, the place where we compassionately weigh the information we know and feel safe to ask questions about the information we don't.

During the Vietnam War, photojournalist Marc Riboud took a powerful photograph in which soldiers are pictured pointing their guns at a young female protester. Standing just inches from the barrels of these guns, this woman, who is holding a flower in her hands, offers it to the soldiers as an emblem of peace. Subsequently, this iconic photograph has become associated with nonviolent resistance amid conflict. Echoing this sentiment, the image on the cover of this book portrays a baby gently placing a flower into a syringe—a metaphor for my plea for peace and understanding as we debate and navigate the future of vaccines.

The place where the syringe and the flower meet represents the beauty of life amid the caustic debates and controversies that often surround vaccine discourse. It evokes the spirit of nonviolent resistance, reminding us that there is room for gentle yet powerful advocacy that fosters understanding and reconciliation, even when it comes to a topic as contentious as vaccine policy. Just as the flower in the barrel of a gun symbolizes a humanizing gesture toward those who hold the instrument of violence—a rejection of war—the flower in the syringe urges us to compassionately weigh public health and individual rights and strive for a resolution that respects personal choice *and* community safety. This cover stands as a visual commitment to fostering a conversation that bridges divides.

As we work toward a healthier future, let's do so together, with open minds, open hearts, and a willingness to continue seeking answers for our children. To every parent reading this who feels stuck between a shot and a hard place, your love, questions, and courage are the galvanizing force shaping the pathway forward and changing the world.

Keep holding up that flower.

APPENDIX A

MOST COMMON QUESTIONS I GET ASKED IN THE OFFICE

This feels like the part of the infomercial where you're told, "But wait, there's more!" Yes, for the price of this book, you get an entire section of frequently asked vaccine questions *at no extra charge*! I will share the questions I most often encounter, clarify common concerns, and provide straightforward, evidence-based information to help you make informed decisions about vaccines.

1. WHICH VACCINES ARE ACTUALLY NECESSARY FOR ME TO GIVE MY CHILD?

It's a good question and one I'm asked at least once a day. Despite its prevalence, I can't answer it, nor should any reasonable practitioner. For medico-ethical-legal reasons, I cannot tell you what to do. I cannot recommend any specific vaccine schedule to you. I don't know your child; I don't know your child's medical history; I don't know you. I understand the decision to vaccinate your child is a monumental one. Nevertheless, it is entirely *yours*, and yours alone to make. Neither I nor any medical professional (or person) can make this decision for you. You must assess your child's unique circumstances and make informed choices that best suit your child's particular needs.

When considering which vaccines to give your child and when to give them, the standard recommendation from health-care professionals typically aligns with the immunization schedule prescribed by the CDC or the local public health organization where you live. Major medical associations carefully crafted the CDC schedule. I picture them sitting inside a macabre castle, situated high atop a menacing cliff. As cartoonish lightning bolts illuminate the room, a voice resembling that of Vincent Price maniachally proclaims, "Yes, yes, two doses of MMR!" Of course, I'm kidding. As Robert Louis Stevenson said, "Nothing like a little judicious levity."

Based on extensive research, the CDC's is the preeminent vaccine schedule. It ensures that, from infancy through adolescence, the timing and sequence of vaccines provide protection against infectious diseases. The schedule was fashioned by scientists far smarter than I—a mere lowly pediatrician. Who am I to suggest you deviate from the schedule these masterminds spent decades forging? Ultimately, the CDC schedule is the only one tested for safety and efficacy. Any departure from it should be carefully contemplated with your pediatrician.

Nevertheless, neither the CDC nor your pediatrician make decisions for your child. Thus, when *you* make this delicate and challenging decision for *your* child, you may wish to weigh several factors so that you can thoughtfully contemplate your child's unique circumstances alongside the broader public health implications:

- *The CDC Schedule (Or Other Local Public Health Recommendations).* The CDC's recommended vaccine schedule is designed to protect children from potentially life-threatening diseases during their most vulnerable years. It outlines when vaccines should be given to provide maximum protection based on expert consensus. Understanding this schedule helps you navigate the reasons specific vaccines are prioritized at certain times. Similarly, for those outside the United States, research the guidelines in your area.

- *Personal and Family Health History.* Your family's health history plays a crucial role in decision-making. Conditions such as autoimmune diseases, genetic conditions, or immune deficiencies may influence the timing or choice of vaccines. Discussing your family's medical history with your pediatrician can help tailor a plan that aligns with your child's needs.

- *Vaccine Reaction History.* Consider whether your child or close family member has had a previous reaction to a vaccine. Mild reactions, such as a fever, are common. However, serious reactions are rare. Your doctor can help determine whether further precautions are necessary.

- *Disease Risk.* Understanding the risks of vaccine-preventable illness is essential. Some diseases, like measles or pertussis, are highly contagious and can be severe in young children. Some vaccines, such as yellow fever, are only recommended for travel.
- *Local Prevalence and Incidence.* Disease prevalence and incidence vary by region. For instance, areas with low vaccination rates may see more outbreaks of diseases like measles, thereby increasing the risk of infection. Your local health department or pediatrician can provide insight into the risks specific to your area.
- *Know the Risks Associated with Vaccines.* Every medical intervention, including vaccines, carries some risk. Reviewing vaccine ingredients, understanding the potential risks, and performing a risk-benefit analysis will help you make an informed decision.

Balancing these factors may feel overwhelming. Yet they offer a comprehensive framework for making thoughtful, informed choices. Every family's journey is different, and working with a trusted pediatrician can ensure that your child's health and safety are prioritized.

2. WHAT ARE THE RISKS AND BENEFITS OF A SLOW VACCINE SCHEDULE?

For a variety of reasons—such as concerns over the number of vaccines given at one time, personal or family health histories, or simply a preference for a more cautious approach to immunization—parents may elect to follow a slow schedule. A slow schedule is, just as it sounds, an alternate approach to vaccination, whereby vaccines are administered over a more extended period than recommended by standard guidelines. Although I cannot explicitly advise you that a slow schedule is beneficial, I can share the risks and theoretical benefits so that you can weigh them for yourself against the known and scientifically supported benefits of the recommended schedule.

The benefits of the recommended CDC schedule include the following:

- *Early protection.* Vaccines given on the recommended timeline protect infants and young children when they are most susceptible to infections like pertussis, measles, and pneumococcus.
- *Herd immunity.* You contribute to broader community immunity, which is critical for protecting those who cannot receive vaccines (i.e., immunocompromised individuals).

- *Reduced office visits*: Minimizing the number of doctor visits for vaccinations can be less disruptive for families and reduce exposure to infections.
- *Compliance with school requirements*: The CDC schedule aligns with school entry requirements across the United States, ensuring children can enroll without delays or complications associated with incomplete vaccination.
- *Efficiency and effectiveness*: Adhering to the CDC schedule assures that vaccinations are administered in a scientifically optimized sequence that maximizes the vaccine's efficacy and reduces the likelihood of vaccine-preventable diseases in your child and the community at large.

When contemplating a slow schedule, you may wish to consider the following risks:

- *Delayed protection.* Slower schedules delay immunity, leaving children vulnerable to serious infections for longer periods.
- *Increased visits.* More frequent medical visits for individual vaccines may increase stress for the child and caregiver, along with exposure to pathogens in clinical settings.
- *Lack of data.* No substantial evidence supports the safety or efficacy of alternative schedules. Since these schedules are not studied or standardized, potential risks and long-term effects are unknown.

A slow schedule may have its theoretical benefits. Despite a lack of empirical evidence to robustly support these views, advocates believe that spreading out vaccinations may offer the following perceived benefits:

- *Parental comfort.* Spreading vaccines over the course of a longer period may ease the concerns of wary parents around administering multiple vaccines in a single visit. This approach may facilitate trust in the vaccination process by aligning with parental comfort levels and personal beliefs about health care.
- *Enhanced observation period.* Parents and health-care providers may feel they can better monitor and manage any adverse reactions that occur. This could potentially identify whether certain reactions are attributable to a specific vaccine.

- *Perceived reduced immune system stress.* Some proponents of a slow vaccine schedule argue that fewer vaccines administered at once may lessen what they view as a burden on the child's immune system. This belief stems from a concern that multiple vaccinations might overwhelm a young immune system.
- *Individualized scheduling.* A slower schedule can be seen as a more individualized approach, which may be appealing to parents looking for tailored health-care solutions that fit their unique concerns or the specific health circumstances of their child.
- *Potential for increased health-care engagement.* When vaccines are spread out, families may have more frequent contact with health-care providers, possibly enhancing overall health-care monitoring and increasing opportunities for health education.

3. HOW DO I CRAFT A SLOW SCHEDULE?

This question is an admittedly difficult one—largely because there is no single answer. Slow schedules are not currently recommended and, therefore, have not been studied for safety or efficacy. As a pediatrician, I cannot endorse any specific schedule that deviates from the standard guidelines without a thorough evaluation of the individual case.

Since timing and spacing are contingent not upon any recommendations other than interval minimums between vaccines, but, rather, are based on individual preference, slow schedules are generally arbitrary and subjective. Alternative vaccine schedules typically fall into two categories: delayed start and extended spacing. Some parents choose to delay the initiation of vaccinations until the child is older, while others opt to administer vaccines one at a time, spreading them out over a longer period than recommended by the CDC. As there are countless ways to implement a slower schedule, each family's approach may vary. It's a little bit like those old choose-your-own-adventure books I used to read when I was in the fourth grade. The lack of guidance in this area relegates slow schedules to that vaccine no-man's-land, where outlaw parents make their own capricious rules. (You can almost hear the main theme from *The Good, the Bad, and the Ugly*.)

A rudimentary internet search for "slow schedule" would likely lead you to Paul Thomas, MD, author of *The Vaccine-Friendly Plan*. Many curious parents look to this seminal book to guide them in fashioning a slow schedule. Notably, Thomas has faced substantial rebuke for advocating for a slower and more selective approach to vaccination. *I must make it abundantly clear that I, in no way, endorse or recommend Thomas's plan. I mention it only for educational purposes.*

In my practice, parents who choose to follow a slower schedule sometimes opt for a single vaccine plan, somewhat similar to the one set forth below, which is comparable to the one proposed in *the vaccine-friendly plan*:

- *Pregnancy*: No vax (no Tdap, influenza)
- *Birth*: No Hep B
- *2M*: Hib, DTaP (no Hep B, RV, IPV)
- *3M*: PCV
- *4M*: Hib, DTaP (no RV, IPV)
- *5M*: PCV
- *6M*: Hib, DTaP (no Hep B, RV, IPV)
- *7–9M*: PCV
- *1Y*: Hib, PCV (no MMR, Hep A, VZV)
- *18M*: DTaP
- *2Y*: No Hep A
- *3Y*: Consider MMR
- *4–6Y*: DTaP (consider VZV, IPV)
- *10Y*: Tdap (boost every 5–10 years)
- *11Y*: MenACWY, VZV
- *12–14Y*: Hep B (3 doses)
- *16–18Y*: MenACWY, consider MenB, Hep A

Below are several additional theoretical slow schedules. I will reiterate that I do *not* advise that you follow these or any schedule other than that recommended by the CDC or your local health authority.

It goes without saying (but I'll say it anyway):

These conceptual sample schedules are purely illustrative and not a substitute for professional medical advice. They are based on schedules that parents have chosen to follow—not upon my recommendation, but upon their election. As always, you must consult with your health-care provider to ensure that any vaccination plan meets the specific health needs of your child and adheres to local health guidelines. (Are you annoyed by the number of times I've repeated this disclaimer yet?)

Conceptual monthly vaccination using combination shots[2]
- *2M:* Pentacel (DTaP/IPV/Hib) (1st dose)
- *3M:* PCV (1st dose)
- *4M:* Pentacel (2nd dose)
- *5M:* PCV (2nd dose)
- *6M:* Pentacel (3rd dose)
- *7M:* PCV (3rd dose)
- *12M:* MMR (1st dose)
- *14M:* Var (1st dose)
- *15M:* Hep A (1st dose)
- *24M:* Hep B (1st dose)

Conceptual monthly vaccination using individual shots
- *1M:* RSV (1st dose)
- *2M:* DTaP (1st dose)
- *3M:* Hib (1st dose)
- *4M:* PCV (1st dose)
- *5M:* IPV (1st dose)
- *6M:* DTaP (2nd dose)
- *7M:* Hib (2nd dose)
- *8M:* PCV (2nd dose)
- *9M:* IPV (2nd dose)
- *10M:*Influenza (1st dose)
- *11M:* Hib (3rd dose)
- *12M:* PCV (3rd dose)
- *13M:* IPV (3rd dose)
- *14M:* MMR (1st dose)
- *15M:* Varicella (1st dose)

---

2   No medical advice is provided anywhere in these conceptual schedules below. These conceptual schedules are not recommendations and are for educational purposes only. Always discuss medical decisions with your medical providers.

Conceptual vaccination every two months, with combination shots
- *2M:* VAXELIS (DTaP/Hib/IPV/Hep B) (1st dose)
- *4M:* PCV (1st dose)
- *6M:* VAXELIS (2nd dose)
- *8M:* PCV (2nd dose)
- *10M:* VAXELIS (3rd dose)
- *12M:* MMR (1st dose)
- *14M:* Varicella (1st dose)
- *16M:* Hep A (1st dose)
- *18M:* Hep B (1st dose)

Conceptual starting at age two, visits every two months, with combination shots
- *2Y:* VAXELIS (DTaP/IPV/Hib/HepB), (1st dose)
- *2Y, 2M:* MMR (1st dose)
- *2Y, 4M:* VAXELIS (2nd dose)
- *2Y, 6M:* PCV (1st dose)
- *2Y, 8M:* Varicella (1st dose)
- *2Y, 10M:* Influenza
- *3Y:* Hep A (1st dose)

As is evident from these mere few theoretical examples, the possibilities are truly limitless. Slow schedules are indeed the Wild West—the place where you may just see a rogue tumbleweed traipse past the exam room door.

4. ARE VACCINE SCHEDULES THE SAME AROUND THE WORLD?

The short answer is, no. While the majority of nations have similar immunization guidelines, variations do exist. Most countries aim to protect against the same preventable diseases. But the timing, specific vaccines used, and number of doses can differ. Not surprisingly, the United States has one of the most comprehensive vaccination schedules in the world. If vaccines were an Olympic sport, the United States would win the gold medal, beating out most other countries in recommending a higher number of doses for infants and children. This approach reflects a proactive stance in preventing diseases early in life; however, it also sparks debate over the intensity and frequency of vaccinations as compared to arguably effective schedules followed in places like Europe or Canada, where the number of recommended doses might be fewer.

Curiously, whereas many other countries recommend a meningococcal vaccine in the first two years of life, the United States does not. Some countries with higher tuberculosis rates recommend the Bacillus Calmette-Guérin (BCG) vaccine early in life, but there are no standard recommendations in the United States unless one is at high risk. Most countries do recommend the MMR, though the timing of the recommended first and second doses vary widely.

Just by way of example, the general recommended Danish childhood vaccination schedule breaks down as follows:

- *3M*: Infants receive the first doses of the combined diphtheria-tetanus-pertussis-polio-Hib vaccine and the pneumococcal conjugate vaccine (PCV).
- *5M*: The second doses of diphtheria-tetanus-pertussis-polio-Hib and PCV are administered.
- *12M*: The third dose of the diphtheria-tetanus-pertussis-polio-Hib and PCV is given.
- *15M*: The first dose of the MMR vaccine is introduced.
- *4Y*: The second dose of the MMR vaccine is administered.
- *5Y*: A booster for diphtheria-tetanus-pertussis-polio is provided.
- *12Y*: Two doses of the HPV vaccine are offered.

In Japan, the recommended childhood vaccination schedule is as follows:
- *2M*: DPT-IPV-Hib (diphtheria, pertussis, tetanus, and polio combination, Haemophilus influenzae type b), pneumococcal, and hepatitis B
- *3M*: Hepatitis B (if not already given), DPT-IPV-Hib (2nd dose), and pneumococcal (2nd dose)
- *4M*: DPT-IPV-Hib (3rd dose) and pneumococcal (3rd dose)
- *5–7M*: BCG
- *7–8M*: Hepatitis B (3rd dose if not already given earlier)
- *12M*: MR (measles and rubella), DPT-IPV-Hib (booster dose), pneumococcal (booster dose), and varicella (1st dose)
- *18M–2Y*: Varicella (2nd dose)

- *2–3Y*: Japanese encephalitis
- *5–6Y*: MR (2nd dose)

Iceland's vaccine schedule is also relatively conservative, with fewer doses required compared to some other countries. They do not require the rotavirus, hepatitis A and hepatitis B vaccines. The MMR is given at eighteen months and twelve years old.

5. DETOXIFICATION FROM VACCINES: IS THERE A NEED FOR IMMUNE SUPPORT, AND WHAT ARE THE THEORETICAL BENEFITS?

The concept of detoxification from vaccines centers on the idea that eliminating or reducing potential toxins will mitigate the adverse effects that some believe can result from vaccination. Despite the mainstream medical consensus that vaccines are safe, many parents remain interested in methods that could enhance the body's natural detoxification processes postvaccination. Little research exists on the subject, underscoring a need for more rigorous scientific investigation.

The following are just a few approaches thought to support the body's immune and detoxification systems, though it is crucial to acknowledge that they are more theoretical than evidence-based. Critics will likely argue that the mere mention of these approaches perpetuates the myth that postvaccine detoxification is necessary. By now you know all too well that certain people will find a reason to be mad about anything I say. To the extent these suggestions provide reassurances to vaccine-hesitant parents who may otherwise opt out of vaccination, I see no harm in including them, particularly as they are lifestyle factors widely accepted as beneficial to overall health.

1. *Hydration.* Adequate water intake is vital for overall health and helps maintain optimal detoxification pathways in the kidneys and liver.
2. *Diet.* Consuming a balanced diet rich in antioxidants, such as fruits and vegetables, can support the body's natural detoxification processes. Foods high in vitamins C and E, as well as selenium and beta-carotene, are considered beneficial.
3. *Probiotics.* These can support gut health, which plays a significant role in immunity and toxin elimination.

4. *Exercise.* Regular physical activity can enhance circulation, promote lymphatic drainage, and help eliminate toxins through sweat.

5. *Sunlight and vitamin D.* Sufficient exposure to sunlight is essential for the body to naturally synthesize Vitamin D, which supports the immune system and plays a role in the detoxification processes. Vitamin D facilitates immune function and can aid in the body's natural detox pathways.

When considering supplements and herbs known to support detoxification, it's important to focus on those that enhance the body's natural processes. Notably, few supplements have been tested on young children. And of course, you should consult your physician before taking any supplements. Nevertheless, some well-regarded options include the following:

1. *Milk thistle.* Often used to support liver health, milk thistle is rich in silymarin, an antioxidant that is thought to help protect the liver from toxins and promote the regeneration of liver cells.

2. *Turmeric.* This spice contains curcumin, a compound with potent anti-inflammatory and antioxidant properties, which can aid in detoxification by supporting liver function.

3. *Dandelion.* Traditionally used for its diuretic properties, dandelion can help the liver and kidneys eliminate toxins more effectively and increase urine production to help flush out waste.

4. *Garlic.* Known for its cardiovascular and immune-boosting benefits, garlic contains sulfur compounds that help activate liver enzymes responsible for expelling toxins from the body.

5. *Chlorella.* This green algae is a potent detoxifier, particularly for heavy metals. Its high chlorophyll content helps cleanse the blood and tissues.

6. *Nettles.* Nettle leaf is a powerful herb known for its detoxification support. It acts as a diuretic, helping to flush harmful chemicals from the body through increased urine output. The anti-inflammatory properties of nettles can further aid in reducing systemic inflammation, promoting overall health and well-being.

7. *Vitamin D.* Enhances immune function and modulates inflammatory responses, which may help the body efficiently manage and recover from the immunological effects of vaccines.

8. *Vitamin C.* A powerful antioxidant that can help reduce oxidative stress and support the immune system, potentially aiding in the recovery process postvaccination.

9. *Zinc.* Supports immune system function and cellular repair, which may be beneficial in helping the body cope with any added stress or immune challenges after vaccination.

10. *B Vitamins (methylated versions).* These help support methylation, a critical detoxification pathway in the body.

11. *Magnesium.* Essential for detoxification and overall cellular function.

12. *Glutathione.* An antioxidant produced by the body, it helps repair cells damaged by pollution, stress, and other harmful influences. It plays a powerful role in eliminating toxins from the liver.

The benefits of employing specific detoxification methods postvaccination have been minimally studied and are currently not evidence-based. For instance, the general benefits of hydration, a balanced diet, and exercise are well-documented in the context of overall health and immune function, but their direct impact on vaccine detoxification is not well-established. The lack of substantial research does not necessarily render these methods ineffective. It simply highlights a gap in our scientific understanding. For now this may be a case of "It may or may not help, but it most likely won't hurt."

6. DO VACCINES SHED, AND IF SO, IS IT DANGEROUS?

The word *shedding* typically conjures images of clothing and couch cushions covered in dog fur. For purposes of our discussion, you can safely don that black sweatshirt. In the context of vaccines, shedding has nothing to do with fur. Rather, shedding refers to the release of weakened, vaccine-derived viruses from individuals who receive live-attenuated vaccines. This phenomenon is specific to vaccines that are designed to replicate in the body to trigger an immune response, such as the OPV and rotavirus vaccines. Yes, your clothing and couch cushions are safe from this type of shedding, but you may not be. I say this mostly in jest, as shedding rarely poses a risk to healthy individuals. However, immunocompromised individuals and newborns may be at greater, albeit still negligible risk, and extra precautions should be taken around them—namely, with respect to the following vaccines:

- *OPV*: Shedding can occur through feces, especially in areas with poor sanitation. In rare cases, the virus can mutate into vaccine-derived poliovirus, leading to outbreaks. Consequently, many countries (including the United States) have switched to the IPV, which does not shed.
- *Rotavirus vaccine*: The virus can be shed in stool for up to ten days postvaccination, posing a theoretical risk to immunocompromised individuals or close contacts, such as caregivers.
- *FluMist*: Shedding is minimal and short-lived (approximately one to two days). Precautions should be taken around severely immunocompromised individuals.
- *MMR vaccine*: Rare cases of shedding have been reported, but the attenuated viruses are so weakened they are unlikely to cause disease, even in immunocompromised individuals.

Notably, shedding can occur *only* with live vaccines, where a weakened form of the virus is administered. For nonlive vaccines, like those containing killed viruses or parts of the virus, shedding cannot occur because these components are not capable of replication.

Distinguishable from viral shedding, excreting inactivated virus or antigen particles through bodily fluids is possible. These components are not infectious and do not pose a risk of disease transmission. They are merely remnants of the vaccine's ingredients clearing from the body.

During the COVID-19 pandemic, some speculated that vaccinated individuals, particularly those who received the mRNA vaccines, were shedding the spike protein. These mRNA vaccines instruct cells to produce a portion of the spike protein, which stimulates an immune response without causing disease. To date, the research does not support the theory that vaccinated individuals can shed or transmit the spike protein in a manner that would pose a risk to others. As far as we know, shedding relates specifically to live vaccines. The mRNA COVID-19 vaccines do not contain a live virus.

7. DO HOMEOPATHIC VACCINES WORK, AND CAN I GIVE THESE INSTEAD OF TRADITIONAL VACCINES?

Homeopathic vaccines, often referred to as nosodes, are preparations made from diluted biological material derived from vaccines, diseased tissues, organs, or cultures. Proponents claim these remedies offer protection against diseases similar to traditional vaccines.

There is no scientific evidence that homeopathic vaccines can stimulate the production of antibodies or provide immunity in the way conventional vaccines do. Conventional vaccines work by introducing antigens that trigger the body to create antibodies, offering protection against specific diseases. In contrast, homeopathic remedies are so diluted that they likely contain no trace of the original substance, rendering them ineffective in generating an immune response.

Most health authorities, including the WHO, caution against using homeopathic vaccines as substitutes for standard immunizations due to the lack of evidence supporting their efficacy in disease prevention.

Homeopathics are not a replacement for conventional vaccines. If you generally favor homeopathy, you may consider using it concomitantly with conventional vaccines.

8. SHOULD I GET TESTED FOR MTHFR?

The potential link between MTHFR gene mutations and vaccine responses has garnered interest and sparked debate. The MTHFR gene produces an enzyme critical for processing folate and regulating homocysteine levels, both of which are vital for methylation and detoxification pathways. Variants of this gene, such as C677T and A1298C, may impair these processes, leading to concerns over the way individuals with such mutations might handle environmental exposures, including vaccines. Some studies, namely, a 2016 meta-analysis published in *Metabolic Brain Disease*, have found associations between MTHFR variants, abnormal methylation, and genetic and developmental conditions. But no definitive causal link has been established between MTHFR mutations and adverse vaccine reactions.

Research has explored this relationship in limited contexts. For instance, a study on the smallpox vaccine found higher rates of adverse events, like fever and rash, among individuals with MTHFR variants. Of course, this vaccine is no longer in routine use, and there is little comprehensive research examining the way these mutations impact responses to vaccines. While some integrative practitioners recommend supporting methylation with supplements like L-methylfolate and methyl-B12 before vaccination, mainstream medical guidelines maintain that there is no evidence to differentiate vaccine recommendations based on MTHFR status.

As interest in pharmacogenomics grows, future research may offer more insights into tailoring vaccine recommendations based on genetic profiles.

9. I'M NOT ANTI-VAX, BUT . . . HOW DO I SPEAK TO MY DOCTOR ABOUT MY VACCINE CONCERNS AND QUESTIONS?

Funny story, my wife tried to wiggle out of our second date because, as a more holistic-minded person, she had been dismissively laughed at by so many doctors that she was apprehensive to date one. Fortunately, I was able to convince her that I was not one of those doctors—though, sadly, her experience is shared by so many. No doctor should ever make his or her patient feel unintelligent. At that, it is one thing to laugh at someone who says she takes echinacea to support her immune system; it is entirely different to berate parents who entrust a doctor with their child's health for asking legitimate questions due merely to the fact that those questions revolve around a topic that the medical establishment has deemed off-limits.

First and foremost, if your doctor is the type who would laugh at you for *any* reason other than you telling a funny joke, he or she may not be the right doctor. Having a trustworthy health-care provider who is willing to engage in meaningful and respectful conversations about vaccines can significantly ease your concerns and help you make informed decisions about your child's health. I hope you have found this doctor. But even assuming you have not, below are some suggestions that may guide you in broaching the vaccine discussion with your doctor with confidence and preparedness:

1. *Be informed.* Before your appointment, gather *reliable* information about your concerns. This will help you to articulate your questions clearly and better understand the responses. (Hopefully, this book has helped).

2. *Prepare specific questions.* Write down your specific vaccine questions (i.e., about side effects, the necessity of certain vaccines, or the timing of the vaccination schedule).

3. *Express concerns with clarity.* Clearly state your concerns. For instance, if you are worried about specific vaccine ingredients or potential side effects, let your doctor know.

4. *Request detailed responses.* Do not hesitate to ask for detailed explanations or evidence supporting your doctor's recommendations. A good health-care provider should be willing to provide the information that makes you feel informed and comfortable.

5. *Seek a partnership approach.* Express your desire to work together with your health-care provider to find the best approach for your child's health.

6. *Be open to dialogue.* Remain open to hearing your doctor's perspectives and explanations. The goal is to participate in a constructive conversation that leads to the best outcomes for your child.

7. *Consider a second opinion.* If your doctor is not amenable to discussing your concerns or if you feel your concerns are not being adequately addressed, you may wish to seek a second opinion from another health-care provider.

Just as you would not allow a cardiothoracic surgeon to perform open-heart surgery on you unless he or she first candidly and respectfully discussed the risks and benefits, so, too, you should not allow any physician to administer a medical intervention to you or your child unless that physician first candidly and respectfully discusses the risks and benefits of that medical intervention. Vaccines are no different from any other medical intervention.

10. IF I CHOOSE NOT TO VACCINATE MY CHILD, WHAT ARE THE RISKS AND WHICH PRECAUTIONS SHOULD I TAKE?

I could write an entire book about the potential risks of not vaccinating . . . Oh, wait . . . Presumably, if you've made it to this section, you've read about these risks (along with the potential risks associated with vaccinating). When contemplating whether or not to vaccinate your child, you must consider all risks and weigh them against the benefits.

Due, in part, to widespread vaccination efforts, many of the diseases prevented by vaccines are now rare—albeit, these diseases have not been eradicated and children may still contract them. While many healthy children may experience only mild or moderate symptoms from these diseases, a small number could suffer from severe complications and, yes, even death. If you read my first book, *Parenting at Your Child's Pace*, you're likely familiar with my recipe, the SEEDS of health—*stress, environment, exercise, diet, and sleep*. SEEDS is an acronym; a seed is also something we plant in the ground. When properly watered, given sunlight, and nurtured, that seed ultimately blossoms into a healthy plant. The double meaning of SEEDS (which my mom tells me is quite clever) reminds us that by focusing on these five foundational principles of health, we grow healthy children:

1. *Stress management.* Reducing stress through mindfulness, adequate rest, and positive family interactions can strengthen the immune system.
2. *Environmental and toxin awareness.* Limit exposure to toxins by using natural products and maintaining a clean living environment.
3. *Exercise.* Regular physical activity boosts overall health and immune function.
4. *Diet.* Whereas a diet rich in fruits, vegetables, healthy proteins, and fats can provide the nutrients necessary for a robust immune system, processed foods that are high in sugar and contain other unpronounceable synthetic ingredients can weaken the immune system and even contribute to infirmity.
5. *Sleep.* Ensuring your child gets enough sleep is crucial for his or her body to repair itself and fight infections.

Although the CDC and other health organizations tell us that the best way to avoid vaccine-preventable diseases is to vaccinate, if you elect not to do so, the SEEDS may help strengthen your child's immune system and overall health, equipping him or her with the necessary strength to fight infections.

APPENDIX B

SUMMARY TABLES

I. VACCINE ABBREVIATIONS AND ACRONYMS

DTaP vaccine: A combination shot that protects against diphtheria, tetanus, and acellular pertussis.

Tdap: A booster vaccine, typically given to older children and adults, that protects against tetanus, diphtheria, and acellular pertussis.

MMR vaccine: A combination shot that protects against measles, mumps, and rubella.

IPV: Inactivated poliovirus vaccine.

OPV: Oral poliovirus vaccine.

Hib vaccine: The vaccine that protects against Haemophilus influenzae type b.

HBV or HepB vaccine: The vaccine that protects against hepatitis B.

HepA vaccine: The vaccine that protects against hepatitis A.

HPV vaccine: The vaccine that protects against human papillomavirus.

RV vaccine: The vaccine that protects against rotavirus.

PCV: Pneumococcal conjugate vaccine.

MCV4 or MenACWY: Meningococcal conjugate vaccine.

MenB vaccine: Meningococcal B vaccine.

Var or VZV: The vaccine that protects against varicella (chicken pox).

Flu vaccine: The vaccine that protects against influenza.

LAIV: Live attenuated influenza vaccine (nasal spray flu vaccine).

CV19 or COVID-19: The vaccine that protects against coronavirus disease 19 SARS-CoV-2 vaccines.

II. CDC VACCINE SCHEDULE

Please visit the CDC website for the most up-to-date schedule.

Vitamin K: Given at birth to prevent bleeding.
RSV: RSV monoclonal antibody recommended for infants in the first RSV season if under 8 months.
Hepatitis B (HepB): Birth, 1–2 months, 6–18 months.
Rotavirus (RV): 2, 4, and 6 months (series depends on the brand).
Diphtheria, tetanus, pertussis (DTaP): 2, 4, 6, 15–18 months, and 4–6 years.
Haemophilus influenzae type b (Hib): 2, 4, 6, and 12–15 months.
Pneumococcal (PCV): 2, 4, 6, and 12–15 months.
Polio (IPV): 2, 4, 6–18 months, and 4–6 years.
Influenza (flu): Annually from 6 months onward (2 doses in first flu season).
Measles, mumps, rubella (MMR): 12–15 months and 4–6 years.
Varicella (chicken pox): 12–15 months and 4–6 years.
Hepatitis A (HepA): 12–23 months (2 doses, 6–18 months apart).
COVID-19: Eligible at 6 months, dose timing varies by vaccine (2–3 dose series depending on brand and annual boosters).

III. MOST COMMONLY USED EARLY CHILDHOOD VACCINES AND MAIN INGREDIENTS

This list includes the most common vaccines in the pediatric schedule, highlighting the diversity of production methods and formulations used:

1. *DTaP (diphtheria, tetanus, and acellular pertussis)*
   - *Brands*: DAPTACEL (Sanofi Pasteur), INFANRIX (GlaxoSmithKline)
   - *Main Ingredients*: Diphtheria toxoid, tetanus toxoid, acellular pertussis antigens
   - *Aluminum*: Yes
   - *Culture*: Grown in modified Mueller and Miller medium (DAPTACEL), synthetic or semisynthetic (INFANRIX)
2. *Hib (Haemophilus influenzae type b)*
   - *Brands*: ActHIB (Sanofi Pasteur), HIBERIX (GlaxoSmithKline), PedvaxHIB (Merck)
   - *Main Ingredients*: Haemophilus influenzae type b polysaccharide conjugated to tetanus toxoid (ActHIB, HIBERIX) or meningococcal protein (PedvaxHIB)

- *Aluminum*: No for ActHIB and HIBERIX; yes for PedvaxHIB
- *Culture*: Grown in semi-synthetic medium

3. *IPV (inactivated poliovirus vaccine)*
    - *Brands*: IPOL (Sanofi Pasteur)
    - *Main Ingredients*: Inactivated polioviruses of types 1, 2, and 3
    - *Aluminum*: No
    - *Culture*: Grown in Vero cells, a continuous line of monkey kidney cells

4. *MMR (measles, mumps, and rubella)*
    - *Brand*: MMR II (Merck)
    - *Main Ingredients*: Live attenuated measles, mumps, and rubella viruses
    - *Aluminum*: No
    - *Culture*: Grown in chick embryo cell culture (measles and mumps), human diploid cell culture (rubella)

5. *Varicella (chicken pox)*
    - *Brand*: VARIVAX (Merck)
    - *Main Ingredients*: Live attenuated varicella virus
    - *Aluminum*: No
    - *Culture*: Grown in human diploid cell cultures (WI-38)

6. *Hepatitis B*
    - *Brands*: ENGERIX-B (GlaxoSmithKline), RECOMBIVAX HB (Merck)
    - *Main Ingredients*: Hepatitis B surface antigen
    - *Aluminum*: Yes
    - *Culture*: Produced by recombinant DNA techniques in yeast cells

7. *PCV (pneumococcal conjugate vaccine)*
    - *Brand*: Prevnar (Pfizer)
    - *Main Ingredients*: Pneumococcal polysaccharides conjugated to a carrier protein
    - *Aluminum*: Yes
    - *Culture*: Bacterial cultures for polysaccharides; carrier protein is produced in E. coli

8. *Rotavirus*
    - *Brands*: ROTARIX (GlaxoSmithKline), RotaTeq (Merck)
    - *Main Ingredients*: Live attenuated rotavirus
    - *Aluminum*: No

- *Culture*: Grown in Vero cells

9. *Influenza*
   - *Brands*: Fluzone (Sanofi Pasteur), Fluarix (GlaxoSmithKline), FluLaval (GlaxoSmithKline), and others
   - *Main Ingredients*: Inactivated influenza viruses
   - *Aluminum*: No
   - *Culture*: Grown in fertilized chicken eggs or cell cultures (specific brands vary)
10. *Hepatitis A*
    - *Brands*: HAVRIX (GlaxoSmithKline), Vaqta (Merck)
    - *Main Ingredients*: Inactivated Hepatitis A virus
    - *Aluminum*: Yes
    - *Culture*: Grown in MRC-5 human diploid cells

IV. DISEASE REDUCTION IN THE UNITED STATES: HISTORICAL AND CURRENT PERSPECTIVES

Disease	Approx. Morbidity in Year Prior to Vaccine Introduction	Year Vaccine Introduced	2023 Cases	% Decrease
Diphtheria	206,000	1920	2	> 99%
Measles	481,530	1963	59	> 99%
Mumps	151,209	1967	436	> 99%
Pertussis	200,752	1914	5,611	97%
Polio	38,476	1955	0	100%
Rubella	57,686	1969	3	> 99%
Tetanus	1,560	1924	15	99%
Haemophilus influenzae b	20,000	1985	27	> 99%

ABOUT THE AUTHOR

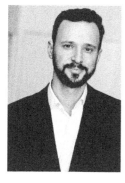

Dr. Joel "Gator" Warsh is a board-certified pediatrician with a passion for integrative medicine. Based in Los Angeles, California, Dr. Warsh blends evidence-based traditional medicine with holistic approaches to help families achieve optimal health. He is the founder of Integrative Pediatrics, where he provides a personalized approach to health care, focusing on prevention, treating the root causes of illness, and fostering lifelong wellness.

Dr. Warsh grew up in Toronto, Canada, and obtained undergraduate degrees in kinesiology and psychology before earning his master's degree in epidemiology from Queen's University. He earned his medical degree from Thomas Jefferson University and completed his pediatric residency at Children's Hospital of Los Angeles.

In addition to his clinical work, Dr. Warsh is a sought-after speaker, podcast guest, and advocate for symbiotically melding conventional and alternative modalities. His work emphasizes the importance of nutrition, exercise, and environmental health in building a strong foundation for kids and families.

A dedicated educator, Dr. Warsh connects with parents through his social media platforms (@DrJoelGator) and as an author of parenting resources like *Parenting at Your Child's Pace: An Integrative Guide to the First Three Years* and *Love, Dad*. His work empowers parents to take an active role in their children's health by offering practical advice rooted in science and compassion.

When he's not caring for patients or writing, Dr. Warsh enjoys spending time with his wife and two children. He is also an ardent foodie and coffee enthusiast.

REFERENCES

Hundreds of references were cited throughout this book and, in the interest of space, are listed online. You may find all the references on the book's website, www.theshotbook.com.

To join our integrative parenting community, keep the conversation alive, stay informed, and access additional resources, scan the QR code below.

You will find ongoing updates, new research, bonus content, courses, and references on our website. Let's continue to explore and learn together.

Join the conversation at *www.theshotbook.com.*

BOOK A ONE-ON-ONE CONSULT

If you have additional questions after reading this book, I offer personalized one-on-one vaccine coaching sessions. Please feel free to book a session to discuss your concerns in detail.

For further information, go to www.theshotbook.com.

Made in United States
Orlando, FL
08 June 2025

61949049R00204